Thriving!
A Manual for Students in the Helping Professions

To our students, both current and past, who have taught us so much about thriving.

Thriving!
A Manual for Students in the Helping Professions

Second Edition

LENNIS G. ECHTERLING
ERIC COWAN
WILLIAM F. EVANS
A. RENEE STATON
J. EDSON McKEE
JACK PRESBURY
ANNE L. STEWART

James Madison University

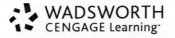

WADSWORTH
CENGAGE Learning·

Australia • Brazil • Japan • Korea • Mexico • Singapore • Spain • United Kingdom • United States

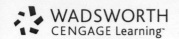
WADSWORTH
CENGAGE Learning

Thriving!: A Manual for Students in the Helping Professions, Second Edition

Lennis G. Echterling, Eric Cowan, William F. Evans, A. Renee Staton, J. Edson McKee, Jack Presbury, and Anne L. Stewart

Publisher: Barry Fetterolf

Senior Marketing Manager: Barbara LeBuhn

Senior Editor: Mary Falcon

Associate Project Editor: Deborah Berkman

Art and Design Manager: Gary Crespo

Cover Design Manager: Anne S. Katzeff

Senior Photo Editor: Jennifer Meyer Dare

Composition Buyer: Chuck Dutton

New Title Project Manager: Susan Brooks-Peltier

Editorial Assistant: Evangeline Bermas

Cover image: © Richard Cummings/CORBIS

For product information and technology assistance, contact us at **Cengage Learning Customer & Sales Support, 1-800-354-9706**

For permission to use material from this text or product, submit all requests online at **www.cengage.com/permissions** Further permissions questions can be emailed to **permissionrequest@cengage.com**

Library of Congress Control Number: 2006939649

ISBN-13: 978-0-618-88214-4

ISBN-10: 0-618-88214-6

Wadsworth
20 Davis Drive
Belmont, CA 94002
USA

Cengage Learning is a leading provider of customized learning solutions with office locations around the globe, including Singapore, the United Kingdom, Australia, Mexico, Brazil, and Japan. Locate your local office at **www.cengage.com/global**

Cengage Learning products are represented in Canada by Nelson Education, Ltd.

To learn more about Wadsworth, visit **www.cengage.com/wadsworth**

Purchase any of our products at your local college store or at our preferred online store **www.cengagebrain.com**

Printed in the United States of America
3 4 5 6 7   17 16 15 14 13

Contents

Preface

What you get from graduate training depends on what you put into it. With hard work, deep commitment to your desired profession, and cooperative interactions with your peers and professors, you will profit greatly from graduate school. If, on the other hand, you adopt the attitude that while you are in school you will be preparing for "real life," you will miss the point. Graduate school *is* real life. So you must resolve to put in your openness to fully being there—in each moment, with each experience, and with each person you encounter.

Back when you were an undergraduate, you probably skated through some of the experiences offered to you, holding your breath and waiting for them to be over. *We* certainly did! You also may have held on to many of the ideas you were taught only long enough to mark the correct answer on the final examination. In graduate school, the ideas that inform you will be those that carry you into a successful professional career.

Graduate school will be amazingly short, and, like a well-crafted short story, nothing in your schooling will be beside the point. Everything will be useful and, indeed, essential to your becoming a skilled counselor. You will find that if you are willing to live each day in the here and now—dropping some of your defenses and opening yourself to new growth—you will, in fact, get much *more* out of your graduate training than you put into it.

This guidebook offers practical and positive strategies that you can use to make the most of your training experience. These strategies are based on six principles for thriving in your graduate training: come well prepared, live your training, learn from others, explore yourself, be open to opportunities, and always act with character. In each chapter, we explore one facet of succeeding in training. The format includes inspirational quotes, personal accounts of students' experiences, practical hints and suggestions, structured activities, recommended resources, and references. The tone of the book is conversational, and we invite you to be actively involved as you read it.

We hope this book will be helpful to you on your training journey. As you encounter obstacles along the way, you will find that rereading these chapters will make more and more sense to you. Pay particular attention to the stories written by students who have traveled the same road that you face. Their experiences will reassure you that you are still on the right path—even though at times you may feel you have lost your way.

A NOTE ABOUT THE SECOND EDITION

Producing a second edition of a book is like renovating an older home. You want to make major improvements, update it with modern features, and even make a few additions, but you also want to preserve the unique character and beguiling charm of the original that you love. So we have taken this opportunity to review the first edition in its entirety, polishing the writing, clarifying points, and adding examples. As we engaged in this task, we found ourselves constantly making small revisions and refinements.

Because this book is about the change that takes place in thriving graduate students, we have added discussions of such concepts as the transtheoretical model of change and the dialectics between self-acceptance and change. We also completely updated the book by incorporating recent literature on training, supervising, and educating counselors and therapists. We have included in the appendices the new ethical codes of both the American Counseling Association and American Psychological Association, both of which were adopted after the first edition came out. Our overhaul included moving up the chapter on managing stress to an earlier part in the book. The reason for this shift was that beginning students face many stressors when they start their training, so they need to apply stress management techniques right away.

Readers of the first edition often commented on how touched they were by the many contributions of current and former students who shared their intimate thoughts and personal experiences. These stories gave readers comfort, hope, and inspiration. Therefore, our additions have included even more student narratives, hands-on suggestions, quotations, and helpful tips for thriving in graduate school. The Internet has continued to be a vital resource for students, so we have added new websites and updated the website addresses that were in the first edition.

ACKNOWLEDGMENTS

We wish to thank the many students and colleagues who generously offered their personal stories so that readers can discover that they are not alone in the doubts and struggles they are experiencing. In fact, having these painful experiences is essential to becoming an enlightened helping professional. These colleagues and students included Robert Anderson, April Bennett, Christine Carmouze, Constance Cromartie, Jane Halonen, Karen Hannam, Christy Hartford, Rachel Heberle, Kasey Hilton, Teresa Hiney, Andrea Hollister, Melissa Lewis, Ellen Neill-Dore, Stan Parcell, Kimberley Payne, Jennifer Phillips, Antoinette Roberts, Grace Viere, A. Renee Wilson, Dara Zafron, and many others who contributed to this renovation.

Producing this book has truly been a team effort. We greatly appreciate the insightful comments of those who reviewed drafts of the first edition of this book, including Alan Caviola, Moumoth University; Ronald S. Kiyuna, Ed.D., California State University, Fresno; Don C. Locke, North Carolina State University; Oliver Morgan, University of Scranton; Greg J. Neimeyer, Ph.D., University of Florida; and Mike Robinson, University of Central Florida. The final version was much better as a result of their feedback.

Like its predecessor, this second edition has been a collaborative labor of love. The reviews for this revision were particularly heartening and beneficial. We are grateful to the individuals who helped us with their detailed comments, ideas and suggestions, including Michael Becker, York College; Marika Ginsburg-Block, University of Delaware; Patricia Goodspeed, SUNY College at Brockport; Lorraine J. Guth, Indiana University of Pennsylvania; Holly J. Hartwig Moorhead, Walsh University; and Merril Simon, California State University Northridge.

Of course, we also want to acknowledge our debt to Barry Fetterolf and Mary Falcon of Cengage Learning for their energetic support and ongoing commitment to our vision of a guide for helping students thrive in their training to become counselors and therapists.

CHAPTER 1

The Thriving Principles

The question is not how to survive, but how to thrive, with passion, compassion, humor, and style.

—Maya Angelou

You must be the change you want to see in the world.

—Mahatma Gandhi

Whether or not you have watched *Survivor*, you've certainly heard of the immensely popular reality TV show. As you may know, the show drops a group of people on a primitive island somewhere in the South Pacific or at a desolate spot in the Australian outback. Week after week, the contestants would have to suffer through ordeals—such as eating rats—that were hatched up by the program's producers. The castaways would hold tribal councils, scheme to form temporary alliances, vote contestants off the program, and compete with one another until only one lone survivor was left standing at the conclusion of the series.

No matter what kind of helping professional you aspire to—counselor, psychologist, clinical social worker, or counselor educator—you must first complete an intensive and rigorous training program. We can guarantee that, whatever program you enter, you'll sometimes feel as if you're a contestant on *Survivor*. Of course, instead of tribal councils, you'll have committee meetings. Instead of foraging for berries, you'll be subsisting on macaroni and cheese. And instead of enduring physical challenges, you'll have tests, papers, and comprehensive exams. In spite of these superficial differences, you'll face ordeals and obstacles in your training that can be just as intimidating and challenging as anything on a reality TV show.

At times, you may feel so overwhelmed by the demands and so plagued with self-doubts that you wonder whether you'll ever make it through the program. One former graduate student used Winston Churchill's words to describe those times as being "full of blood, sweat, and tears." Some trainees may seem to have a knack for picking up the skills almost effortlessly, whereas you may feel that you have to struggle to master even the basics. As you face your first research-methods test or your first client, you may wonder if you're going to survive.

We also guarantee that, as you progress through your training, you will regularly hear a certain phrase, often used with a heavy dose of irony: "Just think of this as a 'learning experience' for you." In other contexts, these words typically suggest an opportunity for enrichment; however, the tone of voice, deep sigh, and shaking head that usually accompany this remark strongly suggest that you're in store for a frustrating, disappointing, and demanding time. After a few difficult experiences, you may begin to suspect that the helping professions use a "no pain, no gain" philosophy of training. We believe, however, that your most productive "learning experiences" can actually be tremendously satisfying, fulfilling, and joyful.

In this chapter, we describe principles that can not only help you *survive* your training experiences, but can help you *thrive*—to succeed, flourish, and even enjoy your training with, as Maya Angelou said, "passion, compassion, humor, and style."

▲▲▲

How Shall We Begin?
Jean's Story

I CAN REMEMBER vividly the first time I opened that door and stepped into the psychology building as one of its newest and freshest trainees. I was so excited! Finally, after years of effort, I had fulfilled my long-standing dream of being accepted into a graduate program with a fine reputation. It was exactly what I wanted, and I couldn't have been happier. Of course, before applying, I had obsessively read all the information I could find about the program. It was credentialed, well-known for its innovative methods, and respected for its commitment to professionalism. I had traveled to the campus, met with a professor, and even talked with several students. After all my research and preparation, I thought I had a pretty good idea of what I was getting into. Boy, was I wrong.

My rude awakening came during my first class. Days before the semester began, I had bought all my textbooks and had even read several chapters in each of them, diligently highlighting nearly every sentence. Back then, I had the delusion that learning took place only by a strange form of osmosis. Somehow, the knowledge contained in the sentences had to travel through the highlighter, up my arm, and finally into my brain. Of course, with this method, I was only turning my black-and-white textbooks into black-yellow-and-white textbooks. For some reason, though, the process seemed comforting to me in its familiarity. That's the way I had studied all through college, so I assumed that I would continue learning in the same tried and true way—by hunting for the absolute truth in a book and pouncing on it with my highlighter.

I attended that first class feeling eager, as well as a bit smug that I had already captured some truth in yellow. I was ready with my sharpened pencils, brand-new spiral-bound notebooks, and an academic-year calendar in pristine condition. I found a desk in front, struck a pose of thoughtful attentiveness, and waited for the professor to begin revealing the hidden truths that would make everything meaningful. My plan was to write those messages neatly in my notebook and later highlight them all in that yellow shade of truth—just to be sure.

That's when it happened, when all my expectations were destroyed. My professor came in, asked us to form our desks into a circle, and sat down with us. That's the thing—she just sat there, smiling and looking at each of us with kind, but penetrating, eyes. What was her problem? Why didn't she begin lecturing?

Finally, one student timidly raised her hand and asked, "Are you the professor?"

"Yes," she replied.

After a pause, the student reluctantly continued, "Well, isn't it time for us to start?"

"Yes, you're right," she answered. "How shall we begin?"

I was sitting there wondering, "What the hell is going on here? Is this woman playing some sadistic joke on us?"

Another student suggested, "Maybe we could introduce ourselves?"

"Sounds good!" the professor said. "Who would like to begin?"

It suddenly dawned on me that I was in new, uncharted territory. I felt like Dorothy landing in Oz and remarking to Toto that "I don't think we're in Kansas any more." I was disoriented but curious, anxious but intrigued, and a little dazed but ready to begin.

▼▼▼

USE IT—DON'T LOSE IT!

The essential of everything you do . . . must be
choice, love, passion.

—Nadia Boulanger

If you are already a trainee, your first experience may not have been as memorable for you as it was for the student who wrote that account, but you probably had some similar feelings. You are likely to find that training to become a counselor or therapist is dramatically different from your undergraduate education.

Huey, Dewey, and Louie, Donald Duck's three nephews, were always on adventures that got them into perplexing and challenging situations. No matter what the problem or circumstance, they immediately got out their trusty *Junior Woodchuck Handbook* and found the precise information and perfect advice for successfully resolving their dilemma. We realize that this book cannot provide *all* the answers, but we hope that you will find it useful as you pursue your own adventure.

As you begin your training, you may sometimes think that you're embarking on a long, arduous journey with seemingly no end in sight. Although you will enjoy many aspects of your training, at times you may feel overwhelmed and disoriented. That is why we have created this book: to serve as a survival guide for you. Because being lost and confused can also make you feel lonely, we hope this book will also be like having a readily available support group. As you read through the book's personal accounts, you may recognize similarities between your own reactions and those of the students' experiences. At times, you may want to set aside this book to take some time to explore your own experiences.

When you read the stories of other students, you may learn from their mistakes and feel encouraged by their successes. Finally, you can use these students' advice and tips as you forge your own training journey.

The earlier in your career training you read this book, the better. And be sure to keep it handy even after you have read it. Throughout your training you may want to refer to it regularly. When a training problem—or opportunity!—catches you off guard, use this book to refresh your memory and review strategies. In other words, "use it, don't lose it." The book provides you with practical information on programs, policies, and procedures and also offers helpful hints on getting the most out of your experiences during your training.

THRIVING

> Life is either a daring adventure or nothing. To keep our faces toward change and behave like free spirits in the presence of fate is strength undefeatable.
>
> —Helen Keller

As you begin your training program, you will most likely discover considerable diversity among your fellow trainees: some of you may have just completed your undergraduate education, whereas others may be embarking on a second career path. Some of you may be from an urban area in Los Angeles, others from suburban Chicago, and still others of you may be from a rural area in the Appalachians. Perhaps you're African American, Caucasian, Latino, Asian American, or Native American. No matter what your background or circumstances may be, you are joining with others who have a common dream—to become a helping professional. As you make this training journey, which we describe in Chapter 2, you can thrive if you use the following simple principles.

Pack Wisely

> What do you pack when you pursue a dream? And what do you leave behind?
>
> —Sandra Sharp

The first principle of thriving involves meeting your basic needs and bringing along the resources you'll require in your training. On any long journey, you'll want to stock provisions, pack the right gear, prepare for emergencies, and travel light.

One resource you bring to your training is time. Unlike money, you cannot bank or buy time. You must learn how to spend your time wisely. One of the ongoing challenges you will face throughout your journey will be how to balance your training opportunities with other important aspects of your life.

It's impossible to eliminate all the stressors you face during your training. These stressors are a lot like Arnold Schwarzenegger's character in *The Terminator*—even when you successfully cope with one, you can almost hear them warning, "I'll . . . be . . . back." In fact, you will continue to deal with stressors throughout your professional career. Therefore, it is vital that you include stress-management skills among the resources you pack for this journey (Kelly, 2005). Chapter 3 explores specific ways to manage your time and successfully handle the stressors that will inevitably confront you in your graduate and professional life.

Taking care of your basic needs enables you to focus your energies on achieving personal and professional growth in your training. In Chapter 4, we present useful information and guidelines for obtaining educational loans, applying for assistantships and scholarships, finding safe and affordable housing, taking care of your nutritional needs, and maintaining an active and healthy lifestyle.

Because you will be preparing to become a counselor and therapist, you will need to bring along some tools of the trade. Of course, a personal computer, notebooks, pens and pencils, a dictionary, the *Publication Manual of the American Psychological Association*, and other reference books are some of the essentials. While you're deciding what to take, keep in mind that how you use this gear is far more important than the equipment itself. For example, you may have a touch of technophobia (many people in the helping professions do), and therefore treat your computer as if it houses an evil entity, like HAL from *2001: A Space Odyssey*. As a result, you may not be taking full advantage of the computer in writing reports, doing presentations, conducting research, exploring resources, and communicating with others. On the other hand, you may be more of a technophile. You may find yourself salivating over any new gadget with all the latest "bells and whistles." In that case, keep in mind that these tools are only as good as your skill in using them.

Of course, a computer and reference books are examples of the obvious tools that you will be using. However, you will want to bring other resources on your training endeavors. These include your academic, time-management, and stress-management skills. Basic academic skills, such as reading and writing, do much more than just help you earn good grades. In fact, they are an indispensable part of being an effective professional helper. Reading broadens and enriches your own experiences by tapping into the minds of healers and thinkers throughout time and from around the world. Writing puts into words your experiences, makes your thoughts known, and clarifies your vague hunches. Keeping your curiosity alive, thinking critically about assumptions, and examining thoughtfully your issues help maintain your professional vitality throughout your career. In Chapter 5, we offer tips on improving your reading, writing, researching, and presentation skills.

Finally, do your best to travel light. If you are bringing a lot of emotional baggage to your training, you will find it hard to stay focused on your clients' needs. One of the best ways to deal with your own emotional issues is to participate in counseling or therapy yourself. Many training programs strongly recommend that their trainees seek counseling and have therefore developed resources to provide this service at little or no cost (Dearing, Maddux, & Tangney, 2005). It makes perfect sense for you to take advantage of this opportunity, even if it's not required. Being a client yourself certainly is a powerful way to appreciate the risks, vulnerabilities, and pain that clients face. More important, however, this level of involvement helps you to truly trust the process of counseling and therapy. Once you have been a client, you are no longer only reading about or observing its benefits; you're experiencing them personally. Besides, if you are encouraging others to seek counseling and therapy, shouldn't you practice what you preach?

Make the Journey Your Destination

To travel hopefully is a better thing than to arrive.

—Robert Louis Stevenson

As with many trips, getting there is half the fun. But when it comes to your personal and professional journey, the trip is *all* there is. You began this journey to become a counselor or therapist long before you entered a training program, and you will continue your journey long after you complete it. The second principle of thriving involves remembering that just as life is not a rehearsal, neither is your training. From day one, your training is the real thing, not merely a ceremonial rite of passage you must endure to become a counselor or a therapist. You actually have chances to practice therapeutic principles in every facet of your training. Consider your helping skills to be like muscles that are strengthened by regular use.

In the nineteenth century, Horace Greeley extolled a "manifest destiny" in the United States by urging people to "go west." Joseph Campbell (1986), on the other hand, recommended, "Follow your bliss." In other words, you will not find your destiny in a particular geographic territory. Instead, it lies in the joy you experience as you fulfill your potential, express your talents, and pursue your dreams *now*.

One of the biggest mistakes you can make on this journey is to view yourself as a customer and your program as merely a service station along the way. When you are truly learning, you are never a passive recipient or merely a consumer of educational goods. Instead, you are a dynamic, full, and equal participant in the learning endeavor (Corey & Corey, 2007).

Your teachers and supervisors will be expecting you to collaborate actively with them by always "bringing something to the table." In virtually every class and training experience, you will have an opportunity to practice counseling—the processes of encountering others, observing interpersonal dynamics, gathering information, conceptualizing, and taking action. You may participate in a structured exercise, respond to a taped segment, act out a role-playing exercise, or engage in some group task that demonstrates a principle you are studying. Actively participating in your readings means more than merely underlining passages or highlighting words. It means involving yourself totally, by jotting down ideas and reactions in the margins, organizing the material into important concepts, critically evaluating the arguments, and talking about the readings before coming to class. It is only when you invest your whole self in such endeavors that you make the most of these learning opportunities. Many of your classes will be small and will have the format of a seminar, which literally means "seedplot." Do your part to tend these gardens so that the seeds will grow and be fruitful.

The depth and breadth of your program's curriculum reflect the high standards that trainers have set for you. Certainly, they expect that you will fulfill all the course requirements, but they also want you to extend yourself, to challenge yourself by pursuing knowledge and skills beyond the minimal course requirements. Coming to each class ready and willing to engage fully in the active, exciting process of learning is a great strategy for success, not only during your training but also throughout your career.

Of course, you'll also want to take full advantage of the many enriching experiences that take place outside the classroom. During virtually any week of the academic year, you are likely to find an exciting array of talented artists, authors, scholars, and performers coming to your campus. Art exhibits, theater performances, poetry readings, invited lecturers, musical performances, and films are just a few of the cultural opportunities you will have available—many of which are free to students.

Truly successful counselors and therapists do not limit their development to their academic careers (Gayle, 2003). Whether you are a trainee or a professional, you need to recognize that you have two simple options: either you can continue to grow personally and professionally by challenging yourself, or you can stagnate. Completing your training with a curiosity about what makes people tick and a zest for discovery will guarantee that your learning will continue long after you earn a diploma. Instead, you will see graduation as another step in the lifelong pursuit of professional mastery. One of the reasons that the counseling and therapy professions are so exciting is that the field is still in its infancy and is wide open for new breakthroughs. You can look forward to a long career of refining your skills, revising your thinking, and pushing the envelope.

Of course, you're familiar with Einstein's formula, $E = MC^2$. However, his friends recalled at his death that Einstein had also developed another formula, as simple and profound as its predecessor, for personal success in life: Personal Success = Work + Play + Not Bragging About Your Success. Einstein's formula sounds like good advice for almost anyone, especially if you're in training to help *others* achieve their personal success. Just remember: it's your tires—not your ego—that should always be inflated.

▲▲▲

The Journey
A Parable

K IONE WAS DISAPPOINTED. The people were having a grand feast to honor the Great Chief, and entire clans were planning to attend. But Kione's village was located on the opposite end of the island. The village's lone outrigger canoe had room for only several local officials, four paddlers, and gifts. He begged his parents to allow him to go—after all, wasn't he named after the Great Chief himself? His father told him that there was not enough room.

"Besides," Kione's mother asked with a smile, "What present could you give the Great Chief?"

But Kione was determined to be a part of such a great occasion. He awoke just before dawn and while the others were still sleeping began the long trek to the Chief's village. He carried only some dried mullet and fruit wrapped tightly in a large cassava leaf, his bamboo knife, and a pouch containing his favorite seashell.

When the sun god was directly over his head, the boy stopped to eat beside a cool stream. As he was eating, an old man sat down beside him. Politely, Kione offered to share his meager fare with the stranger, who carefully consumed his portion. Thanking the boy, the old man said, "I want to offer you something in return, but all I have is my wisdom. People can be like a pack of monkeys—chattering, mimicking one another, and fighting for a better place in their pack. Or they can be like a pride of lions—sharing food, caring for one another, and protecting both the old and the young. You have been a lion with me. Can you be a lion surrounded by monkeys?" Kione did not know what the old man meant, but he politely thanked him for the advice and continued on his way.

In the early evening, Kione reached the village, which was full of music and revelers. He quietly joined the line of people waiting in front of the *bai* (council house) to offer their gifts. When his turn came, Kione bowed and solemnly handed his only treasure to the Chief, who showed it to everyone within sight and exclaimed rather loudly that this boy had brought a seashell to honor him! The crowd laughed uproariously, and Kione felt his face grow hot with shame. The laughter quickly subsided, however, as three distinguished looking older women, moving quietly, gracefully, and majestically, gathered beside the Chief. They spoke quietly but intently to him while the festivities halted. Even the children and animals became quiet, for these women were very powerful—they decided who was to be chief and when it was time for a chief to be replaced. The women beckoned Kione to them and began gently asking him questions about his village and his trip. After a few minutes, the trio went back to the Chief, spoke briefly, and moved back into the small group of elder women at the *bai*.

The Great Chief beckoned Kione to come and sit beside him. Then he announced in a humble voice, "This boy is a hero.

He was willing to give us his only possession, but his long, hard journey here made his present the most magnificent gift of all."

The story has been told and retold throughout the years, and the message is always the same at the end. The gift *is* the journey.

▼▼▼

Have Traveling Companions

When we can share—that is the poetry in the prose of life.

—Sigmund Freud

Every culture has its folktales and myths about a heroic figure on a quest. No matter how talented and strong a protagonist may be, a hero neither travels nor triumphs alone. Before the journey, the heroic figure may recruit traveling companions or may encounter strangers along the way who become comrades. Jason had his Argonauts. Dorothy had the Cowardly Lion, Tin Man, and Scarecrow. Luke Skywalker had Obi-Wan Kenobi, Princess Leia, and Han Solo. As the journey progresses, these companions serve vital roles by giving guidance to the traveler, using special powers to help overcome obstacles, or offering useful gifts to provide physical and emotional sustenance.

Like the protagonists in those archetypal stories, you will also encounter others—peers, mentors, instructors, supervisors, and clients—who will have a profound impact on your training journey. The third principle of thriving in your program is being open to the resources others offer you. This openness is essential because you cannot be trained as successfully, as completely, or even as joyfully on your own. Of course, you need to engage in the solitary work of reading, writing, reflecting, and studying if you expect to be successful in any training program. But to become an effective counselor or therapist, you also need to come together with others to engage collaboratively in observing, discussing, practicing, offering feedback, challenging, and encouraging one another.

Our society emphasizes individual achievement and competition. In fact, most of your previous educational experiences probably reinforced a "do it yourself" approach to learning. Homework involved assignments that you completed on your own. Group activities, from elementary school spelling bees to high school debates, emphasized competition. Even your class ranking determined whether you'd receive scholarship offers or rejection letters. In the game of education, having winners also means that there must be losers.

Because you were probably a successful student, it may be a challenge for you to participate in a program designed to train *helping* professionals—counselors and therapists who work effectively with others. Now your learning experiences will emphasize relating, listening, communicating, and collaborating. Although it may be hard for you to admit, it's absolutely true: you are not an island unto yourself in this kind of training—you cannot learn it all on your own.

As a matter of fact, such a collaborative approach to learning is closer to the roots of a true college experience. The word *college* comes from the same Latin word as *colleague—collega*, which means "one chosen to work with another." In other words, you need trainers, supervisors, fellow learners, and clients to inform, inspire, prod, and even provoke you to refine your thinking, develop your skills, and make discoveries about yourself and others. For example, you will be receiving feedback from others on a regular basis. In every instance, you have the chance to be open to their observations, reactions, and suggestions. Just remind yourself that your mind is like a parachute—it works best when it's open.

Based on this principle of having traveling companions on your training journey, you have two daunting, but crucial, tasks. First, with each of your instructors, supervisors, fellow trainees, and clients, you need to develop a working relationship that is based on honesty, understanding, and acceptance. It is essential that you get to know, trust, and respect others if you are going to work well with them. Your second and equally important task is to do your part to contribute to developing your program into a learning community. Instead of competing with one another for individual accolades, members of a learning community make a commitment to share information and ideas. They respect—and even value—different points of view. And they support one another in the formidable enterprise of becoming helping professionals. That way, *everybody* wins.

Because you learn by example, the heart of a training program is not the curriculum, but its people. Actions do speak louder than words, so it is vital that you seek out trainers and supervisors who exemplify the knowledge and skills you want to learn. You want to be with those whom you respect and admire, because the most important lessons in this line of work are not taught, but caught. Like chicken pox at a day-care center, openness to feedback, commitment to helping, and curiosity about the human heart can be highly contagious. So take a close look at the people in a training program. What do you want to catch from them? Is it obvious that they are enthusiastic about training new professionals? Are they dedicated to the art of doing counseling and therapy? Do they have a sense of awe about the mysteries of the mind? Instead of looking for trainers who merely spoon-feed simplistic answers, seek out those who truly educate by demonstrating their professionalism and who challenge you to do likewise. The counseling profession, like a fidgety kid, is never still—it is a living, breathing, kicking, and constantly evolving entity. Look for mentors and trainers who personify the kind of professional you want to become (Johnson & Huwe, 2002).

Of course, you can also serve as an example to others. You can demonstrate the fundamental helping attitudes of genuineness, caring, and openness. You can practice the skills that you are developing. In class discussions, you can share your own discoveries and observations. Whatever the situation, you bring a wealth of experience and ideas to this training, and your colleagues will appreciate your generosity in sharing it. Keep in mind that your training program has changed in one important way since you applied to it—you are now a member of it! A vibrant, thriving training program, like the entire profession, is continually changing and growing as members like you contribute to its vitality. The African Mbuti have a ritualized song that is a wonderful example of what every learning community should aspire to achieve. In the song, individual singers are responsible for specific notes, but no one carries the entire melody. As a result, only the community can sing the song (Turnbull, 1990). You can follow the spirit of this song by adding your voice to your learning community. Practice making a difference by volunteering for committees, offering suggestions, and making your program a better one by the time you leave it.

When you join a community, one of the things you need to do is communicate with other members. Of course, effective communication is important to any organization, but it is particularly essential to one that is dedicated to training counselors. Virtually every day, you will have opportunities to engage in all sorts of stimulating, intriguing, encouraging, and challenging interactions with your teachers, supervisors, and colleagues. In Chapter 7, we offer suggestions for ways you can connect with others in your program, broaden your experiences with diverse populations, and network with your professional colleagues. We also explore how the personal changes you experience will have an impact on your relationships with significant others, friends, and relatives.

▲▲▲

Worst Parents of the Year
Jen's Story

Y OU WOULD have thought by the look on their faces that I had just handed them the award for "Worst Parents of the Year." They sat looking confused, hurt, and angry. On my left, my father was perched on his chair, waiting for me to give him a better explanation for all of this. To my right was my mother, fighting back tears as she struggled to understand what I had just told them. I was in the middle, feeling like the conversation I was having in my living room was just about the worst mistake I had ever made.

My intentions had been so noble, so heartfelt. I wanted to share with my parents my desire for a closer relationship with them. I wanted our conversations to reach beyond everyday chitchat and into depths of who we were. I wanted to know my parents as people, and I wanted the same from them in return. And why not? After the first three months in my counseling program, I was having conversations like this on a daily basis. My whole world was about sharing, listening, reflecting, and accepting the ideas of others. As classmates, we laughed together, cried together, and poured out our souls to one another. I thought for sure I could take home all the treasures I had learned and initiate the same discourse with my parents.

Unfortunately, like some baseball pitchers, my windup was great, but my delivery stunk. In my naïveté, I had assumed that, because I had been living in a counselor's world, everyone else had been doing the same. I had forgotten that most people aren't having intimate discussions about the meaning of life on a daily basis. Therefore, when I brought my request to my parents, I chose words that had worked so well with my peers and professors but had a different effect on my parents. As you might think, their reactions were not what I had expected. They couldn't understand how, after all the love and support they had given me, I could ask for something more. How could I suggest that we were not close enough, or that we didn't talk enough about the right things? The more I tried to explain, the unhappier they got. By the end of the conversation, I truly felt like I was speaking a different language. Needless to say, what started out as the perfect plan ended up as a complete failure. Or was it?

After I returned to school, strange things started happening. I began to get calls from my mom for no particular reason. My dad stopped asking me if I had gotten my oil changed and started inquiring what I wanted to do after graduation. E-mails began to appear from them, filling me in on how they were feeling about different things. I even went home out of the blue to spend the weekend with them.

What started out as a disaster turned into something amazing. I learned that we are all on a journey to find intimacy with our loved ones, but not all of us go about it at the same pace. Those who are in training must resist the urge to carry those who prefer to walk. In this way, we will all feel comfortable when we reach the finish line.

▼▼▼

Keep Your Bearings

> Our life's journey of self-discovery is not a straight line.
>
> —Stuart Wilde

The fourth principle of thriving is based on your need for solitude, which is as important as having company on your training journey. You need time alone to check your bearings, process your experiences, and reflect on the discoveries you are making. As Paul Tournier (1957) explained, "The real meaning of travel . . . is the discovery of oneself" (p. 57). No matter what classes you take, you're likely to learn the most about yourself. As a result, your training experiences will be like your fingerprints—uniquely your own.

Your school catalog and student handbook probably have information about your program's policies and procedures. However, because embarking on any important journey is neither a certain nor an easy venture, you need to rely on more than this information to gain your bearings. As with any trip, you need to remember where you've been, determine where you are now, and envision where you're heading. In other words, you need to explore within yourself to find your internal compass that can give you a sense of direction, to develop a training time line and map, and to assess your progress regularly.

Keeping a journal is an excellent way to recollect important events, explore ideas, sort out reactions, and work through personal issues. Your journal then becomes a reservoir of discoveries, the place in which you face and answer your own questions by having an ongoing written conversation with yourself. You can use your journal to reflect on and tie together all of your learning experiences: readings you encounter, relationships you establish, observations you make, and skills you practice. You may even find that your journal entry can take the form of a poem, such as the following.

Tears of Cleansing, *Constance's Poem*

Water . . .
I drink it.
I bathe with it.
I was baptized in it.
And I need to be cleansed by it—
Oh, not just physically, but emotionally.
The kind of cleansing that only comes through tears.

But tears do not come easily for me.
I don't remember Mama crying. I remember
    strength.
I don't remember being comforted when I had
    tears, so I learned to keep them in.

Now that I am journeying down this pathway
To help others find their light
I find that I must let go of the need
To be the one who has it all together.

As I struggle with myself like a tug of war
Wanting to be free, yet afraid to soar . . .
Free to experience the pain, sorrow, and joy
I've got to know it's okay
To let the tears of cleansing flow

No one knows better than I,
That I cannot expect from others what I cannot do
    myself.
Tears of cleansing, please come so that I can be
    set free.

At the very least, it is vital that you set aside personal time for yourself—to meditate, ponder, speculate, pray, relax, or simply *be*. Throughout your training, from admissions interview to graduation ceremony, you will have countless opportunities for personal growth and greater self-awareness. It is up to you to take full advantage of these opportunities and to make meaning of these experiences. You will find that the most important discoveries you make in your training—the greatest learning experiences you have—take place when you are truly open to looking at yourself.

Training programs repeatedly invite you to explore yourself, because in no other profession is the adage, "Know thyself," more important or more central. The many recordings you will watch, the extensive feedback you will receive, and the countless occasions for introspection you will have can help you tremendously in knowing your most important tool as a counselor—yourself. However, the process is neither easy nor pain free. For example, you may begin a course on multiculturalism feeling pretty self-satisfied, confident that you do not have a racist or sexist bone in your entire body, only to discover quickly that you need to confront your own ethnocentrism and racism (Kiselica, 1999).

In life, it's sometimes tempting to stay right where you are, remaining in familiar territory, avoiding the troubling questions, and not breaking out of your routine. But remember: when you have both feet firmly planted on solid ground, you're not moving. You only advance when you lean forward enough to become momentarily imbalanced and then take a step. Simply put, progress is knocking yourself off balance and regaining it in a new position. Nobody can become a counselor or therapist without a spirit of adventure, without the willingness to try something different, take a few risks, and make lots of mistakes along the way. You might as well abandon any perfectionistic tendencies you may have, because they will do you no good in this field. There's an Inuit saying that expresses this spirit of adventure: "Only the air-spirits know what lies beyond the hills, yet I urge my team farther on."

As you engage in this process, remember to focus on your strengths, too. It's easy to ruminate on your mistakes, limitations, and blunders. If that is your inclination, then you are bound to keep yourself restless, troubled, and awake on many a night. Of course, many trainees occasionally feel demoralized (Watkins, 1996). At these times, it may be helpful to remind yourself that you were selected for training because of your strengths, talents, and potential—and that you also chose to accept this challenge. So give yourself credit for having the chutzpah to think that perhaps you have what it takes to enter what Janet Malcolm (1982) called "the impossible profession."

▲▲▲

You'll Go Far in Life
Andrea's Story

LIKE MOST graduate students, I've had my share of moments of self-doubt. At times I've wondered how I ever got to graduate school in the first place. I sometimes believed that my acceptance to graduate school was a fluke and that I got in by the skin of my teeth. It was during one of these low points that I had what I consider a moment of clarity.

I was in one of my first graduate courses, and the professor was explaining to my class that his course was not part of the admissions process. I remember thinking, "Admissions process, what the heck is he talking about? What would this course have to do with the admissions process anyway?" Sensing our confusion, he went on to explain that his class was not designed to "weed out" any of us. He said that being accepted into graduate school was a difficult undertaking, but it was a task that we had already accomplished. He told us that he firmly believed that each and every one of us deserved to be there. He explained that he expected a lot out of us, because he believed that we were all quite capable. He concluded by telling us that as long as we were willing to work hard, he would do whatever he could to help us in our graduate careers. I left class that day feeling as though my professor had a personal investment in each of us. I also knew that not living up to his expectations would make me feel as though I had personally let him down.

Reflecting on that particular class experience helped me to understand graduate school overall. I began to realize that it isn't about proving myself over and over again. I finally understood that everyone assumed that I deserved to be here. Furthermore, I realized that my professors were all willing to do whatever they could to help me succeed. And as I began to look around, I became aware of the feeling that they all had a personal investment in me.

On the last day of that particular class, my professor told me how much he had enjoyed having me in his class. I thanked him and told him that I had thoroughly enjoyed his class. He went on to say that he knew that I would go far in life. Not being one to accept a compliment easily, I brushed his comment aside with a little bit of humor. Days later, though, I could not get his words out of my head. What did I ever do to deserve such a compliment?

This man, one of the most brilliant people I have ever met, believes that I am going to go far in life? Those words still echo in my mind at times, and I know that I will spend the rest of my life trying to do just that.

▼▼▼

Of course, you're going to encounter roadblocks along your training journey, but how you view them can turn stumbling blocks into stepping stones. It was during a particularly tough time that one student, Christine, found it helpful to give herself this motivational nudge: "If I look at challenges as only obstacles, then I'll have trouble handling them, but if I look at them as opportunities, I'll be enriched."

Another way to cope with this turmoil is to appreciate the humor in your situation, particularly if the joke is *yourself*—your own hang-ups, idiosyncrasies, limitations, and foibles. For example, during one class, when students were discussing their consultation projects, one participant, John, instead of presenting a successful experience, decided to talk about a session in which he "blew it." During a meeting with his consultees, John found himself making one mistake after another. His description of his frantic but futile attempts to salvage his image made the discussion a memorable learning experience. It was not only a hilarious story, but John's willingness to share his predicament was liberating for everyone in the class. They realized that they did not have to be perfect in their work and that they could safely talk about their mistakes with one another.

An important part of keeping your bearings is knowing where you're heading. One of the simplest ways to achieve a goal is to envision it vividly. You will find that your vision of yourself as an emerging professional will help you to start acting as if you already have achieved that goal. All thriving counselors and therapists share certain fundamental qualities (Conyne & Bemak, 2005). First, they are committed to providing competent, caring, and ethical services. Second, they are professionals who engage in a lifelong process of learning and refining these helping skills. Finally, they are actively involved in advancing the profession through research, innovation, training, or service. What particular kind of helper do you want to become? To answer that question, you first must explore who you are *now*. In Chapter 6, we invite you to examine your belief system, your values, your paradigms, and your attitudes toward others who may differ significantly from you.

■ ■ ■

EXERCISE 1.1 **Whatcha Gonna Be?**
A Magic Mirror Exercise

The purpose of this activity is for you to relax, reflect, and envision your future. Find a comfortable spot by yourself, away from distractions, and let yourself relax. You may find yourself relaxing by lying down, closing your eyes, letting your muscles unwind, breathing more deeply and evenly, and allowing your mind to drift along. Once you're in a nice state of relaxation, imagine that you are about to step in front of a nearby magic mirror. Like any ordinary mirror, this one shows your reflection, but this magic mirror reflects how you will look and what you will do in the future. Now go ahead and gaze into this magic mirror to see how you will appear when you have become a professional helper. Look carefully at your face. What does that expression communicate about the person you will become? Notice what you are doing. What skills are you demonstrating? What services are you providing? Pay attention to where you are in the future. Where are you working? Notice the other people around you. Who are your clients? Who are your colleagues? After you have completed this activity, use your journal to describe your vision of the future.

By the way, although you used an imaginary mirror in this exercise, you may be interested in reading how Michael Mahoney (1991) used an actual mirror with clients to evoke powerful emotions and encourage self-exploration.

■ ■ ■

Let the Trip Take You

If you surrender to the wind, you can ride it.

—Toni Morrison

As you move along your training journey, you'll also discover that, in spite of all your careful planning, you'll find yourself being pulled in surprising directions. In *Travels with Charley*, John Steinbeck (1962) wrote, "We do not take a trip; a trip takes us" (p. 6). Your progress will build its own momentum, and you'll find yourself taking an unexpected turn and discovering new territories. This thriving principle invites you to let yourself be carried along by the flow of your training and to be open to the possibilities of your own transformation.

Learning is one of the most challenging, and most fulfilling, of life's adventures. As you examine ideas that may threaten your preconceived notions, as you grope through periods of confusion, and as you read, reflect, synthesize, speculate, and brainstorm, you will forge a new personal and professional identity. As a successful graduate, you will not be the person who originally entered the training program. Along the way, you will gain a sense of self-efficacy, confidence, and trust in your own resources as a counselor or therapist (Sipps, Sugden, & Favier, 1988). Eventually, you will be "replacing an external supervisor with an internal one" (Granello, Beamish, & Davis, 1997, p. 305).

By the time you complete your program, you will be more seasoned and have a greater insight into and a deeper appreciation for the clutter, confusion, and complexity of people's lives. Through this learning, you will acquire essential knowledge and develop valuable skills (Schaefle, Smaby, Maddux, & Cates, 2005). Moreover, at a fundamental level, you will transform yourself from a student into a professional. In other words, just as participating in counseling and therapy changes clients, becoming a helping professional will change *you*.

Chapter 8 helps you identify important sources of knowledge and emotional support to help you venture out, take risks, and grow in your practicum, field placement, or internship. These experiences give you the opportunity to translate your theoretical knowledge into effective clinical work and to gain confidence in yourself as an emerging professional.

▲▲▲

I'm going in. Want to join me?
Lennie's Story

LONG AFTER receiving my diploma, my friends from graduate school are still helping me learn the most important lessons of life—and death. A group of us gather regularly for informal reunions. We share a beach house for a weekend, where we retell old stories, catch up on each other's lives, play together, and take delight in these special relationships that have aged so well and endured so long.

A couple of years ago, one friend was determined to attend our gathering. Stan had been dealing with cancer and undergoing treatment that included radiation and chemotherapy—the whole poisonous works. Hit hard by the side effects, Stan was hairless, fatigued, and tormented by aches and pains, but he joined us for that weekend. In spite of his life-threatening illness, Stan was still Stan, a counselor who never lost his idealism, a former Eagle Scout who thrived on nature, and a fun-loving guy who was ready for any adventure. On our outings together over the years, Stan had always been willing to run in challenging races, hike steep mountain trails, and bodysurf the roughest waves.

My final excursion with Stan on that weekend began with a slow, laborious walk from the house to the nearby beach. He had been a tall and graceful runner, so it was heartbreaking for me to see Stan moving so stiffly, swinging his arms in awkward arcs as his body lurched along. When he finally reached the water's edge, he gazed across the ocean's heaving surface and breathed deeply of the pungent, salty air. At that very moment, Stan became transformed. He flashed that mischievous grin I had seen so many times before and declared, "I'm going in. Want to join me?"

Before I knew it, we were both swimming on that late fall afternoon. For nearly half an hour, we rode the gently cascading waves, floated on our backs to watch seagulls swoop overhead, and let the powerful ocean current carry us along on its inevitable course. Together, we savored the experience of being immersed in the deep, dark, mysterious, living sea.

Three decades earlier, Stan and I had been immersed in graduate school, which had its own mysterious undercurrents, rhythms, tides, and surges. Stan was in a different program, but when we became friends, we found that we brought to our training a similar mixture of rough edges and potential, doubts and dreams, hangups and hopes. We told each other our life stories, gave each other feedback on our work, and threw ourselves into heart-felt discussions that lasted late into the night. After we had solved, to our satisfaction, all the world's problems, revamped all the tired old theories with intriguing new concepts, and articulated the true meaning of life, we rejoiced by partying together. You won't find "parties well" on any checklist assessing graduate student performance, but Stan taught me how essential it was not only to work hard with your colleagues, but also to celebrate with them.

In spite of his love for sharing stories, debating issues, and telling jokes, Stan was an expert at detecting BS. Time after time, when I would find myself becoming inauthentic, spouting some counseling jargon, or acting the least bit pretentious, Stan would grimace and, without hesitation or diplomacy, give me his blunt two-syllable assessment. Then, my whole phony house of cards would begin to collapse, no matter how elaborate my self-deceptions. Even when I protested and argued, I knew in my heart that he was right and it was only a matter of time before I would be answering his challenge to be my true self. In my graduate training, I was fortunate to have supervisors and mentors who could sense my defenses and invite me to set them aside, but their style had tact, subtlety, and discretion. I was truly blessed to also have a friend who may have been crude every now and then, but who always spoke to me straight from the heart.

After graduation, our careers took us in different directions. I entered academia, where I now train counselors. Stan went on to work with adolescents who were court-ordered into counseling. Although many other counselors burned out quickly in this setting, Stan continued to thrive year after year, keeping his idealism, working with integrity, and becoming a master counselor. He was at the peak of his powers and in the prime of his life when a routine medical examination found disturbing evidence of malignant and aggressive tumors.

However, alongside me on that October afternoon in the Atlantic Ocean, Stan was swimming with grace, laughing once again with gusto, and relishing his chance to feel in harmony with nature. The cancer seemed to be pacified, tamed—at least for the moment. Far off, the still ocean surface had a mirrorlike sheen that melded imperceptibly into the sky. There was no horizon, no separation between the sea below and the heavens above. The whole universe seemed balanced, harmonious, and unified. When Stan and I finally emerged from the water, I looked down and noticed a nearly translucent pebble that the churning waves had polished over the centuries. I picked it up and put it in my pocket as a memento of our swim together.

Stan died several months later, but I still have that pebble. In fact, I carry it in my pocket. When my counseling work is particularly challenging, I find myself noticing that pebble by my side. It reminds me of important lessons that Stan taught me: dive in, trust the process, go with the flow, and always remember that, just like in graduate school, you are never truly all on your own.

▼▼▼

Always Take the High Road

> On life's journey . . . virtuous deeds are a shelter,
> wisdom is the light by day, and right mindfulness
> is the protection by night.
>
> —Buddha

The final principle for thriving during your training recognizes that the helping professions are based on more than knowledge, skills, and self-awareness. They are also based on values. In fact, you cannot become a competent therapist or counselor unless you're also an ethical one (Cohen & Cohen, 1999). As an emerging professional trainee, you'll sharpen your moral compass by learning your professional code of ethics (see the appendices) and following it in *all* situations.

When you become a helping professional, you will have to comply with myriad state and federal laws, follow your profession's ethical standards, and observe the policies of your agency or school. As an enrolled student, you are expected to behave legally, ethically, and honorably in all your course work. Whenever you are unsure about what conduct is allowed by the law, the ethical standards of your profession, or the honor code of your university, immediately consult your trainer or supervisor. A violation can be grounds for failing a course and being expelled from the program.

Finally, taking the high road also means challenging yourself to maintain high professional standards. For example, you need to avoid the temptation to merely act out Hollywood's version of a counselor or therapist—using jargon, spouting simplistic slogans, and blindly following the latest therapeutic fads. At times, you may find yourself attracted to the certainty and confidence that this posturing seems to offer.

Randy, for example, was a beginning trainee who found himself enamored of his expanding vocabulary of terms culled from courses on counseling theories, interpersonal dynamics, and abnormal psychology. At parties, he would liberally sprinkle these phrases throughout his conversations. Finally, one of his friends took Randy aside, gently pointed out these affectations, and told him how she missed the "real," unpretentious person she once knew. When he brought up this issue in his own counseling, Randy began to recognize how he was harboring serious doubts that he would ever be able to master the complex skills of helping. He discovered that he found some consolation in at least sounding like an expert.

When Zelda looked back on how she began her training, she realized that she was counting on her trainers to tell her exactly what to say to her clients. She had the notion that providing good counseling and therapy could be reduced to following a script or relying on "chicken soup" inspirational maxims. But her supervisor challenged her to discover and develop her own therapeutic voice. Zelda remembered vividly how much she wrote in her journal that night about her doubts of ever becoming a therapist. As she read over her anguished journal entry, she realized that her words rang strong and true. Her voice, and no one else's, was emerging on her journal pages. With a sense of determination, Zelda wrote, "Hey, I'm here to become a therapist—not a ventriloquist's dummy!"

Of course, it's only natural to succumb to some of these temptations as you take on a professional identity. You are, after all, entering a tough, challenging, and nebulous line of work, so taking refuge in jargon, labels, and fads can be very appealing. However, you will come to realize that a true professional speaks and writes with clarity in an effort to enlighten others, not to impress them. A real helping professional avoids slapping on labels like a grocery clerk and, instead, recognizes the uniqueness and complexity of each client. Finally, a true counselor or therapist thinks critically and develops a healthy skepticism regarding fads, misinformation, and biases in the field. Sure, as a helping professional, you may be softhearted toward people, but you also have to be hardnosed about the evidence needed to validate the effectiveness of therapy and counseling techniques. Taking the high road isn't the easy way, but it's the only way if you plan to be a successful helping professional.

SUMMARY

In this chapter, we presented six principles to follow on your training journey. Observing these guidelines will help you succeed not only as a student but also as a helping professional. The first principle is to pack wisely for the trip. Making provisions to meet basic needs and bringing along important resources are vital for your success. Second, make the journey your destination. Your training is not a rehearsal—it is an integral part of your lifelong commitment to professional development. The third principle of thriving is to have traveling companions. Be open to what your peers, mentors, instructors, supervisors, and clients can offer you because it is impossible to become a helping professional on your own. Fourth, keep your bearings. You will find that the most important discoveries you make in your training—the greatest learning experiences you have—take place when you are truly open to looking within yourself. Fifth, let the trip take you. Allow your progress to build its own momentum, and you'll find yourself taking an unexpected turn and discovering new territories. Finally, always take the high road. You can't become a competent counselor or therapist unless you also become an ethical one.

RESOURCES

One of the best ways to develop a professional identity is to join the club. All helping professions have state, regional, and national organizations. Below is contact information for five national associations in the helping professions. All five have websites that provide excellent information on resources, training, and employment opportunities and current issues in the profession.

American Association for Marriage and Family Therapy
112 South Alfred Street
Alexandria, VA 22314-3061
703-838-9808
www.aamft.org

American Counseling Association
5999 Stevenson Avenue
Alexandria, VA 22304-3300
800-347-6647
www.counseling.org

American Mental Health Counselors Association
801 N. Fairfax Street, Suite 304
Alexandria, VA 22314
800-326-2642
www.amhca.org

American Psychological Association
750 First Street, NE
Washington, DC 20002-4242
800-374-2721
www.apa.org

American Psychological Association Graduate Students (APAGS)

www.apa.org/students

APAGS is the support organization for psychology graduate students. It offers members opportunities to enhance their development towards a career in psychology and to shape the future of the discipline. The website lists a variety of services that address the needs of graduate students in psychology.

Graduate Student Association (GSA) of ACA

www.counseling.org/students

The American Counseling Association recently developed a professional organization for graduate students. The purpose of GSA is to advocate for the specific needs and interests of students in counselor education graduate programs. The website offers resources and opportunities for students, including contests and scholarships.

National Association of Social Workers

750 First St., NE, Suite 700

Washington, DC 20002-4241

202-408-8600 or 800-638-8799

www.naswdc.org

REFERENCES

Campbell, J. (1986). *The inner reaches of outer space: Metaphor as myth and as religion.* New York: van der Marck.

Cohen, E. D., & Cohen, G. S. (1999). *The virtuous therapist: Ethical practice of counseling and psychotherapy.* Belmont, CA: Wadsworth.

Conyne, R. K., & Bemak, F. (2005). *Journeys to professional excellence: Lessons from leading counselor educators and practitioners.* Alexandria, VA: American Counseling Association.

Corey, M. S., & Corey, G. (2007). *Becoming a helper* (5th ed.). Belmont, CA: Brooks/Cole.

Dearing, R. L., Maddux, J. E., & Tangney, J. P. (2005). Predictors of psychological help seeking in clinical and counseling psychology graduate students. *Professional Psychology: Research and Practice, 36,* 323–329.

Gayle, B. J. (2003). The graduate school experience: One faculty member's perspective. *Behavior Therapist, 26,* 245–247.

Granello, D. H., Beamish, P. M., & Davis, T. E. (1997). Supervisee empowerment: Does gender make a difference? *Counselor Education and Supervision, 36,* 305–317.

Johnson, W. B., & Huwe, J. M. (2002). *Getting mentored in graduate school.* Washington, DC: American Psychological Association.

Kelly, M. M. (2005). Psychological adaptation to graduate school: How to smell the roses while burning the midnight oil. *Behavior Therapist, 28,* 57–59.

Kiselica, M. S. (1999). Confronting my own ethnocentrism and racism: A process of pain and growth. *Journal of Counseling and Development, 77,* 14–17.

Mahoney, M. J. (1991). *Human change processes: The scientific foundations of psychotherapy.* New York: Basic Books.

Malcolm, J. (1982). *Psychoanalysis: The impossible profession.* New York: Random House.

Schaefle, S., Smaby, M. H., Maddux, C. D., & Cates, J. (2005). Counseling skills attainment, retention, and transfer as measured by the Skilled Counseling Scale. *Counselor Edsucation and Supervision, 44,* 280–292.

Sipps, G. J., Sugden, G. J., & Favier, C. M. (1988). Counselor training level and verbal response type: Their relationship to efficacy and outcome expectations. *Journal of Counseling Psychology, 35,* 397–401.

Steinbeck, J. (1962). *Travels with Charley.* New York: Bantam Books.

Tournier, P. (1957). *The meaning of persons.* New York: Harper & Row.

Turnbull, C. (1990). Luminality: A synthesis of subjective and objective experience. In R. Schechner & W. Appel (Eds.), *By means of performance* (pp. 50–81). New York: Cambridge University Press.

Watkins, C. E. (1996). On demoralization and awe in psychotherapy supervision. *Clinical Supervisor, 14,* 139–148.

CHAPTER 2

Making Your Training Journey

When one travels, the first step is the beginning of
the arrival.

—Seng-Chao

Our task is to make ourselves architects of the
future.

—Jomo Kenyatta

After receiving his doctoral degree, one of our colleagues said that
during his journey through graduate school he saw himself taking on the characteristics of each of the Seven Dwarfs. "At the start of
my training," he said, "I felt so naïve and shy that I was Dopey and
Bashful. By the second year, I felt so sick, exhausted, and frustrated
with everything that I was either Sneezy, Sleepy, or Grumpy. Finally,
when I got my Ph.D., I was thrilled that I was at last both Doc and
Happy."

Although our friend offered this description as merely a cute story,
you can expect to undergo profound transformations in your own identity. Whether you pursue a master's, educational specialist, or doctoral
degree, you take on four distinct roles as you enter and make your
way through a program. These roles are applicant, novice, apprentice,
and emerging professional. This chapter is organized according to
those four roles that you assume as you chart the course of your training
journey.

You also encounter important milestones—such as selection, orientation, comprehensive examination, capstone experiences, and
graduation—that mark the crucial turning points you face along the

way. In this chapter, we describe how to proceed through a training program's rites of passage. In many ways, the milestones involved in becoming a helping professional parallel your development from childhood into adulthood. Just as children learn to crawl before they can walk, you will learn basic theories and techniques before you can practice counseling and therapy. And just as children discover and explore their unique sense of self as they grow and mature, you will also learn about yourself as you forge a new identity that will emerge and crystallize at each stage of your own professional development.

By thriving in your training, you also go through major changes in how you think. Mark Young (2005) described the successful process of becoming a helper as a personal journey with identifiable developmental stages. Basing his observations on Perry's (1970) research on adult development, Young considered three stages—dualistic, multiplistic, and relativistic thinking—to be applicable to most graduate students learning a new profession (Simpson, Dalgaard, & O'Brien, 1986). These developmental stages can provide a useful framework for reflecting on your own training journey. But do not view this developmental process as a predictable sequence of steps. In reality, your development involves much ebb and flow, and at any point in your training, you probably incorporate elements from all three stages, even though one may dominate.

The following sections, in addition to offering practical advice about handling the "nuts and bolts" of completing your training requirements, also suggest ways you can thrive at each stage of your development. For example, by creating a portfolio, keeping a journal, and using rituals, you can support your development, document your achievements, celebrate your progress, and foster a sense of community with your colleagues.

▲▲▲

Why Not Enjoy the Ride?
Cathy's Story

A T THE END of this semester, I'm going to be graduating. Of course I'm excited about finishing up and a little nervous about finding a job. While I'm pretty busy completing my internship and sending out résumés, at times I've found myself just skimming through the journals I've written over the past three years. It reminds me of when I was a senior in high school. I was excited about all the changes in my life, but I also had a need to look through my yearbooks and relive a little of my earlier high-school days.

I'm not sure why, but my reactions to my journal entries have changed incredibly. When I used to read over my entries just after writing them down, I would often feel embarrassed and supercritical. I would think to myself, "Those words don't capture my experiences at all. They're so lame, superficial, and trite!" Now when I read over those same entries that I had written at the start of my training, I feel like I'm encountering another person.

Like an indulgent older sister, now I am quick to forgive this person's mistakes, find her awkward phrases endearing, and am charmed by her naïve views. In fact, I feel protective of her, wanting to offer her some nurturance and encouragement, saying something like, "You go, girl!" I'm proud of how that person hung in there through some tough times.

I haven't really counted, but I bet that the number of words I wrote in an entry was a pretty good measure of the turmoil I was in at the time. Last year, there were lots of entries about my comps. I was so afraid that I was going to fail that exam! One week, I had spent every free minute in the library doing this marathon review of all the comps material. When I finally finished studying, I was convinced that there was no way that I could pass.

When I came home that night, my partner innocently asked me about my day and the next thing I remember is sobbing uncontrollably in her arms, saying that it was no use because passing was impossible. She was great—she didn't give me any silly reassurances or inspirational slogans. She just stayed with me until I was ready to move on to making a plan of action. Reading that journal entry reminded me of just how lucky I've been to have her and others in my life.

I'm at a different place now—more confident of myself, more seasoned, and on my way to becoming a good counselor. As I reread what I've just written, I recognize that my words still don't capture fully what I'm experiencing right now, but I'm a lot more tolerant and charitable toward myself than I used to be. Sure, I haven't arrived—I still have a long way to go, but why not enjoy the ride?

▼▼▼

BEING AN APPLICANT

Change is not made without inconvenience, even
from worse to better.

—Richard Hooker

In any graduate program, the first role you take on is that of applicant—someone who wishes to become a member of that learning community. As an applicant, you are participating in the phase of your training that is typically called the "admissions process." We prefer, however, to use the term "selection" instead of "admissions" because it emphasizes that the process involves a *mutual* decision. While a program's selection committee is deciding whether to admit you, you are deciding if that program would help you to meet your personal and professional goals. As in considering any committed relationship, one of your most important obligations in graduate training is finding the best match for you. In fact, the best predictor of completing your training successfully is the quality of the match between you and the program faculty regarding goals and expectations (Hoskins & Goldberg, 2005).

Here we highlight only some of the major strategies you'll want to use to become a successful applicant. There are several fine guides you can read for detailed information regarding program selection (e.g., Walfish & Hess, 2001). In the Resources section of this chapter, we recommend one that is especially relevant to counseling and psychology (Keith-Spiegel & Wiederman, 2000). The selection process is a tough and difficult one that involves literally years of preparation. To succeed, you should take the following steps:

Gain Experience

Your first task is to gain relevant experience. This experience may be volunteer work or paid employment, but any experience in which you engaged in developing helping relationships would certainly be relevant to counseling and therapy. You may have been, for example, a Big Brother or Big Sister, an advocate for sexual assault survivors, or a volunteer at a crisis hotline.

Many college graduates work for a year or two before returning to graduate school. Many bachelor's-level positions in education, community service, and mental health can offer you invaluable experience to prepare you for graduate training. Some of these positions include teacher, case manager, psychiatric aide, mentor, advocate, and outreach worker.

Gaining experience in helping others is essential for a number of important reasons. First, these activities help you develop some fundamental skills in establishing and maintaining a trusting relationship with someone in need of assistance. Second, you gain a sense of the realities of a helping profession. Becoming involved in this work can help you confirm your hunch that counseling and therapy may be your life's calling. Third, selection committees examine thoroughly your application materials for evidence of relevant experience. Applicants who have extensive experience, whether it's paid or volunteer, are more likely to be selected for graduate training programs.

Complete the Academic Prerequisites

One of your fundamental responsibilities is to meet the educational requirements for entering a graduate program. Although academic excellence has not been found to predict a counselor's effectiveness (Markert & Monke, 1990), selection committees do expect that you have successfully completed academic course work that has prepared you well for graduate training. If you are one of the increasing numbers of older people who have decided to pursue a graduate degree in counseling and therapy, you may need to complete some undergraduate courses before you can qualify.

Explore Your Training Options

Buskist and Mixon (1998) have written a useful guide that lists many training programs in counseling and psychology. Sayette, Mayne, and Norcross (2004) have provided detailed descriptions of all APA-accredited clinical, counseling, and combined-integrated programs, offering helpful advice on selecting schools based on your training goals. Read brochures, check directories, search graduate program websites. Be sure to talk to both professors and students in the programs that particularly interest you. You'll soon discover that program descriptions can differ considerably from the reality. Remember that old saying, "You can't tell a book by its cover."

Take the Required Standardized Tests

Another important task is to take the standardized tests required by the programs to which you are applying. The Graduate Record Examination (GRE) has, at best, only a small correlation with grades in graduate school (Morrison & Morrison, 1995; Sternberg & Williams, 1997). In particular, directors of counselor education programs have rated the GRE as the least effective component of their admissions procedures (Leverett-Main, 2004). Nevertheless, most counselor training programs require the GRE general test, which has three scores. The Verbal Reasoning test items involve analogies, sentence completion, antonyms, and reading comprehension. Quantitative Reasoning items involve basic concepts of arithmetic, algebra, geometry, quantitative comparisons, and data interpretation. The Analytical Writing test requires that you provide a sampling of your writing abilities. Doctoral programs in counseling psychology typically require that you also take the GRE Subject Test in Psychology.

A few graduate programs give you the choice of taking either the GRE or the Miller Analogies Test (MAT). The MAT is a fifty-minute test consisting of 100 items, all involving analogies. For example: Rose is to flower as chihuahua is to

    a. chalupa.

    b. Mexico.

    c. dog.

    d. Taco Bell.

To help you do your best on these standardized tests, you can read preparation manuals, take practice tests, and even participate in workshops to enhance your scores (Finkle, 1999). Many of these practice tests are available as computer software. At the end of this chapter, you will find useful websites that have detailed information about these resources.

Arrange for References

Most training programs expect you to provide at least three references from people who know you well and can confidently comment on your readiness to become a counselor or therapist. These people will need to complete a form or write a letter of support for each school to which you are applying.

You can help make this task as simple as possible for the people who will be writing your letters of reference. For example, provide each of them with a cover sheet listing all the schools to which you are applying. You should also organize the reference forms and other materials—and be generous with the paper clips to keep each school's forms together! Provide all the necessary envelopes, appropriately addressed and stamped. These people are already offering you their time and attention to serve as your references—they shouldn't have to worry about details such as postage. It is also helpful to offer them a résumé and other specific information about your qualifications and interests. Finally, follow up with a thank-you note and keep them updated on the results of your applications.

Write a Personal Statement

Most programs also require that you submit a personal statement as part of your application. Keith-Spiegel and Wiederman (2000) examined 360 essay questions that were included on the application forms for master's and doctoral programs in psychology and related fields. Typically, the questions concern your career plans, interests, and experiences. The personal statement is the least structured part of your application; be sure, however, to answer the specific question that has been asked. Writing one generic statement to use on all your applications may save you time but can sabotage your chances of getting accepted into a program. So make sure your statement does not appear as if you did not pay attention to the question—a bad sign for potential counselors and therapists!

Also be sure that you use the personal statement as an opportunity to supplement the other information you already have provided. For example, you can make a truly *personal* statement by sharing your own individuality: experiences that have formed your character, dreams you hope to realize, and personal qualities that you bring to the program.

Along with providing the mandatory content, take care that your statement is well written. As we discuss in Chapter 5, writing is one of the basic academic skills you need to succeed in graduate school. Selection committees read these statements for evidence that you possess this skill.

Participate in a Selection Interview

Many programs include an interview as a final step in the selection process. In fact, the majority of counselor education program directors have rated the interview as the most valuable part of the admission procedure (Leverett-Main, 2004). Some applicants make the mistake of trying to prepare for an interview by developing a template of prepared answers. Keep in mind that you're not interviewing for drama school. In counseling and therapy, there are no scripts. Instead, make a commitment to be open, genuine, and engaged throughout the interview—to be yourself. The interview is also your chance to learn more about the program, so take advantage of your opportunities to ask questions. You need information in order to make *your* selection decision, too.

Consider Your Options Carefully

If you are offered admission to one or more programs, take some time to carefully weigh all the important factors as you come to a decision. Remember that you're investing several years of your life in this training, so don't take this decision lightly.

You need to consider a number of important issues. Two fundamental questions concern the third thriving principle, having traveling companions. Do faculty members personify the helping professional you hope to become? Do you look forward to working with the other students? Other questions, however, are just as important. Are you enthusiastic about the quality, depth, and breadth of the curriculum? Do you like the location of the school? What are the possibilities of financial assistance?

Once you have made your selection, contact the program as soon as possible. After you have confirmed your entrance into the program of your choice, you should quickly notify any other programs that have selected you. These programs can then offer admission to someone on their waiting lists.

BEING A NOVICE

A dream [is] the bearer of a new possibility,
the enlarged horizon, the great hope.

—Howard Thurman

When you successfully complete the selection process, your counseling identity makes a major shift from that of an applicant to that of a graduate student. You are now a member—albeit the "new kid on the block"—of a community dedicated to training helping professionals. As a novice, you probably feel a thrilling combination of excitement and worry, eagerness and apprehension (Kersting, 2005).

When you enter a program, you receive information regarding program policies, requirements, options, and procedures. In fact, it is likely that you have access to an overwhelming amount of data. Just sifting through it all, along with skimming through your new textbooks, can leave you confused and intimidated, reaffirming just how little you actually do know—and just how much you still need to learn. But take it easy on yourself. Your basic goal as a novice is to embark on your training journey successfully.

In Chapter 5, we describe in detail how you can enhance your abilities to perform well academically. In the meantime, we invite you to focus on the broader themes of your novice experience—becoming oriented, learning the basics, connecting with others, and becoming fully involved in the training process (McAuliffe & Eriksen, 2000). As you participate in your beginning courses, you begin to develop a foundation—the basic knowledge, skills, and attitudes—necessary for you to move into the apprenticeship phase of your training.

When you first become a novice, you may feel like a kid who has just climbed up the ladder to the high diving board for the first time. You think that everyone is looking at you, while you stand up there wondering what in the world you were thinking when you decided to make this dive. A belly flop would be painful enough, but also, to add insult to injury, everyone would see you fail. Well, if you want to thrive in your training, your best option is to go ahead and dive right into this new endeavor.

To help you leap into your training and succeed as a novice, just remember the thriving principles—come well prepared, live your training, learn from others, explore yourself, be open to opportunities, and always act with character. In the following section, we discuss how you can use rituals to engage deeply in your training experiences right from the start.

Opening Rituals

Rituals are ceremonial activities that give expression to beliefs, values, and concepts. Baptisms, bar mitzvahs, Hindu samsaras, vision quests, walkabouts, and marriage ceremonies are only a few of the countless religious and cultural rituals that enrich people's lives (Bell, 1997). Many counselors, especially those who work with couples and families, have found that rituals can be powerful intervention techniques (Becvar & Becvar, 2006). Rituals can also enrich your own training experience, strengthen your sense of community, celebrate your accomplishments, and give voice to your fundamental values (McKee, Smith, Hayes, Stewart, & Echterling, 1999).

All counselor and therapist training programs have orientation meetings or social gatherings to welcome new students and mark the beginning of a new academic year. These opening rituals are nice ways to introduce everyone to one another and to familiarize newcomers with the workings of their new community. For example, recognizing the emotional and bonding power of rituals, one counseling program added an initiation ceremony to its orientation. The ceremony involved faculty and students forming a circle, lighting candles, declaring personal goals, and pledging support to one another. However, even if your program does not offer any initiation ceremony, you can develop your own ritual to mark this occasion.

▨ ▨ ▨

EXERCISE 2.1 **Traditions**
A Reminiscing and Planning Exercise

Rituals that are repeated become traditions. In this exercise, we invite you first to think about two important traditions that have already enriched your life. Select one tradition that is closely connected to your family life and another that reflects your religious or cultural heritage.

Spend a little time reminiscing about each tradition. What were the circumstances? Who was involved? What was your role? When you're ready, go ahead and describe each tradition.

Looking back on this tradition, write about the meaning it holds for you now.

FAMILY

Tradition:

_____

_____

_____

Meaning:

_____

_____

_____

_____

_____

RELIGION OR CULTURE

Tradition:

_____

_____

_____

Meaning:

_____

_____

_____

_____

_____

The second part of this exercise is a planning task. Think of a ritual that you would like to make a tradition connected with your training. It could be a personal ritual that only you would perform, a family ceremony that involves your relatives, or a community activity that includes everyone in the program. Describe the activity and explore its meaning for you.

TRAINING

Tradition:

_____

_____

_____

Meaning:

_____

_____

_____

_____

We encourage you to perform an individual or shared initiation ritual at the start of your training and at the start of every academic year. Describe your experience in your training journal so that you can refer to it each year to reflect on your progress. Such an initiation ritual, like morning rituals of brushing your teeth and taking a shower, can be invigorating and awakening experiences. Besides, you may be surprised by the powerful emotions and meaningful discoveries that your ritual can evoke.

■ ■ ■

Communication

If you are to thrive in your new learning community, you need to be communicating with others. As you've heard so many times, communication is a two-way street. Be ready to do your part to be both an active listener and an open communicator in your program. Stay in touch. Keep your program administrators up-to-date on your current postal address, telephone number, and E-mail address. Be sure to let people know what's on your mind. Both you and the program will be the better for it.

Most training programs have developed a number of ways for their members to share information, ideas, and feedback with one another.

Bulletin boards Even the most high-tech programs still have plenty of physical bulletin boards hanging in the hallways for students to post paper copies of announcements, newsletters, brochures, and other information. Check these boards regularly and use them to post interesting and useful information.

E-mail Electronic mail has become a great way to communicate quickly and easily with others. You can share information about employment possibilities, social events, or other opportunities. Of course, E-mail is useless if you don't check your messages regularly.

Meetings with your advisor Every graduate student has an assigned faculty advisor, and you should be meeting regularly with yours. Consider your advisor as a ready and reliable source of information and support. Yes, of course, your faculty advisor is a busy person, but remember that advising is an integral part of teaching—and an essential resource for you.

Newsletters A program newsletter provides an overview of recent developments and a preview of upcoming events. It may, for example, introduce you to new members, update you on the accomplishments of students and faculty, and announce program changes. It also offers information on important deadlines, meetings, and conferences.

When you receive a newsletter, take some time to jot down immediately the important dates and times in your calendar. Then keep the most recent edition handy in case you need to refer to it. It is a valuable tool to help you stay up-to-date and involved. Also feel free to suggest items for inclusion in your program's newsletter.

Formal assessment procedures All graduate training programs have developed several formal assessment procedures in order to obtain your feedback and suggestions. In your courses, your faculty members will ask you to assess their teaching performance and class activities. We encourage you to offer constructive feedback and practical suggestions when faculty and supervisors request your assessment of training experiences.

Program-committee meetings All counselor training programs have regular meetings to review procedures, develop policies, and address concerns. Most programs include student representatives as members of these committees. We encourage you to consider volunteering to be a student representative at these meetings. It's a great way to see how the organization operates and to participate in the planning process.

Progress reviews One accreditation standard is that the faculty must review the overall progress each student is making every semester. Near the end of each semester, you can also conduct your own review by taking some time to think about all that you have discovered, learned, and experienced during the semester. Record these evaluations in your journal and write your ideas for making continued progress. The end of the semester is an especially busy time, but reviewing your progress and planning your future will be time well spent!

Handling Personal Problems

Because you were selected for admission from among many candidates, you will likely do well in your training and make satisfactory progress throughout the program. However, it's also possible that, at some point in your training, you could face serious academic or personal difficulties. If these difficulties threaten to impair your performance as a trainee, then you have the responsibility to take positive steps to address the concerns. You can pursue several practical, specific strategies. These steps may include taking a remedial course, repeating a course, entering personal counseling or therapy, or taking a leave of absence.

If you are dealing with concerns that seem overwhelming, then talk to your advisor about your options. In Chapter 3, we explore in detail how to deal with the stressors of graduate training, and in Chapter 6 we elaborate on the value of receiving counseling or therapy. There's no need for you to be struggling through your training like one of the walking wounded. Take care of yourself and seek help at the first sign of impairment.

Keeping a Portfolio

A portfolio is a collection of your work that tells the story of your efforts, progress, and achievement in your training (Carney, Cobia, & Shannon, 1996). As part of their evaluation procedures, many programs now require students to assemble certain materials into a portfolio (Cobia, Carney, Buckhalt, Middleton, Shannon, Trippany, & Kunkel, 2005). Even if your program does not require a portfolio, we encourage you to begin one to take advantage of its many benefits.

Your portfolio offers a composite picture of your professional development. It allows you to demonstrate what you know in a way that reflects the complexity of particular topics and how you have integrated your skills and knowledge to create useful counseling tools. There are no specific rules for what goes into your counseling portfolio. In fact, you can include different items in your portfolio depending on how you're going to use it. For example, if you plan to document your progress or to evaluate the effectiveness of your program, then certain materials will be required. However, if you intend to use it at a job interview, then you can design your portfolio to fit the position's requirements. A portfolio is also often used to record your personal growth and reflection. Consider your training journal to be an essential piece of your portfolio, even though you are unlikely to share it with others. Your journal, however, is your personal forum for noting your reflections and observations regarding the experiences documented in your portfolio.

What are some possible items for your portfolio? Obvious choices include written samples of your work, such as assessment reports, diagnostic reports, intervention plans, term papers, handouts for presentations, published articles, and important correspondence. Of course, you need to take care to protect the confidentiality of the clients you describe in these work samples. You also may want to have a section of works in progress, such as your philosophy of intervention, your evolving counseling and therapy theory, and ongoing projects. It can be useful to include a list of conferences and workshops you have attended, class presentations you have given, professional service activities, and awards. It's also a great idea to add scrapbook items, such as photographs, newspaper clippings, and program announcements, concerning your professional activities. Include drawings and comments by clients, notes from colleagues, and performance assessments from professors and supervisors.

Dualistic Thinking

As a novice, you are likely to be at Perry's first stage of adult development, which is characterized by a dualistic, right-or-wrong attitude (Young, 2005). At this stage, you tend to approach your learning in a somewhat perfectionistic manner. You may find yourself trying to determine which of the theories of counseling you are learning is *the* correct one. You may, for example, be attracted to a person-centered approach or a cognitive-behavioral theory, and you feel you must choose one or the other. After all, they can't both be right … can they?

▲ ▲ ▲

The One
Juanita's Story

As a beginning counselor, I went through a series of infatuations with various counseling fads. The process later reminded me of the series of boyfriends I had had in high school. At first, I was completely fascinated with a particular counseling approach, certain that I had finally found "The One." However, as reality began to set in and I began to notice the imperfections and limitations of the technique, I quickly became disenchanted, "dumped" it, and went on to another counseling approach.

It was only later in my training, when I began to look closely at myself and to value what I brought to the counseling relationship, that I realized that I could set aside my desperate search for "The One."

▼ ▼ ▼

Perfectionism

Besides embarking on a quest for the perfect theory, as a novice, you're likely to be demanding perfection from yourself in your performance. You may come to your class in basic counseling skills believing that your performance must be impeccable—otherwise, you will be an absolute failure. With so much at stake, instead of really listening to the person who sits before you as your client, you are focusing on what to say next. You feel queasy as you attempt to make sense of what your client is saying. Nervous mannerisms, such as rhythmically kicking your foot or saying "uh-huh," begin to pop up. You're under pressure to come up with the answer to your client's problem, and if you don't, you believe that you have not been helpful at all. So you wind up saying something ineffectual like, "Have you tried talking to your roommate?"

As you reflect on your feelings of incompetence at the beginning of your program, you might secretly believe that you are a fraud, and that, sooner or later, you will be found out and excommunicated from the ranks. This is what Harvey and Katz (1985) called the "impostor phenomenon." Don't become too worried about it. Most trainees feel that way at the beginning of their program. In fact, we'll let you in on a little secret in the counseling and therapy training profession. We warn one another, "Be afraid, be very afraid!" about any beginning trainee who is supremely confident that he or she is already a genuine master of the art of counseling and therapy. People who think that they've already arrived see no point in going on a journey—and they make terrible travelers.

BEING AN APPRENTICE

We work to become, not to acquire.

—Elbert Hubbard

When you have completed your basic courses, you are no longer a novice. As you proceed to the next level of your training program, you begin to take on more responsibilities as you assume a new identity—that of an apprentice. As an apprentice, you are under close supervision, but you now have opportunities to practice your professional skills. For example, you may be assisting a professor on a research project, offering counseling services at a practicum site, presenting a guidance unit at a school, or cofacilitating a personal growth group with an intern.

Once you have demonstrated that you can succeed in a graduate program, you can, for example, apply for membership in Chi Sigma Iota, an honor society for the counseling profession. This society recognizes excellence in counseling and helps create an atmosphere of professional commitment. You are invited to apply for membership each semester. Activities often include philanthropic projects, presentations, and social events.

Multiplistic Thinking

As you shift from a novice to an apprentice, you progress from a dualistic to a multiplistic way of thinking. At this point in your development, you begin to give up the idea that there is one correct answer or a single right way to work with people. Furthermore, you begin to see that your standard of right and wrong is not shared by all the people you meet and that their views have merit. You feel less threatened by ideas that once seemed strange—or just plain wrong—to you, and you become more accepting of other lifestyles. Instead of wanting to argue with people who see things differently, you become interested in their way of experiencing the world. Now, you spend less of your energy attempting to figure out what your professors expect of you and begin to operate more on your inner sense of how to carry out a project.

Still, at this stage of your development, you may be overwhelmed by all the new possibilities that are presented to you and a bit suspicious of those who attempt to persuade you to go in new directions. You may find that you become irritable, as well as regularly confused, during this phase of your training. Young (2005) stated that students at this stage

> often report being frustrated and defensive with supervisors who "correct" them because they do not yet know how to select the most helpful course of action. All roads seem to be equally valid (p. 6).

▲▲▲

A Deer Caught in the Headlights
Bill's Story

"YOU'RE THE FIRST counseling graduate student I've ever met who's atheoretical!"

After recovering from the initial shock of that statement from my practicum supervisor, I rather dumbly replied, "Oh, I guess I have a theory, I just don't know what it is yet."

"Maybe it's time you found out," he responded. "You are trying to counsel from your personality alone, just being a nice person. I think your clients may be looking for more than that from you," he concluded.

He was right. My secret was out. I was a deer caught in the headlights. I really didn't have a clue about integrating theory into practice. Oh, I had completed several theory and technique classes, even received great grades in them, but somehow the content of those classes had not yet become a reality for either my counseling work or for me. It was time to begin the quest for a theory I could claim as my own.

It was not an easy journey. I had to work more, read more, question more. Being "eclectic" seemed like a cop-out to me. I really wanted to discover a theory that made sense to me, that worked for me in helping relationships and allowed me to be me at the same time. After two practicum experiences and a year-long internship, I landed on what I now call "holistic-integrative" counseling. It includes many aspects from well-known theories, such as those of Albert Ellis, Salvador Minuchin, Fritz Perls, Carl Rogers, and Virginia Satir, yet it also became uniquely mine—an integration of my personality, experiences, and worldview. The really neat part is that it is open-ended, allowing for constant adjustments based on new discoveries I make. In other words, I'm still growing, and so is my theory.

▼▼▼

The "Sophomore Slump"

Gregory Neimeyer (personal communication, March 12, 2001) has observed that many graduate students become disillusioned during their second year of training. During your first year, you probably had an intensive, challenging time and made some steady progress. You may, however, be disappointed if you did not make the dramatic advances that you had hoped in your professional development. You also may feel somewhat disenchanted because even though you gained many personal insights, you have not yet achieved any extraordinary breakthroughs in your own self-awareness.

As a novice, you not only demanded a great deal from yourself, but you also had high expectations of faculty and supervisors. Such expectations do not match the realities of faculty life. During your undergraduate days, you may not have worked closely with faculty members. Consequently, you may not have realized that the average university faculty member works well over fifty hours a week, with direct teaching duties accounting for only a small fraction of this time. Now that you are working more closely with the training faculty, you may notice that they are often heavily overcommitted, with work schedules that are, like a middle-aged man's old blue jeans, dangerously tight.

Certainly, faculty members want to collaborate with you as you progress through the training program. However, they also have to juggle the demands of a challenging teaching load, supervisory meetings, multiple scholarly projects, never-ending committee work, and service to the profession and community. There will be times during which they do not respond quickly to your frantic E-mail messages, seem distracted when you share a concern, or are unavailable when you have an important question. In short, faculty members will not always be there for you. However, take care not to assume that they are disengaged or unconcerned about your well-being. The more likely reason is that they are stretched too thin and overburdened—sound familiar?

Whatever you do, watch out that your minor frustrations and disappointments don't crystallize into resentment against the faculty. It's a common dynamic in counseling groups. People are tempted to find a "scapegoat" to blame for their unfulfilled needs. If you find yourself regularly grousing and griping about the faculty with your fellow students, it's time to deal productively with the hostility before it gathers momentum. Recognize that your feelings are normal and that you can communicate your concerns in direct and respectful ways with your teachers, supervisors, and mentors.

Comprehensive Examination

Near the end of the apprenticeship period of your training, you complete a comprehensive examination. Its purpose is to document that you have integrated essential knowledge of counseling and psychological theories, research, and practice.

The format of the comprehensive examination differs from program to program. One popular format is the Counselor Preparation Comprehensive Examination (CPCE). The CPCE is a knowledge-based multiple-choice examination that reflects the eight core curriculum areas approved by the Council for Accreditation of Counseling and Related Educational Programs (CACREP). Another common format for the comprehensive examination is a series of essay questions.

Some programs require a portfolio of documents that demonstrate the student's knowledge. In a few programs, students provide a sample of their counseling work, such as a recording of a counseling session and other supporting documents, for the comprehensive examination. A number of programs use some combination of written and oral examinations.

Whatever its format, a successful comprehensive examination involves more than merely passing. Your comprehensive examination serves as an important rite of passage for you. You can use this experience to help you pull together useful information and ideas from your earlier courses and therapeutic experiences. In meeting the challenge of the examination, you also discover a great deal about yourself, both personally and professionally. The comprehensive examination experience gives you a chance to demonstrate not only to faculty members but also to yourself that you are ready to become a professional. You can thrive during this rite of passage, emerging from this process with a greater sense of personal and professional confidence.

The following strategies can be helpful in preparing for the examination:

- **Be confident.** The comprehensive examination is your opportunity to demonstrate what you have learned from your hard work and long preparation. Come to the examination looking forward to your chance to demonstrate your knowledge and readiness to be a professional.

- **Focus on yourself.** Use the examination preparation to reflect on your own theoretical perspectives, personal issues, competencies, and limitations as a beginning counselor or therapist. Take time to explore your own personal and professional development.

- **Join an informal support group.** Sharing concerns and encouragement can be helpful. It is also reassuring to find out that you are not the only one to have doubts and worries about your performance.

- **Review previous course material.** You will find it helpful to look over all the information, concepts, and issues that you have addressed in your earlier classes.

- **Take care of yourself.** You can do this by taking time to relax and rest. On looking back after successfully completing the examination, most students report wishing that they had not worried so much.

- **Train well from the start.** From the start, be actively involved in all facets of your training. The best way to prepare for a successful comprehensive examination is to be a successful trainee in the program.

- **Work long and hard.** There is no quick and easy way to be successful in your examination. It requires intense preparation involving hours of study and review. Once you have laid the groundwork, however, you're more likely to come to the examination feeling equal to the task and confident.

Although you will only complete this examination once, we encourage you to do your part to make this a thriving experience for other students. You can help by supporting your fellow students as they embark on this rite of passage, encouraging them as they confront their own doubts, and congratulating them on their successes.

AN EMERGING PROFESSIONAL

One's work may be finished someday, but one's
education never.

—Alexandre Dumas

The final stage of your graduate training involves the completion of two important capstone experiences—your internship and your research project. *Capstone* refers to the finishing stone of a structure. In your training, your capstone experiences are the culmination of all your work and preparation. You began the program as a novice, progressed to become an apprentice, and have now developed into an emerging professional. Although you will continue to need supervision and advising, you have demonstrated your readiness to successfully complete your formal training and to graduate (Leach, Stoltenberg, McNeil, & Eichenfield, 1997).

Your internship gives you an opportunity to practice an important dimension of your emerging professional role. In Chapter 8, we discuss internships in detail.

Relativistic Thinking

As an emerging professional who is nearing the successful completion of your program, your thinking continues to evolve, from multiplistic to relativistic. At the last of Perry's (1970) stages, you begin to tailor your responses to the circumstance at hand, realizing that there are "different strokes for different folks." During this period of development, you probably use one kind of intervention with people who present with specific phobias and another kind of approach with those who seem "existentially lost." As you learn more about the various theoretical approaches, you begin to see commonalities among them. You may begin to become more eclectic or transtheoretical in your attitudes. Instead of viewing your clients as ignorant or misguided, you begin to understand the circumstances that have brought them to their current situation. As you enhance your therapeutic skills, you also become more cognitively complex (Little, Packman, Smaby, & Maddux, 2005).

You judge your own responses in sessions based on whether they seem to produce the desired effects in the client. You grow less preoccupied with your own performance and become much more focused on helping your client achieve his or her goals. In your classes, you begin to notice that you are no longer working for the grade as much as you are working for self-improvement. Your learning shifts from "outside in" to "inside out."

As Young (2005) put it, "The main value of thinking about stages of development is that it can help you recognize that your struggles are part of a normal progression" (p. 8). Throughout your program, you are continually progressing. If you are recording your counseling work, you may want to save your first recording—provided that this is not a breach of confidentiality and that you have the permission of your client. Saving this recording can be helpful to you because your progress is often gradual and imperceptible. If you have a recording, you can look back and be amazed at how much you have improved over the course of your training.

As we have mentioned earlier, keeping a journal is helpful in tracking the metamorphosis you are experiencing. However, no matter how long your training program may be, you must remember that this journey is lifelong (Kottler, 2002). You may have expected that you would graduate and leave your training as a more-or-less finished product. Once you realize just how much more you have to learn, you may at first feel inadequate, disappointed in yourself, or disillusioned with your training. These reactions are simply more of those normal, typical, and common feelings that you'll experience in your professional development.

Keep in mind that in order to become a master counselor, you will need years of practice, intense supervision, and many varied experiences (Etringer, Hillerbrand, & Claiborn, 1995). It has been said that it takes as many as ten years and the accumulation of at least 50,000 bits of information to achieve mastery (Hoffman, Shadbolt, Burton, & Klein, 1995). Right now, that may seem a long time and an overwhelming amount of learning, but if you are truly committed to the helping profession, you *will* get there. The information in this book will help you keep your journey in perspective. There will be times, however, when you judge yourself harshly for not being good enough. Remember to trust in yourself and in the process. Wherever you are right now in your progress through Perry's stages, just be there! Go with the flow. You'll get where you want to go.

Research Project

The purpose of the thesis or dissertation is to provide you with an opportunity to complete an intensive and comprehensive scholarly project that makes an original contribution to the profession (Cone & Foster, 2006). In most programs, you have a wide variety of possible topics that are acceptable for a thesis or dissertation, as long as you demonstrate relevance to the field. Your final report will include a review of the professional literature and a discussion of implications. It may take one of the following forms:

- **Applied study.** An applied study may involve assessing the needs of a population or evaluating the effectiveness of an intervention or program.
- **Critical review.** A critical review of the literature regarding an issue in counseling and therapy would be more than merely a summary of the literature. The critical review should offer new and creative ways of looking at an issue, develop a useful conceptual framework, or give a well-reasoned critique of the material.
- **Research report.** The research report involves collecting and analyzing quantitative or qualitative data to answer a particular research question.
- **Technique or program development.** Your research project may involve developing an innovative therapeutic technique or program.

You may have been using a journal to explore the emotional nuances of your training, but you can also use it in your research to jot down your hunches, speculate on possible topics, or sketch out your plans. You can get much more out of keeping a journal if you do more than merely summarize your experiences. For example, consider what is particularly interesting, meaningful, unusual, or even puzzling about the research you are doing. Date your entries and write regularly, at least two or three times a week. Use your journal to explore your thoughts, sort through your feelings, recollect memories, and develop ideas. You can use a variety of strategies—questioning, synthesizing, speculating, and brainstorming.

Selecting a Committee You need to select a faculty committee for your thesis or dissertation. Typically, your committee consists of one chairperson and at least two members. You may be able to elect to have an additional reader if this person has expertise relevant to your research project.

As you work on your project, keep in mind that it is your responsibility to keep your chairperson and committee members informed of your progress. Typically, you will have at least two meetings with the entire committee—one at the beginning of the project and another at its completion. At the first meeting, the committee considers your proposal. The purpose of the second is to discuss your final report, recommend revisions, and make a final decision on whether to accept it.

Completing Your Final Draft The format for the final report should follow the guidelines presented in your institution's handbook for theses and dissertations and in the *Publication Manual of the American Psychological Association* (American Psychological Association, 2001). The institutional guidelines impose stringent conditions on the format, such as quality of paper, size of margins, font type, and legibility requirements.

Evaluating Criteria The chairperson and readers of your thesis or dissertation will be evaluating your performance based on several criteria. First, the report must be a thorough consideration of the topic that you have selected. No matter what type of research you perform, you must present a comprehensive review of pertinent professional literature. Another criterion is originality. You must offer a contribution to the professional literature that is based on your own ideas and work. Your report must be more than a summary of the thoughts and efforts of others—it must have the distinction of presenting your individual notions and views. Finally, the most fundamental criterion is the extent to which you are successful in accomplishing what you set out to do in your proposal. Whether it was to perform an empirical study, to develop an innovative program, or to write a critical review, your final report will be assessed in terms of your attainment of that goal.

Graduation and Commencement

The graduation and commencement exercise is a widespread and long-standing tradition. We invite you to personalize this final ritual by saying good-bye to one another as students and professors and greeting one another as professional colleagues. Savor the moment, and soon you will begin to see that the intuition that brought you to the training program in the first place is still valid. You really are a professional helper!

SUMMARY

Your training journey is a metamorphosis from student to professional. This transformation involves much more than gaining knowledge and acquiring skills. You take on new roles, progress through developmental stages, and pass important milestones. Successfully completing this journey sets the stage for launching your career as a professional.

RESOURCES

Several books are available that can help you begin your training journey. If you are applying to programs, then read *The Complete Guide to Graduate School Admission: Psychology, Counseling, and Related Professions* (Keith-Spiegel and Wiederman, 2000). It's a comprehensive and practical guide on everything you need to know to enhance your chances of admission, make choices that are right for you, and successfully navigate through the admissions process.

Another helpful resource at this stage of your journey is the *Getting In: A Step-by-Step Plan for Gaining Admission to Graduate School in Psychology*, published by the American Psychological Association (1997). You'll find detailed information on models of training, tips for interviews, and a timetable for planning.

We also recommend *Becoming a Therapist: A Workbook for Personal Exploration*, by Kerr (2000). This workbook includes activities for helping you to experience therapy processes, such as empathy, change, and feelings. Other activities invite you to explore personal topics, such as enhancing your relationships, expressing your feelings, and taking care of yourself.

As its title states, the second edition of *Dissertations and Theses from Start to Finish: Psychology and Related Fields* (Cone and Foster, 2006) helps you plan and complete your research project from beginning to end. The authors offer useful suggestions on getting organized, finding a topic, developing a proposal, and selecting a chairperson.

Websites also offer information, advice, and links to resources. Here are a few of what we consider to be best:

Center for Credentialing & Education, Inc. (CCE)

3 Terrace Way, Suite D

Greensboro, NC 27403–3660

336-547-0607 or fax, 336-547-0017

Council for Accreditation of Counseling and Related Educational Programs (CACREP)

5999 Stevenson Avenue

Alexandria, VA 22304

703–823-9800, ext. 301

www.cacrep.org

Gradschools.com
www.gradschools.com

This popular site offers the most comprehensive on-line source of graduate school information, with links to thousands of program listings. It contains information on graduate programs, standardized tests, financial aid, and graduate school events.

Kaplan
www.kaptest.com

The Info Center of the world's leader in test preparation has the available option of taking test preparation courses on-line. Information on the site includes strategies for selecting and applying to graduate schools. There is an online bookstore, updates on changes in the GRE, an overview of the MAT, and information on study skills, financial aid, and career planning.

Peterson's Graduate Planner: Student Edition
iiswinprd01.petersons.com/GradChannel/code/search.asp?

This site has links to information on finding schools, preparing for the GRE and MAT, discovering the program that matches your interests, and strategies for managing your education expenses. It has an online advice center and a bookstore.

REFERENCES

American Psychological Association. (1997). *Getting in: A step-by-step plan for gaining admission to graduate school in psychology.* Washington, DC: Author.

American Psychological Association. (2001). *Publication manual of the American Psychological Association* (5th ed.). Washington, DC: Author.

Becvar, D. S., & Becvar, R. J. (2006). *Family therapy: A systemic integration* (6th ed.). Boston: Allyn & Bacon.

Bell, C. (1997). *Ritual: Perspectives and dimensions.* New York: Oxford University Press.

Buskist, W., & Mixon, A. (1998). *Guide to master's programs in psychology and counseling psychology.* Boston: Allyn & Bacon.

Carney, J. S., Cobia, D. C., & Shannon, D. M. (1996). The use of portfolios in the clinical and comprehensive evaluation of counselors-in-training. *Counselor Education and Supervision, 36,* 122–132.

Cobia, D. C., Carney, J. S., Buckhalt, J. A., Middleton, R. A., Shannon, D. M., Trippany, R., & Kunkel, E. (2005). The doctoral portfolio: Centerpiece of a comprehensive system of evaluation. *Counselor Education and Supervision, 44,* 242–254.

Cone, J. D., & Foster, S. L. (2006). *Dissertations and theses from start to finish: Psychology and related fields* (2nd ed.). Washington, DC: American Psychological Association.

Etringer, B. D., Hillerbrand, E., & Claiborn, C. D. (1995). The transition from novice to expert counselor. *Counselor Education and Supervision, 35,* 4–17.

Finkle, J. (1999). *Graduate school.* Seattle, WA: Resource Pathways.

Harvey, C., & Katz, C. (1985). *If I'm so successful, why do I feel like a fake? The impostor phenomenon.* New York: St. Martin's.

Hoffman, R. R., Shadbolt, N. R., Burton, A. M., & Klein, G. (1995). Eliciting knowledge from experts: A methodological analysis. *Organizational Behavior and Human Decision Processes, 62,* 129–158.

Hoskins, C. M., & Goldberg, A. D. (2005). Doctoral student persistence in counselor education programs: Student-program match. *Counselor Education and Supervision, 44,* 175–188.

Keith-Spiegel, P., & Wiederman, M. W. (2000). *The complete guide to graduate school admission: Psychology, counseling, and related professions* (2nd ed.). Mahwah, NJ: Erlbaum.

Kerr, D. R. (2000). *Becoming a therapist: A workbook for personal exploration.* Prospect Heights, IL: Waveland Press.

Kersting, K. (2005). First-year hurdles: Make the most of your initial year in graduate school. *gradPSYCH, 3,* 14–16.

Kottler, J. A. (Ed.). (2002). *Counselors finding their way.* Alexandria, VA: American Counseling Association.

Leach, M. M., Stoltenberg, C. D., McNeil, B. W., & Eichenfield, G. A. (1997). Self-efficacy and counselor development: Testing the integrated developmental model. *Counselor Education and Supervision, 37,* 115–124.

Leverett-Main, S. (2004). Program directors' perceptions of admission screening measures and indicators of student success. *Counselor Education and Supervision, 43,* 207–219.

Little, C., Packman, J., Smaby, M. H., & Maddux, C. D. (2005). The skilled counselor training model: Skill acquisition, self-assessment, and cognitive complexity. *Counselor Education and Supervision, 44,* 189–200.

Markert, L., & Monke, R. (1990). Changes in counselor education admissions criteria. *Counselor Education and Supervision, 30,* 48–57.

McAuliffe, G., & Eriksen, K. (2000). *Preparing counselors and therapists: Creating constructivist and developmental programs.* Virginia Beach, VA: Donning.

McKee, J. E., Smith, L. W., Hayes, B. G., Stewart, A., & Echterling, I. G. (1999). Rites and rituals in counselor education. *Journal of Humanistic Education, 38,* 3–12.

Morrison, T., & Morrison, M. (1995). A meta-analytic assessment of the predictive validity of the quantitative and verbal components of the Graduate Record Examination with graduate grade point average representing the criterion of graduate success. *Educational and Psychological Measurement, 55,* 309–316.

Perry, W. G., Jr. (1970). *Forms of intellectual and ethical development in the college years.* New York: Holt, Rinehart & Winston.

Sayette, M. A., Mayne, T. J., & Norcross, J. C. (2004). *Insider's guide to graduate programs in clinical and counseling psychology.* New York: Guilford Press.

Simpson, D. E., Dalgaard, K. A., & O'Brien, D. K. (1986). Student
    and faculty assumptions about the nature of uncertainty in
    medicine and medical education. *Journal of Family Practice,*
    23(5), 468–472.

Sternberg, R. J., & Williams, W. M. (1997). Does the Graduate
    Record Examination predict meaningful success in the graduate
    training of psychologists? *American Psychologist, 52,* 630–641.

Walfish, S., & Hess, A. (Eds.). (2001). *Succeeding in graduate school:*
    The career guide for psychology students. Mahwah, NJ: Lawrence
    Erlbaum.

Young, M. E. (2005). *Learning the art of helping: Building blocks and*
    techniques (3rd ed.). Upper Saddle River, NJ: Merrill/Prentice-
    Hall.

CHAPTER 3

Embracing Your Stress

There were only two times when I felt stress in
graduate school—night and day.

—A colleague

What man needs is not a tensionless state but the
striving and struggling for something worth
longing and groping for.

—Viktor Frankl

At this stage of your life journey, you've probably heard a lot about
stress management. You may even think you already know enough
about stress and the need to take care of yourself. However, before you
are tempted to skip this chapter with the assumption that you've heard
it all before, consider this: Have you ever considered *embracing* your
stress? Yes, we're serious! After all, this book is a manual on how to
thrive in graduate school. Developing resilience under stress is an excellent way to thrive throughout your training as well as your career.

Let's be honest; training is stressful. In fact, all forms of training—
athletic, academic, or occupational—involve increasingly demanding
and challenging tasks. Physical exercises, essay exams, and field placements are all different sources of stress. Of course, successful training
also includes plenty of support and guidance as you gradually progress
through achievable steps. As an athlete, you can overstress your body by
exercising too much or too quickly. If you don't take care, you can put
yourself at risk for fatigue, injuries, and physical breakdown.

As a trainee in a helping profession, you can also become overstressed. You may often feel as if you are living by the law of supply and demand. You have limitations on your "supply"—resources such as time, energy, money, and information. Meanwhile, your training, as well as life in general, continues to place seemingly limitless demands on you—tests, reading assignments, work obligations, and family responsibilities. It's no wonder that you may feel overwhelmed and depleted! As stress is an essential part of your training, why not learn how to welcome it? Just as an athlete relishes a vigorous workout, you can approach challenging experiences with enthusiasm because they can help you grow stronger as a counselor and therapist.

In the first half of this chapter, we offer specific tips for successfully managing the stressors that you will face in graduate school and your professional life. We also present important principles for dealing with stress. Maintaining balance, harmony, an even pace, and a healthy perspective can help you keep your bearings along your journey (Rollins, 2005). Remember that if many of our recommendations may seem obvious, then why do most people—probably even you, yourself—fail to use them regularly? How obvious are they really? Isn't it ironic that, as counselors and therapists, we want to help *others* deal with stress, but we're often reluctant, unwilling, or unable to handle our own?

Once we have examined these practical approaches to managing stress—the "how" questions—we turn to the meaning of stress—the "why" questions. In the second half of this chapter, we encourage you to do much more than merely manage your stress as you pursue your desire to become a helping professional. We invite you to make your stress meaningful. In his book, *Psychotherapy and Existentialism*, Viktor Frankl (1967) asserted, "What man really needs is a sound amount of tension aroused by the challenge of a meaning he has to fulfill" (pp. 87–88).

What meaning are *you* fulfilling by completing this challenging and rigorous training program? You're going to graduate school because you desire to become a helping professional. You know it is not an easy journey, but what meaning has it for you right now? Certainly, you realize that attending graduate school adds stress to your life. You have made a public commitment by embarking on this adventure, but you have no guarantee that you will succeed. How will you make the stress you experience worthwhile? What is the point of the inevitable struggles and frustrations you will encounter in your training?

How would your life experiences change if you actually anticipated—even looked forward to—the stress that is inevitably part of a productive training and professional career? We believe the outcome would be considerably different! Just as an oyster transforms an irritating grain of sand into a beautiful pearl, you can embrace stress and turn it into something of great value.

▲▲▲

Stressed Out
Bill's Story

THE YEAR 1991 was a very stressful time in my life. I had just returned home after serving several months in Saudi Arabia with the Air National Guard during the Persian Gulf War. My mother died very suddenly of a massive stroke. My marriage of eleven years was crumbling. On top of all that, I had just started a graduate program in counselor education. The demands on my life were overwhelming!

By October of that year, I was completely stressed out. I began the painful journey of a separation and divorce, moved into an apartment, started visitation with my son every other weekend, and watched helplessly as my bank account dwindled into nothingness. I found myself feeling isolated, alienated from others, depressed, and lifeless.

How did I survive? Faith and hope helped tremendously. I believed that the stressful time would not last forever and that I would become stronger, wiser, and more compassionate for enduring the pain of those life events. A few very close friends and family members also enabled me to keep going because they accepted my situation, supported and encouraged me, and truly lightened my load as I made this difficult journey. I am very thankful for the people who allowed me to vent my anger, shed my tears, and express my fears. I am also grateful that I had the courage to seek professional therapy, and the therapeutic relationship empowered and strengthened me to move on with my life.

I learned to take responsibility for my own life (and my thoughts, feelings, and actions) and intentionally began eating better, sleeping more, and exercising regularly to regain my energy and relieve some of the pressure in my life. The people who really cared about me never gave up on me, and as a result, I learned to never give up on myself.

▼▼▼

STRESS

We learn the rope of life by untying its knots.

—Jean Toomer

Do you ever watch nature programs on television? Every one of those shows seems to feature some hapless insect, bird, or mammal being eaten by something else. On one recent program, the narrator calmly explained how the world is divided into predators and prey. To illustrate the concept, a mink was shown dragging home a reluctant muskrat for dinner—presumably as the main course, rather than as a guest. While a cow was shown grazing, the narrator pointed out that some creatures are herbivores. The program went on to present a sampling of carnivores—a weasel enthusiastically chewing on a mouse—and omnivores—a raccoon eating a fish and, for dessert, a plant. The narrator concluded by asserting that at the top of nature's food chain are humans, who are the only species on the planet without a natural enemy.

So humans have *no* natural enemy? If that's the case, then why are so many of us dying before our time every year? For many of us, the answer may be found in a line from "Pogo," an old newspaper comic strip—"We have met the enemy, and he is us." Suicide and murder are among the top ten causes of death. Our own behaviors—smoking, poor nutrition, and lack of exercise—are also major contributors to our early deaths. One factor, however, is a common thread among all the major causes of death. That factor is stress. Many researchers now believe that stress is involved in more illnesses than any other single contributor known to science. As human beings, our problem is that even though we are at the top of the food chain, what seems to be eating us is stress.

In this section, we discuss stress and recommend some practical ways to prevent the negative physiological consequences of stress. In the second half of the chapter, we move beyond coping strategies to explore what you can learn and gain from stressful encounters so that you can thrive in your training.

In a very real sense, stress is a natural part of living. Stressors are any demands placed on you by life events and circumstances that require your attention, time, and energy. Not all stress is bad. In fact, you may feel bored, empty, and unfulfilled without enough stress in your life. As you will read in Chapter 5, a certain amount of stress can enable you to perform at your best, but too much may deplete and overwhelm you. Would you ever study for a big test and put in all the necessary time for an important paper if you didn't feel some stress about your performance? Yet when exams, papers, relationships, and work are all clamoring for your attention, you can quickly feel overwhelmed. At these times, you are in distress. Life's demands are far exceeding your personal resources, and the experience may feel anything but positive.

The Stress of Helping

One cannot be deeply responsive to the world without being saddened very often.

—Erich Fromm

As occupations, the helping professions are very stressful. The responsibility inherent in counseling and therapy, combined with the professional isolation that often occurs, can cause many practitioners to become so physically and emotionally distressed that they burn out. The results of one study (Sowa, May, & Niles, 1994) are, however, promising: The researchers found that people with higher coping abilities, such as recreational activities, and social supports, reported lower levels of occupational stress. Furthermore, graduate students who had completed stress-management courses reported greater coping skills than those who had not completed such a course. This research also suggests that graduate school is an ideal time for you to improve your stress-deflecting skills and to take positive steps toward handling stress and preventing burnout.

Distress

The process of living is the process of reacting to stress.

—Stanley Sarnoff

When you begin to feel overwhelmed by particularly stressful events or circumstances, you may notice some physical symptoms of distress. You may have a faster heartbeat, a dry mouth, and increased sweating and urination. You may also develop indigestion, feel nauseated, develop migraine headaches, and have pain in your neck and shoulders. You may discover that you are having more colds and viruses. On an emotional level, you may feel more irritable, tired, sad, or apprehensive. You may discover that you laugh nervously or that you have the urge to cry, scream, hide, or argue more than usual. On a cognitive level, you may find that you have more difficulty concentrating and making decisions. Finally, on a behavioral level, you may notice that you are more impulsive, more accident prone, or have the need to smoke, drink, or medicate yourself. You may find it difficult to relax or sleep.

Prolonged symptoms of distress may include high blood pressure, chronic indigestion, and decreased immunity to disease. The more of these symptoms you notice in yourself, the more aggressively you will need to use healthy stress management strategies.

Stressful Events

What you can do is learn to take better care of yourself, now and in the future. Life is filled with events, both large and small, joyful and tragic. Any of those events can cause stress or, when multiplied together, distress. The Social Readjustment Rating Scale (Holmes & Rahe, 1967) measures some of these life events and their impact on us. Take a few moments to go to www.teachhealth.com/#stressscale, and take the inventory. As the number of stressful life events you have encountered over the past year begin to mount up, ask yourself how you've handled them. Researchers suggest that unresolved stress may accumulate over time, multiplying the pressure on your life. The higher your score, the more you'll want to incorporate healthy stress approaches into your life.

▲▲▲

When It "Hurts Good"
Rachel's Story

WHEN I ENTERED my graduate counseling program, I anticipated a great deal of stress. However, in a smug sort of way, I thought that I was prepared for it. I had been a massage therapist, so I was already accustomed to dealing with stress. I ate well, exercised every day, and practiced deep breathing and meditation. I wrote in my journal, sought solitude, prayed, listened to soft music, and all while the sweet fragrance of aromatherapy infused my house.

These stress reducers worked very well for a while. What I did not foresee was the stress that came from getting to know myself in a more in-depth and revealing way. That first semester, not only did I worry and stress out about the normal things—grades, finances, and relationships—but also my program required me to take a very close look at myself. "This is not what it's supposed to be about," I thought, "I'm here to help *other* people."

Later, a professor explained to me, "You can't expect clients to confide in you their flaws and imperfections, if you are not willing to do the same work yourself." This made sense, but I thought, "I'm not sure that I'm prepared to deal with this *and* worry about writing papers."

I stopped exercising because I felt that the time would be better spent studying. I started eating a lot of those little snacks from machines to quell my anxiety. Meditating was out because statistics problems kept popping into my "white space." Stress was beginning to consume me.

Fortunately, in my second semester, as I became more familiar and in tune with the therapeutic process of counseling others, I also benefited. I began to discover better ways of looking at things and more effective ways of expressing myself. I was also learning, through my experiences, all of the things that I would want to provide potential clients. Of course, there were growing pains, but they were like the soreness that is felt when I am getting a massage and the therapist is working directly on a painful spot. It is a hedonistic pain that hurts—but it "hurts good." I was gaining more from my counseling program than just a master's degree; I was gaining the ability to function more productively in the world.

All this is not to say that I have no more stressful days—for there are plenty. I have come to learn how to balance my schoolwork with exercise, meditation, and time for myself. However, it has been the personal growth through the trials and tribulations of my program that has helped me to become a stronger, healthier person.

RESPONDING TO STRESS

> You can out-distance that which is running after you, but not what is running inside you.
>
> —Rwandan Proverb

The ability to respond effectively to stress, like many other abilities, varies tremendously among individuals. Some people feel they're falling to pieces if they break a fingernail, but those people are not likely to be admitted to graduate programs in the helping professions. It's a safe bet that you've been able to manage stress pretty well. In fact, you probably can face looming deadlines, car breakdowns, and financial woes without being overwhelmed. However, you cannot put your life "on hold" when you enter training, so the added pressures of graduate school can be a tremendous strain. Therefore, now's the time to consider specific steps you can take to better handle stress.

Research has suggested that there may be differences in the ways in which women and men respond to stress (Taylor, Klein, Lewis, Gruenewald, Gurung, & Updegraff, 2000). The "fight or flight" response, which has been a widely accepted model for depicting reactions to stress, may now be supplemented by the "tend and befriend" response. This response describes the tendency of many women to reach out to others during stressful times. The researchers found that previous research on stress focused primarily on men, and the "fight or flight" response may be an accurate description of how most men react to stress. Women, however, are more likely to reach out to others in their social network and to care for others around them during times of stress.

This research does not necessarily suggest that all men respond to stress in one way and all women respond in another. You may want to think about how you typically respond to stressful situations. The "tend and befriend" response can remind you that you do have options in how you choose to react, live, and be. If you've maximized your "fight or flight" response, perhaps those perpetual butterflies in your stomach are a reminder of just how good you've gotten at this. Maybe it's time to consider new ways to make the most of the energy that stress generates within you. Reaching out to others, drawing strength from relationships, and contributing to your community are fine ways to channel your stress into connections and creativity. The key is to recognize the possibilities and then use your own ingenuity to adaptively respond to stress.

Whether you worry, fight, flee, tend, or befriend, you can develop a wide range of adaptive responses as you manage stress. Consider the following suggestions, recalling the personal examples illustrated in the stories earlier in this chapter. As you read through this section, assess your own stress-response strategies.

- **Resting.** This may not be as easy as it sounds, but do find ways to relax and "let go" of each day's events so that you can get the rest you need. Many people under stress may say they are sleeping "like babies," but what that really means is that they are waking up and crying every couple of hours!

  Adults need between seven and nine hours of sleep to function well. Many cultures also have rest or "nap" times during the middle of the day. Perhaps our parents, caretakers, and kindergarten teachers were on to something. Your body must rest to replenish your energy supply. Yet you may be sleep deprived at the times when you need rest the most. Are you getting the rest you need?

- **Eating well.** Good nutrition provides your body with the fuel it needs to deal with the daily hassles and struggles of life. Especially because you're leading a hectic life, you need to eat more fruits and vegetables to function well.

  When under stress, you may be tempted to grab quick foods on the run or to skip meals altogether, but eating nothing or eating foods with little nutritional value, such as Pop Tarts, potato chips, and pizza, will not supply critical energy when you need it most. Also, be careful about using caffeinated beverages to compensate for too little sleep and alcohol to cope with stress. Such quick fixes will never replace bona fide remedies, and alcohol is actually a depressant, which is just what you *don't* need when you're under a lot of stress! Moderation and balance are the key. How do your nutritional habits measure up?

- **Exercising.** Walking, jogging, biking, swimming, aerobic classes, and weight training are fun ways to improve your physical fitness and sense of well-being. What's more, exercise relieves stress and provides you with additional energy to persevere in your training. People who exercise regularly find that they usually rest better at night. Make it a part of your daily routine to exercise moderately for at least 30 minutes.

  Have you ever noticed that when you're under stress, you find it hard to remember things? People under prolonged stress show a marked degeneration of the hippocampus, which can lead to memory loss (LeDoux, 1996). On the other hand, physical exercise can actually help generate new cells in the hippocampus (van Praag & van Praag, 2000). Apparently, spending time in the gym can do more than relieve stress and improve muscle tone; it may also improve your memory and help you "bulk up" your brain!

Of course, what you do for exercise is up to you, but make sure that you're having fun. A word of caution here—if you have not exercised for quite some time, getting a health screening is the best place to start. And take care! A few precautions, such as stretching your muscles and wearing safety gear, can help you avoid injury. Remember that your primary goal is to feel better, not tear yourself up. How would you assess your physical fitness at this time?

- **Using humor.** There is much truth in the expression, "Laughter is the best medicine." Laughter releases endorphins in your brain that help relax and calm you. Humor can also be a powerful therapeutic tool for developing rapport with your clients and promoting their resilience (Goldin & Bordan, 1999). Being able to laugh at yourself is probably the best indication of a healthy self-concept.

  Of course you can add some humor to your life by renting a comedy, watching something funny on television, or reading something that will make you laugh. You can also make a point of being with people who add laughter to your life. Even more important than appreciating humor is actually creating it yourself. You're probably not a professional comedian, but you definitely have the potential to see humor in life's daily aggravations, nuisances, and hassles. By putting a funny "spin" on such annoyances, you can "thumb your nose" at them and laugh some of your stress away. As Langston Hughes said, "Humor is your unconscious therapy." How's your humor quotient?

- **Relaxing and renewing.** Do something just for *you*—a trip to a hair salon or getting a therapeutic massage can work wonders when you are under a lot of pressure. Yoga, prayer, meditation, tai chi, or biofeedback can help promote relaxation responses. Learning to breathe deeply and slowly can enable you to slow yourself down and allow your soul time to replenish itself.

- **Seeking professional help.** Talking with someone you can trust, whether it is a therapist, nutritionist, or personal trainer, can provide you with some guidelines for leading a healthier lifestyle. If you're feeling overwhelmed by stress, consider asking for help at a counseling or health center on campus. Professional helpers can guide and support you through difficult times. Seeking help for prolonged stress, anxiety, or depression should not be postponed indefinitely. An added benefit to seeking professional help is that you get the experience of knowing what it's like to be a client, which will enhance your empathic skills once you begin working with others.

- **Reflecting.** Confucius once said, "The person who wants too much will always be in need." You may find that much of your stress comes from wanting too much. Determine what you may think you want from what you really *need* to live well. For too many Americans, enough is rarely sufficient. Watch what you are striving for, and be aware of your thoughts and attitudes. Negative attitudes can drain you of valuable energy and add insult to injury when you are under duress. An anonymous writer once cautioned, "Watch your thoughts; they become your words. Watch your words; they become your actions. Watch your actions; they become your habits. Watch your habits; they become your character. Watch your character; it becomes your destiny."

  Is your definition of success driving you toward perfectionism? Compare your definition to this one commonly attributed to Ralph Waldo Emerson:

  > To laugh often and much; to win the respect of intelligent people and the affection of children; to earn the appreciation of honest critics and endure the betrayal of false friends; to appreciate beauty; to find the best in others; to leave the world a bit better, whether by a healthy child, a garden patch, or a redeemed social condition; to know even one life has breathed easier because you have lived—this is to have succeeded.

- **Managing your time.** Set realistic goals and prioritize your responsibilities. Because you cannot do everything or please everyone in your life, you must learn how to say "No" to some things and make room to say "Yes" to your higher priorities (Covey, Merrill, & Merrill, 1994). You can practice ways of saying "No" and "Yes" in the following exercise.

EXERCISE 3.1 **Your Success with Stress**

You cannot have made it as far as you have in your life without encountering a variety of stressors. Take a few minutes to reflect on how you have successfully dealt with stress by answering these questions.

1. What were the major stressors you faced during the past year?

_____

_____

_____

_____

2. What reactions do you recall having to those stressors?

_____

_____

_____

_____

3. How did you handle your stress?

_____

_____

_____

_____

4. What important lessons did you learn from these experiences?

_____

_____

_____

_____

Keep in mind your successful coping skills as you read the following suggestions on managing stress. As Rachel did in the preceding story, you may need to remind yourself of the strategies you have successfully used in the past.

■ ■ ■

■ ■ ■

EXERCISE 3.2 Ways to Say "No" and "Yes!"

Saying "no" to others is probably difficult for you. After all, you want to become a professional *helper*. Here are some different variations on the theme of declining requests.

- **The polite no.** "I'm sorry, but I really have to pass on your request."
- **The postponement no.** "I might be able to do this in the future, but I can't right now."
- **The considerate no.** "It was very nice of you to think of me, and I'm honored you asked. But I won't be able to help you with that right now."
- **The backpedaling no.** "I'm sorry, I made a mistake. I shouldn't have committed myself so soon. I must either reschedule or back out this time."
- **The forthright no.** "I'm sorry, but I have no desire, time, energy, or inclination to do anything like that. Catch you later!"

Let's face it: Saying "no" can be disheartening if you don't consider what priorities you're also affirming when you turn down a request. Each time you say "no" to an opportunity, you're saying "yes" to another, so be sure that every "no" counts for something important. Here are some ways to remind yourself of the positive values and goals you are pursuing.

- **The committed yes.** "I'm determined to do my best in my practicum class."
- **The dedicated yes.** "I want to be sure that I stay a vital contributor to my family's well-being."
- **The playful yes.** "I'm making time for some recreation in my busy schedule."

- **The spiritual yes.** "I'm preserving my time for meditation, reflection, and prayer."
- **The compromise yes.** "Instead of what you're requesting, I can help out in a smaller way."

Think about the last time that somebody made a request that you wished you had declined. In the space below, write out a couple of answers you could have given by combining one type of "no" with one type of "yes."

_____

_____

_____

_____

_____

_____

_____

                                                    ■ ■ ■

Beyond Stress

Life is at its best when it's shaken and stirred.

—F. Paul Facult

The idea of stress has inspired a great deal of productive thinking, fruitful research, and useful interventions in the helping professions. However, the concept does have its limitations. For one thing, its physiological emphasis fails to capture the complexities and depth of the human experience. When we must confront challenges or endure difficult conditions, we do have physiological reactions. But, as human beings, we are also reaching out to others, creatively coping with threats, courageously sacrificing ourselves, or experiencing spiritual transcendence. Labeling these responses as merely reactions to stress is like using the concept of arousal to capture the essence of romantic passion. It's foolish to reduce our mysterious strivings and deeply powerful emotions to only physical functioning.

Another limitation to the concept of stress is that it does not take into account the creative, transformative powers that human beings can demonstrate under challenging and difficult circumstances. This mechanistic model suggests that humans may be able to reduce the negative impact of stress but can never actually gain positive transcendence through stress. Think about the most important achievements you have accomplished, the greatest lessons about life that you've learned, and the times in your life that you went through the most dramatic positive changes. Our bet is that you did not make these gains without some stress.

Rather than running from stress, consider turning to face it and learn from it. Taking this action now, while you're in graduate school, will strengthen your ability to take good care of yourself later in your career. You'll find that the personal exploration that you engage in during your training experience will remind you of your own resilience and strengths. Embracing your stress can lead to surprising discoveries and delightful rewards. After all, "stressed" spelled backwards is "desserts"!

Resilience Under Stress

Life does not happen to us, it happens from us.

—Michael Wickett

Resilience, the ability to bounce back from life's blows, has been the subject of recent exciting research (Echterling, Presbury, & McKee, 2005). By focusing on those people who can be amazingly resilient in times of stress, researchers have uncovered promising results that question the traditional views of stress. For example, some children are incredibly hardy and actually thrive in such severe circumstances as grim poverty, domestic violence, and negligent institutional settings (Masten & Coatsworth, 1998). In fact, resilience is the norm, not the exception, for people in stressful circumstances. When Antonovsky (1990) observed so many people learning how to devise such successful strategies to handle stressful adversities, he coined the phrase "learned resourcefulness" to describe this valuable trait. Marilyn Bowman (1997) made a convincing case that even most traumatic stress survivors show remarkable resilience.

Another promising line of research offers even more encouraging news regarding our resilience during times of stress. Many people actually achieve a positive transformation as they make their way through difficult and threatening situations. Tedeschi and Calhoun (1995), as well as other writers, have documented the dramatic changes and significant personal growth many people achieve under stressful circumstances. As Grotberg (1999) affirmed:

> Being resilient does not protect you from pain and suffering. Pain and suffering, however, can trigger resilience responses that help you face, overcome, and be transformed by ... adversity. (p. 26)

The important implication of these findings is that you are not merely the product of your environment—even if the environment is stressful and challenging. You have the potential not only to survive hard times but also to actually thrive and prosper under stressful conditions.

Of course, when you're feeling overwhelmed by stressors, you're less in touch with your own personal strengths and not as aware of the resources available to you. These feelings can undermine your confidence, sap your motivation, and cloud the once-clear vision you had of your future. At these times, you need to make a special effort to consciously look for your strengths and resources—to search for those clues that point to a successful strategy of thriving.

Making Meaning of Stress

Meaning, not raw facts, is what humanity seeks.

—Alvin Kernan

What makes you resilient under fire? Why aren't you a passive victim of your environment? Fundamentally, you are the master of your own fate because you can choose how to make meaning of your circumstances. Even if you lose everything else, according to Frankl (1969), you still have "the last of human freedoms—the ability to choose one's attitude in a given set of circumstances" (p. 73).

If you decide to find positive meaning in your stress, then you are likely to prevent its typical negative consequences. Thompson (1985) found that survivors of a variety of traumas who identified some positive meaning in their traumatic stress were able to cope better. In another study, those people who were able to find meaning in the death of a loved one reported less intense grief reactions (Schwartzberg & Janoff-Bulman, 1991). Likewise, those who report a greater sense of meaning also experience less distress (McIntosh, Cohen, & Wortman, 1993).

Telling Your Story

You are the hero of your own story.

—Mary McCarthy

What makes humans unique is our ability to create meaning by weaving the raw material of our lives into a fabric of stories (Atkinson, 1995). But your narratives do much more than organize your experiences. The stories that you spin to give coherence and meaning to your life also help form your own identity. They encourage you to take on certain roles, play out particular expectations, and choose some options over others. Yes, you have stories to tell, but your stories also tell you.

Recently, researchers have found that writing about the stressful events you have experienced can produce a wide range of benefits (Lepore & Smyth, 2002). People who wrote about some traumatic stress experience had significant improvements in their health, emotional well-being, and physiological functioning compared with control participants who wrote only about neutral events.

Once again, we find support for the tremendous value of keeping a journal of your training experiences. The process of telling your story helps you to find some meaning in the challenges you are enduring. One student, Cathy, noticed that the length of her journal entries were an accurate barometer of the stress she felt. The more stressful her day, the longer her journal entry was. She also found herself returning to write about particularly stressful times.

The mindfulness you bring to your studies can be especially helpful in seeking understanding and insight into your own experiences. As you shift through the rubble of a setback or failure, be on the lookout for those golden nuggets of strengths and resources among the disappointments and mistakes. By looking carefully, you can find plenty of examples of your own resilience, determination, creativity, and courage. Remember, it's also okay to compliment yourself in your journal. When you're under stress, your self-esteem and confidence may suffer, so at these times you can benefit from some reminders of your strengths and abilities.

▦ ▦ ▦

EXERCISE 3.3 The Embracing Attitudes
A Quick Check Exercise

Here are some quick tips for embracing stress successfully along your journey:

- Look for puzzles that intrigue you.
- Involve yourself in meaningful causes.
- Strive for progress—not perfection.
- Forgive yourself and others.
- Take the Serenity Prayer to heart: "Grant me the serenity to accept the things I cannot change, the courage to change the things I can, and the wisdom to know the difference."
- Start a "feel good" file. Keep encouraging notes, cards, letters, and E-mails people send you. Even if you don't have immediate access to these important people in your life, you can find consolation in their words. When you're having a particularly difficult day, pull out your file and read the words these persons have written about you. It will amaze you how uplifting a few of these can be on a stressful day!

▦ ▦ ▦

THRIVING UNDER STRESS

> Power is the ability to achieve purpose.
>
> —Martin Luther King, Jr.

Most approaches to managing stress begin by assessing your stressors. For example, Sowa (1992) developed a process by which you carefully list all the stressors in your life, assess how much each is under your control, decide how important each stressor is, and then consider your options. But focusing on all your stressors at once can seem both daunting and disheartening—especially for counseling trainees, who feel demoralized too often already (Watkins, 1996).

Envisioning Your Goals

To truly thrive under stress, begin on a positive note by envisioning your goals. Remember, you are always a work in progress—extending, evolving, and expanding. Therefore, you want to regularly orient yourself to where you are heading—especially when you are going through stressful episodes. During these dark times, your goals can serve as beacons to light your way and keep you on track.

■ ■ ■

EXERCISE 3.4 **Mission Possible:**
An Exercise in Envisioning

What do you hope to accomplish once you've completed your graduate program? Reflect on your training hopes and dreams. Once your vision of the future has come into focus, write down your training mission statement. Be sure to develop goals that are positive, specific, and achievable. Knowing why you are going through stressful times can enable you to thrive under stress.

My Training Mission

_____

_____

_____

_____

_____

_____

_____

■ ■ ■

Using Your Strengths

You are going to be relying on your personal talents to succeed in your venture. Now is the time to bring your positive qualities to the foreground as you begin planning your strategies for thriving under stress. Earlier in this chapter, for example, you reflected on your success experiences in dealing with stressful events and circumstances.

■ ■ ■

EXERCISE 3.5 **Panning for Gold:**
            Uncovering Strengths and Resources

Recalling your accomplishments is a great way to recognize special talents that you may be taking for granted and to remember important people that you may be forgetting. Write an inventory of your strengths and resources.

_____

_____

_____

_____

_____

_____

_____

_____

■ ■ ■

Connecting with Others

Remember, we all stumble, every one of us. That's
why it's a comfort to go hand in hand.

—Emily Kimbrough

Over and over again, researchers have found that social support serves as an important buffer against stress (Berscheid, 2003). Having traveling companions, the third principle of thriving, is particularly valuable if you're feeling overwhelmed with stress.

A supportive network of friends, relatives, peers, and others can make a world of difference when you're going through an ordeal. In fact, one of the surest ways to thrive in tough times is to reach out to others and face the stressors together. Cultures throughout the world have developed rituals in which family members and friends congregate to deal with difficult events—everything in life from births to deaths.

Talking to a trusted friend or family member, sharing time together, or joining others for a meal can lead you to the truth of the proverb: "A sorrow shared is half the sorrow; a joy shared is twice the joy." Even if your stressful circumstances involve only you, by telling your story to others, your experience becomes an episode of your network's shared history—a piece added to the communal mosaic. Sharing your turmoil helps to reconnect you, during a time when you may feel all alone and alienated, to others who can offer support.

▨ ▨ ▨

EXERCISE 3.6 **The Sea Star I:**
A Transcending Exercise

Using the image of a sea star, or starfish, we invite you to take a look at how well you are thriving on each of these five dimensions: relational, spiritual, physical, emotional, and mental. Using a scale of 1–10, with 1 representing the absence of any sense of thriving and 10 representing your highest level of thriving, rate your current level in each area.

Whatever rating you give to each dimension of thriving, take some time to consider carefully what you can do to move from your present score to the next higher number. Describe the specific steps you can take. As you imagine possible strategies, you may discover that you have more capabilities and resources than you realize. Share your ratings and plan with a friend.

RELATIONAL THRIVING

My current level is a _____ . I can move higher by . . .

_____

_____

_____

SPIRITUAL THRIVING

My current level is a _____ . I can move higher by . . .

_____

_____

_____

PHYSICAL THRIVING

My current level is a _____ . I can move higher by . . .

_____

_____

_____

EMOTIONAL THRIVING

My current level is a _____ . I can move higher by . . .

_____

_____

_____

MENTAL THRIVING

My current level is a _____ . I can move higher by . . .

_____

_____

_____

▨ ▨ ▨

STRESS AND CHARACTER

> Character cannot be developed in ease and quiet.
> Only through experience of trial and suffering can
> the soul be strengthened, vision cleared, ambition
> inspired, and success achieved.
>
> —Helen Keller

Loosely translating the words of Buddha, life is not for sissies. You get knocked around quite a bit by just trying to get on with living, much less striving to realize your cherished dreams. Though advertisements would have you believe otherwise, you cannot avoid all of life's bruises and stresses. Advertisers try to sell the idea that, with the right car, the right body, the right *something*, you will magically be insulated from stress, loss, disappointment, and discomfort. For example, in a once-popular luxury automobile advertisement, the caption under the car said simply, "Fire your therapist." For many people, particularly those who live in Western cultures, achieving personal happiness requires the absence of all suffering and stress.

It is likely, because you are attracted to the helping professions, that you do not believe personal fulfillment can be found either in static, Eden-like bliss or in a double overhead cam V-8 engine with a turbocharger. It is also likely that your journey toward becoming a counselor or therapist began as you struggled to respond to difficulties and painful stumbling blocks in your own life. You are interested in what makes you "tick," and curious about how you are "put together." Perhaps there is something that draws you to looking at your own life head-on—even the stressful and unsettling experiences that you sometimes would just as soon forget.

Regardless of how well you may have been shielded by benevolent circumstances, you have faced stressors and endured pain while growing up. Each of us has experienced injuries from important care-giving relationships, in traumatic experiences with peers, in unanticipated losses that seemed overwhelming or unbearable at the time. Sometimes, our injuries are less discrete or identifiable but emerge from harmful long-term relationships or stressful living situations.

You will be reminded again and again in your training that, though you can never expect to be completely free of painful life events, you can choose how to respond to them. A particular trauma or wound does not determine who you are. Rather, it is how you cope with those painful experiences that shape your process of "becoming" (Rogers, 1961). Even painful and agonizing times can be rewarding if they enable you to mature and increase your empathy for the anguish of others. As Frankl affirmed, "Through the right attitude, unavoidable suffering is transmitted into a heroic and victorious achievement" (1969, p. 88).

Converting suffering into wisdom and the possibility for new choices is the work of personal transformation. Booker T. Washington once said, "Success is to be measured not so much by the position that one has reached in life as by the obstacles . . . overcome while trying to succeed." Always hard won, never trivial, the process is metaphorically represented by the structure and color of the yin-yang symbol. One side represents crisis, the other side opportunity. The dot in the center of each side means that each experience is embedded in the other. Our personal wounds are such an expression of crisis and opportunity. As a counselor in training, you will find that they are a two-ingredient recipe for transformation and change.

Of course, this transformation is ongoing throughout your life. The work of fully integrating and understanding yourself is never finished, and you have sustained injuries and faced difficulties in life that are still "alive" in you now. These experiences are often well hidden, but sometimes they become open wounds that show up in your relations with others, in your particular sensitivities and needs, and in your unique ways of protecting yourself from new painful events.

Your graduate training will include many courses with a variety of academic and experiential exercises to give you a firm understanding of the counseling field. You may find, however, that your training evokes a parallel process of self-examination and exploration that more fully reveals your areas of sensitivity and defensiveness (Adams, 2006). These are the "sore spots" that seem to keep getting nudged as you move through your program, especially in work with clients and supervisors. If it's any consolation, you can be sure that you are not the only one whose old wounds are resurfacing during this intensive training. If you are able to skate through your program without the experience bringing up charged issues in your own life, then you haven't fully engaged in your training.

STRESS INTO STRENGTH

> Life is a grindstone. Whether it grinds us down or polishes us up depends on us.
>
> —Thomas L. Holdcroft

The poet William Stafford once observed that, unless one had experienced difficulty and personal distress, it would be impossible to be a poet. The same can be said of becoming a counselor. The trick, he observed, was to suffer intelligently and then to share that suffering with others. By this, he meant that you can mine the experiences of your own life for the valuable images, feelings, and responses that characterize you as uniquely human. You can then communicate with others about a shared human situation. In this sense, the particular psychological and emotional stresses that have attended your own growth and development and through which you have suffered intelligently represent personal strengths. These are your true areas of expertise. One form of communicating in the counseling situation is by understanding these areas in others.

The idea that your personal struggles have the potential to be your areas of greatest strength is not some cozy notion that we offer to reassure you. The words "What does not kill you makes you stronger" express something of the experience of having to develop some new talent or strength in response to a particular life wound. History is replete with examples of persons whose genius and wounds were inextricably linked. Winston Churchill, whose oratorial skills galvanized the Allies against Hitler's aggression, stuttered as a child. Django Rheinhart, the first great jazz guitarist, known for his astonishingly unique phrasings, had only two working fingers on his left hand (Hillman, 1996). Maya Angelou, the lyrical writer of transcendent prose and poetry, was mute for nearly five years after she was raped as a child. She transformed her struggles into works of beauty, such as her first work of literature, *I Know Why the Caged Bird Sings* (1970), and has become a marvelously powerful and inspirational speaker.

Carl Rogers, whose work changed the practice of counseling and therapy by emphasizing interpersonal authenticity, warmth, and empathy, observed that his early years were characterized by an "unconscious, arrogant separateness" that emerged from his family's strict religious conservatism and fear of outsiders (Rogers, 1980, p. 28). Reflecting on his inauthentic relationships with other family members, Rogers admitted that "it would never have occurred to me to share with them any of my personal or private thoughts or feelings, because I knew these would have been judged and found wanting" (p. 28).

Think about your own life. In what ways have you transformed the "slings and arrows of outrageous fortune" into your personal character? Perhaps you have used your stress as a teacher. You may have learned valuable lessons about life as the result of these experiences. It may be that you have used your stress as an empathic bridge to help you connect with the anguish and suffering of clients. Or you may have used stress to gain an appreciation for the creativity, resourcefulness, and resilience of humans. However you have used stress, you have done so by embracing it, engaging in the struggle of making it meaningful, and finally emerging from that encounter as a better person and counselor.

SUMMARY

In this chapter, we discuss how stress is an essential part of any successful training program. We describe a variety of strategies, such as relaxation and exercise, you can use to manage stress. We also encourage you to embrace stress as a means of thriving in your training. Relying on your resilience, connecting with others, learning from your stress, and envisioning your goals are ways in which you can transform stress into wisdom, empathy, and character. Finally, we end this chapter with words from Viktor Frankl: You are "called upon to make the best use of any moment and the right choice at any time: it is assumed that [you know] what to do, or whom to love, or how to suffer" (1967, p. 93).

RESOURCES

The writings of Victor Frankl are a wonderful resource for reflecting on the meaning of life's stress and suffering. We suggest you start with *Man's Search for Meaning: An Introduction to Logotherapy.* Frankl describes his experiences in a Nazi concentration camp. In his painfully honest and unsentimental account, Frankl (who had intended to write it anonymously, using only his prison camp number) explores the psychology of suffering and our struggle to find meaning. His approach to therapy, which is an outgrowth of his concentration camp experiences, challenges us to confront the essence of our existence and to create a meaningful life through faith and love.

Association for Support of Graduate Students (ASGS)
www.asgs.org

This site provides the following services for graduate students coping with the stressful demands of research and scholarship: thesis news, DOC-Talk, professional consultant directory, and computer template disks for APA style.

Medical Basis of Stress
www.teachhealth.com/#stressscale

At this site, you can take either the adult or youth forms of an updated version of the Holmes and Rahe Stress Scale. Steve Burns and Kimberley Burns, who are health educators, also provide helpful and basic information about stress.

ResilienceNet
www.resilnet.uiuc.edu

This site offers information on resilience, including guides and teaching materials, program descriptions, and evaluative reports. There is a virtual library with full-text publications of articles and reports. An onsite discussion group gives you an opportunity to interact with others interested in resilience.

REFERENCES

Adams, D. (2006, May). How I lost my voice and found it again. *Counseling Today, 48,* 12–13.

Angelou, M. (1970). *I know why the caged bird sings.* New York: Random House.

Antonovsky, A. (1990). Pathways leading to successful coping and health. In M. Rosenbaum (Ed.), *Learned resourcefulness: On coping skills, self control, and adaptive behavior* (pp. 31–63). New York: Springer-Verlag.

Atkinson, R. (1995). *The gift of stories.* Westport, CT: Bergin & Garvey.

Berscheid, E. (2003). The human's greatest strength: Other humans. In L. G. Aspinwall & U. M. Staudinger (Eds.), *A psychology of human strengths: Fundamental questions and future directions for a positive psychology* (pp. 37–47). Washington, DC: American Psychological Association.

Bowman, M. (1997). *Individual differences in posttraumatic response: Problems with the adversity-distress connection.* Mahwah, NJ: Erlbaum.

Echterling, L. G., Presbury, J., & McKee, J. E. (2005). *Crisis intervention: Promoting resilience and resolve in troubled times.* Upper Saddle River, NJ: Merrill/Prentice Hall.

Frankl, V. E. (1967). *Psychotherapy and existentialism: Selected papers on logotherapy.* New York: Pocket Books.

Frankl, V. E. (1969). *The will to meaning.* New York: New American Library.

Frankl, V. E. (1984). *Man's search for meaning: An introduction to logotherapy.* New York: Simon & Shuster.

Goldin, E., & Bordan, T. (1999). The use of humor in counseling: The laughing cure. *Journal of Counseling and Development, 77,* 405–410.

Grotberg, E. H. (1999). *Tapping your inner strength: How to find the resilience to deal with anything.* Oakland, CA: New Harbinger.

Hillman, J. (1996). *The soul's code: In search of character and calling.* New York: Random House.

Holmes, T. H., & Rahe, R. H. (1967). The social readjustment rating scale. *Journal of Psychosomatic Research, 11,* 213–218.

LeDoux, J. (1996). *The emotional brain: The mysterious underpinnings of emotional life.* New York: Simon & Schuster.

Lepore, S. J., & Smyth, J. M. (2002). *The writing cure: How expressive writing promotes health and emotional well-being.* Washington, DC: American Psychological Association.

Masten, A. S., & Coatsworth, J. D. (1998). The development of competence in favorable and unfavorable environments: Lessons from research on successful children. *American Psychologist, 53,* 205–220.

McIntosh, D. N., Cohen, R., & Wortman, C. B. (1993). Religion's role in adjustment to a negative life event: Coping with the loss of a child. *Journal of Personality and Social Psychology, 65,* 812–821.

Rogers, C. R. (1961). *On becoming a person.* Boston: Houghton Mifflin.

Rogers, C. R. (1980). *A way of being.* Boston: Houghton Mifflin.

Rollins, J. (2005, October). A campaign for counselor wellness. *Counseling Today, 47,* 22, 23, 42.

Schwartzberg, S. S., & Janoff-Bulman, R. (1991). Grief and the search for meaning: Exploring the assumptive worlds of bereaved college students. *Journal of Social and Clinical Psychology, 10,* 270–288.

Sowa, C. J. (1992). Understanding clients' perceptions of stress. *Journal of Counseling and Development, 71,* 179–183.

Sowa, C. J., May, K. M., & Niles, S. G. (1994). Occupational stress within the counseling profession: Implications for counselor training. *Counselor Education and Supervision, 34,* 19–29.

Taylor, S. E., Klein, L. C., Lewis, B. P., Gruenewald, T. L., Gurung, R. A., & Updegraff, J. A. (2000). Biobehavioral responses to stress in females: Tend-and-befriend, not fight-or-flight. *Psychological Review, 107,* 411–429.

Tedeschi, R. G., & Calhoun, L. G. (1995). *Trauma and transformation: Growing in the aftermath of suffering.* Thousand Oaks, CA: Sage.

Thompson, S. C. (1985). Finding positive meaning in a stressful event and coping. *Basic and Applied Social Psychology, 6,* 279–295.

Watkins, C. E. (1996). On demoralization and awe in psychotherapy supervision. *Clinical Supervisor, 14,* 139–148.

Van Praag, F., & van Praag, H. (Producers). (2000, November 21). *Scientific American Frontiers.* New York and Washington, DC: PBS.

CHAPTER 4

Meeting Your Basic Needs

One of the oldest human needs is to have someone to wonder where you are when you don't
come home at night.

—Margaret Mead

Dance like no one is watching, love like you'll
never be hurt, sing like no one is listening, and live
like it's heaven on earth.

—William Purkey

We receive love . . . not in proportion to our
demands or sacrifices or needs, but roughly in
proportion to our own capacity to love.

—Rollo May

Many cultures have addressed the question of what constitutes our "basic needs." A Navajo legend, for example, tells of the Spirit Being, who created People to share the beauty of the world with all other living things. The Spirit Being then spent a summer with the People to teach them what they needed to know to survive in the earth world. They were taught to build shelters, hunt game, and grow crops. The Spirit Being's most important teachings were the songs and chants that would keep the People healthy and in harmony with their world. The lesson here is that our basic needs are not confined to food, clothing, and shelter. In fact, our needs for meaning, beauty, and balance are just as fundamental.

Bread and Roses, founded in 1974 by Mimi Farina, a folk singer and social activist, has taken that lesson to heart. Bread and Roses presents free, live entertainment to institutionalized and isolated people. Well-known performers, who usually demand big money for their talents, have performed without pay in hundreds of concerts. One of Mimi Farina's songs was inspired by a James Oppenheim poem, written in 1912 to protest the miserable conditions of textile workers. One stanza, in particular, is a powerful statement about fundamental human needs:

> Our lives shall not be sweated from birth until life closes;
> Hearts starve as well as bodies; give us bread but give us roses!

As the poem said, you need more than bread. Of course, you need shelter, food, and clothing, as well as books and the various other necessities of academic life. But remember to meet your other needs, which will always be present. Be sure to nourish your heart during your time in graduate school. Stop to plant, nurture, give, receive, savor, and, of course, *smell* the roses.

In this chapter, we present suggestions and strategies to help you satisfy all your basic needs while you are a graduate student. Contrary to the typical view, it is possible not only to take care of yourself but also to succeed in your training program. You don't have to sacrifice your health and well-being to become a counselor or therapist. In fact, meeting your needs with flexibility, creativity, and sensitivity can actually help you to thrive.

As you perceive them, your "needs" are, in part, a reflection of your values. They have come from your parents and extended family, religious beliefs, education, and the media—in short, your culture. When people move from one culture to another, they often experience "culture shock." You are entering a graduate training program in which you may encounter unfamiliar language, awkward situations, and atypical behavior. You are likely to feel off balance, self-conscious, and, perhaps, defensive because you find this new environment to be somewhat strange. You are entering the culture of counseling and therapy. As you become acculturated, you will not only begin to feel more comfortable with this new community but also carefully examine and change many of your values and assumptions about human needs.

YOUR PERSONAL HIERARCHY OF NEEDS

The things that matter most must never be at the
mercy of the things that matter least.

—Goethe

Any discussion of your basic needs would be incomplete without referencing the work of Abraham Maslow. Maslow (1970) identified a hierarchy of needs—usually depicted as a pyramid—that motivates humans to strive toward self-actualization, which is at the top of the pyramid. People first strive to satisfy their needs at the bottom of the pyramid before moving on to the next higher need area. Maslow named the following five levels of need that must be fulfilled for psychological well-being.

Physiological needs are basic for survival and include such necessities as drinking, eating, and sleeping.

Safety and security include the need to be safe from physical harm and to have adequate shelter.

Love and belonging are the needs for affiliation and for giving and receiving love.

Self-esteem refers to the need for self-confidence, for self-worth, and for truly believing in your own value and capabilities.

Self-actualization is at the top of the pyramid and refers to the fulfillment and realization of your potential. Finding ways to fully express your creativity and feel a sense of accomplishment are meeting your self-actualization needs.

Maslow's hierarchy actually bears a striking resemblance to a model of the soul that Plato proposed more than 2,000 years earlier (Leahey, 2000). The lowest level is the "desiring soul" that resides in the belly and below. This level includes selfish desires for food, money, and sex. Today, you may recognize people at this level on many popular daytime talk shows or court programs. The next level up is the "spirited soul," which resides in the chest. This level is motivated by fame and glory, exemplified today by many professional athletes, politicians, and movie stars. The highest level is the "rational soul," centered in the head, which seeks Goodness and Truth, even at the expense of lower-level desires. We hope to find people who have achieved this highest level in our spiritual leaders, mentors, and sages.

We offer Plato's model because it emphasizes a vital point that has been lost in most discussions of Maslow's hierarchy of needs. Although Plato's model is inaccurate in its understanding of human physiology, it does hit the mark regarding our essential ability to *choose* which desires we fulfill, to determine our own personal hierarchy to reflect our fundamental values. We are not condemned to remain at the lower levels until those needs are met. Instead, we can decide to strive for higher values—to forgo satisfying all our lower needs as we reach for the stars.

In this chapter, you will explore how Maslow's paradigm can be a useful perspective for coping in graduate school. For example, you can meet your physiological and safety needs by finding and creating a home, investigating options for financial assistance, and maintaining your physical wellness. However, Plato's emphasis on choice can alert you to opportunities for thriving even in times of scarcity. Therefore, we discuss how you can fulfill your self-actualization needs in spite of other deprivations in your life. Let's begin by exploring ways in which you can not only fulfill your needs but also thrive in this unfamiliar culture.

▲▲▲

A Constant Challenge
Ellen's Story

MEETING BASIC NEEDS is a constant challenge! I find I do well for some time, but then I look up and realize I've neglected them again. I have trouble remembering to take time for myself. With a husband, kids, and a job, it is easy for me to feel like school is "my time." Even though it's rewarding, it is not the same as having time to myself for meditation, reflection, journaling, or just having fun! My goal is to create some time for *me* every day—some days it will be ten minutes, other days an hour.

The other basic need that I often neglect is getting enough sleep. I run close to empty most days of the week. I have come to realize that I often use my fatigue as an excuse—for yelling at my kids, for saying "no," for not being intimate with my husband, and for having an extra glass of wine at night to unwind. I think I have become addicted to the cycle of being exhausted, getting one or two nights of good sleep, and then feeling so good I stay up late. Then it all begins again.

I realize as I write this that so much of counseling is about meeting our basic needs, such as intimacy and love. I know that when I am sleep deprived and leave no time for myself, I have a difficult time meeting those basic needs. When I am well-rested and deeply connected with myself, I am in a good place to give and receive love and to create the kind of relationships I want in my life—relationships that I need to be a healthy, fulfilled person.

▼▼▼

Shirley MacLaine (2000) wrote an account of her pilgrimage across the Santiago de Compostela Camino, a grueling 500-mile trek through northern Spain that people have undertaken for centuries. Like a true pilgrim, MacLaine traveled alone on her month-long journey and took only what she could carry in her backpack. She discovered that she needed little more beyond water, good shoes, and a floppy hat. By discarding all the distracting unessentials that can clutter one's life and embarking on a demanding quest, she gained an important new perspective.

As you enter graduate school, you are traveling on new terrain, and, as MacLaine's pilgrimage illustrates, you need to decide what is truly essential. You may find that some seemingly pressing needs will fade or even disappear. You may be a little confused and perhaps feel pressured—mostly out of habit—to respond to old needs. At the very least, you're likely to be uncomfortable at first, so consider reframing this situation as an invitation to explore your fundamental motivations and values in life. You see, we don't notice when our needs are met. It's only when we believe our needs are not satisfied that we are motivated to reflect, decide, and act.

BASIC NEEDS AND SELF-ACTUALIZATION

> Life is easier to take than you think; all that is
> necessary is to accept the impossible, do without
> the indispensable and bear the intolerable.
>
> —Kathleen Norris

In the previous story, Ellen engaged in two very important steps toward self-actualization—taking time to identify just what is important to her and then finding ways to meet those basic needs. What needs were truly essential to her? How was she able to organize her day to satisfy them? Most students, faculty, and staff—in fact, most people—face similar challenges in trying to balance needs and demands in their daily lives. At first, successfully juggling all your family commitments, personal needs, and graduate-school requirements can seem utterly hopeless.

Remember the old riddle about a farmer who had to figure out how to safely transport a fox, a chicken, and a sack of grain to an island? The farmer could only take one of them at a time in a small boat. However, the fox couldn't be left alone with the chicken, because the fox would eat it. By the same token, the chicken couldn't be left alone with the grain. The farmer solved the problem by deploying resources and manipulating the conditions in a creative way. (An answer to how the farmer resolved this dilemma appears at the end of this chapter.)

Like the farmer in the riddle, you face a similar conundrum: how to adequately meet your basic needs, personal obligations, and training demands. Leading a reasonably fulfilling life while learning to be a counselor or therapist requires ingenuity, quick wits, and lots of energy. This balancing act is challenging enough, but the idea of meeting your self-actualizing needs seems like a Catch-22. You entered into training to realize your potential, but the stresses and deprivations inherent to life as an impoverished graduate student seem to make scaling the pyramid impossible.

A quick reading of Maslow may lead you to assume that meeting your self-actualization needs is achievable only when you are financially secure and relatively stress free. Self-actualization, like caviar, may seem to be a delicacy that only the fortunate and affluent can afford to experience. How in the world can graduate students—in debt up to their ears with student loans, living in austere accommodations, and trying to cut corners everywhere—seek self-actualization? And what about people who are returning to school after raising a family or who are beginning a second career after already achieving financially success in another profession? Aren't they moving *down* several rungs?

Maslow (1962) himself criticized the simplistic interpretation that regards personal growth as merely "progression toward self-actualization in which the basic needs are completely gratified, one by one, before the next higher need emerges" (p. 24). As Plato pointed out, humans are not slaves to their desires. We can choose to seek self-actualization even though our pursuit may deprive us of basic comforts, take away our financial security, and threaten our personal safety.

▨ ▨ ▨

EXERCISE 4.1 **Take That Job and . . .**
A Guided Fantasy Exercise

Imagine that instead of going to graduate school for the next few years you accepted a high-paying job that offered excellent benefits, the ability to buy a beautiful home, job security, a close-knit group of colleagues, and plenty of recognition for your accomplishments. In short, this job would satisfy every conceivable physical and emotional need. The only catch is that you could not fulfill your personal potential for self-actualization.

As you consider this possibility, describe the needs you would be sacrificing.

_____

_____

_____

_____

_____

Now, describe your plans for ensuring that you will address these self-actualization needs in your training.

_____

_____

_____

_____

_____

▨ ▨ ▨

CONDUCTING A NEEDS INVENTORY

The hardest thing to learn in life is which bridge to cross and which to burn.

—David Russell

Below, Renee shares her story of leaving a successful career and enrolling in a training program in which she had to live away from her home and family for several days a week. In her story, she conducts an informal needs inventory for herself.

▲▲▲

Touch the Sun
Renee's Story

WHEN TACKLING this portion of my training journey, I first had to identify my basic needs. I cheated a little and borrowed my hierarchy of needs from Maslow, as he seemed to have the right idea, although his may not be basic enough for this point in my life.

According to my mother and my kids, I am not doing a good job meeting my physical needs. Sleep would indeed be a wonderful thing, but I haven't figured out how to work that in yet.

A need for safety has become very important. My family home is in a nice residential area where signs are regularly posted proclaiming "Neighborhood Watch in Effect." While at school, I try to handle my fear of living alone by leaving lots of lights on.

Being part of a family has fulfilled my belonging and love needs; however, right now it seems like distance doesn't make the heart grow fonder—it just makes communication harder. My husband and I are maintaining a long-distance relationship, and we're sure our love can stand the test of time, as the songs say. But I really miss him and my family.

I find I need a social circle here, too. Friendships are beginning to develop, as I tentatively move past the point of "socialized" hellos into more meaningful relationships.

I am working on feeling competent, independent, successful, respected, and worthwhile to improve my self-esteem. At the moment, though, I feel I have lost my sense of self, and because I am not successfully satisfying the preceding needs, I have to fall short somewhere. Can a "high-maintenance, emotionally needy" person ever hope to reach this goal?

If I cannot successfully meet my need for good self-esteem, I can't even begin to imagine where I stand with self-actualization. Isn't that the thing we're all supposed to be striving for, anyway? I'd hate to touch the sun too soon.

▼▼▼

As you read Renee's story, with what parts did you find yourself identifying? Did you notice that Renee was dealing with needs at several different levels? Assessing your needs and taking action to meet them are effective methods of coping. But what about thriving? Renee suggests that she cannot address her self-actualization needs until she has met her self-esteem needs. What do you think? Would Renee be "touching the sun" too soon? How could Renee use her struggle to help her thrive in her training?

Dealing with the challenges of satisfying your personal needs in graduate school can actually enhance your training in two fundamental ways. First, your own strivings are far better than "book knowledge" in helping you to understand and appreciate the struggles that all people face in their lives. So, as you try to balance your needs, remain aware of your fatigue, yearnings, and sense of deprivation. These experiences can help you build an empathic bridge to clients whose concerns may be different but who are, nevertheless, struggling. Second, your own successful endeavors to live a full and balanced life can help remind you of the perseverance, creativity, and resilience that your clients have. Even though you have felt overwhelmed at times, you've discovered personal strengths and social resources that have helped you through these difficulties. With your assistance, your clients can also uncover their own hidden abilities and sources of support.

If you stay on the alert for learning opportunities, you are likely to gain surprising insights regarding your needs. For example, students conducting a parenting group often found that some sessions offered valuable lessons for themselves, too. Below is an experiential exercise that has routinely helped student group leaders as much as it did the group members.

One student who completed this exercise found, to her dismay, that decorating the sea star was the most fun she had had in a long time. She realized that she had been neglecting her need for creative activities. By the way, you can vary this activity for use with couples and families in counseling. For example, have them first come up with a thriving list that is completely unrestricted by finances, time, family, or work constraints. Then they can look over the options and circle ones they can help each other to do, given their current circumstances.

EXERCISE 4.2 **The Sea Star II**
        A Balancing Exercise

Returning to the image of a sea star, you can learn a lesson about being responsive to your needs. A sea star has five distinct arms that work together gracefully. Even if an appendage breaks off, a sea star regenerates its lost limb to ensure that it can thrive in its environment. Your thriving needs, like a sea star's arms, can work together in harmony, but some of your "arms" may be better developed than others. In fact, most people are able to satisfy certain needs more successfully than other needs. This exercise reminds you of the different types of needs and how you can address each of them.

On a large sheet of paper, draw a sea star and label each arm with a thriving need: physical, mental, emotional, relational, and spiritual.

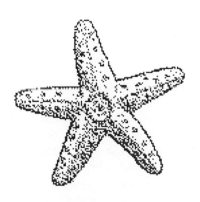

Consider how well you are currently fulfilling these thriving needs. Draw a line on each arm to indicate your satisfaction with that particular need—the larger the area within that arm, the greater your fulfillment. Your sea star figure will now have a line at some point across each of its five arms.

Now, using the area that you have set aside on each arm, draw the ways in which you are meeting that need. The more you are fulfilling a certain need, the more room you have to draw. Feel free to decorate each area anyway you would like. For example, you might draw certain people, activities, or symbols to portray how you thrive in that area.

You may be surprised at how successfully you are satisfying some needs and how little you are attending to others. What did you discover about the balance of your thriving needs?

CRAFTING A BALANCED LIFE

> Happiness is not a state to arrive at, but a manner of traveling.
>
> —Margaret Lee Runbeck

A cow is a ruminative animal; it chews its cud but gains no nourishment from the process. When you ruminate, you may obsess or worry for hours on end but gain no benefit from this activity. Well, if you're a ruminator, then it's time to put aside the ways of the cow and bring balance to your life. Fully commit yourself to the task of the moment, but when you have completed it, then set it aside. Returning to reflect on your work, ponder its meaning, and sort through it to find nuggets of success can certainly be nourishing. However, take care not to become so caught up in your work that you can never set it aside and just *be*.

In another ancient Navajo story, when Spider Woman gave Weaving Woman her ability to weave, she also instructed her to walk the Middle Way by keeping her life in balance. Weaving Woman was able to maintain this harmony at first, but then she began to weave night and day until she collapsed, unable to move or speak. She had woven her spirit into her work and could not escape it. Like Weaving Woman, you may be learning important skills but may also be having a very difficult time keeping your life in balance. Regularly pulling "all-nighters," ignoring relationships, and never taking any breaks from work all indicate that you are losing yourself in the role of a student. Here is how Beth achieved a satisfying balance and avoided weaving herself into her work.

▲ ▲ ▲

We Have Nothing to Fear But ...
Beth's Story

RECENTLY, I sat down and wrote about my greatest fear. I was afraid that, as a student, mother, wife, teacher, daughter, and friend, I couldn't balance all my roles and responsibilities. I worried that my children would suffer. I was the one who stayed home from my part-time job when they were sick. My part-time job required enormous energy and frequent attendance at meetings. Would there be enough time? My marriage was shaky at best. How much would it suffer? How would I take care of everything? How would I take care of me? Finally, I told myself that if I couldn't keep a healthy balance, I could quit graduate school. Telling myself that it's okay to stop my training if it wasn't working calmed me.

▼ ▼ ▼

Beth found that reminding herself that she had the power to bring balance to her life helped her gain a sense of peace. Feeling overwhelmed by unmet needs is a concern that you will hear from your clients, fellow students, and significant others. Why can it seem so challenging to create a balance, to satisfy all these needs? Using your list from the sea star exercise may provide a different perspective.

■ ■ ■

EXERCISE 4.3 Your Needs in Context
A Systemic Exercise

On a separate sheet of paper, draw three small sea stars. One of the stars represents you, so quickly draw a simple, miniature version of your previous star, by just adding the lines indicating how well you are satisfying the five thriving needs: physical, mental, emotional, relational, and spiritual. Now select two people who have a deep emotional connection to you. You may choose a partner, family member, best friend, or roommate. Put their names at the top of each of the other stars and, to your best guess, draw lines to reflect the extent to which they are meeting their own thriving needs.

Draw walls and a roof around the three stars to group them in a single house. If you like, you can add other details and decorations to make it more like home. This picture illustrates two important points. First, meeting your needs can sometimes feel overwhelming because you live under the same emotional roof with relatives, friends, and colleagues who have their own needs. In what ways do their unmet needs complicate your life? At the same time, your picture also portrays the second important point—these people are also excellent resources! You cannot achieve self-actualization by yourself. In fact, you can join with others synergistically to fulfill many of your thriving needs. How can these people help you?

■ ■ ■

Pathways to Balance

Paint as you like and die happy.

—Henry Miller

So, what can you do? A useful psychological construct for situations such as yours is termed *equifinality*. *Equifinality* means that there are multiple pathways to the same end. Beth's pathway was to deliberately acknowledge that attending graduate school was a choice that, for the time being, she was saying "Yes." At some time in the future, she may choose to say "No."

Another pathway to achieving balance is described in the conclusion of the legend of Weaving Woman. According to the story, to free Weaving Woman's spirit from her work, Spider Woman made the blanket Weaving Woman had woven less perfect. By pulling out a thread, Spider Woman created a pathway for Weaving Woman's spirit to leave the blanket and return to her. Weaving Woman thankfully said she had learned her lesson and began to teach others the importance of not trying to make their weavings perfect. She taught them how to make spirit trails in their weavings so their spirits would not be trapped in their work.

Weaving Woman learned to meaningfully engage in the work of creating beauty, but not at the risk of losing herself in the process. You may notice similar themes in your own life. Do you try to make your work absolutely perfect? Do you ask for help when you feel you may be getting trapped? Who lets you know when you are "weaving" too much?

As you continue to enter the culture of counseling and learn more about yourself, you can periodically conduct an inventory of your needs and, using all of who you are and what you know, create pathways to a more meaningful and satisfying life. In the next section, we discuss the base from which you will operate—your home.

Housing

Home is where the heart is and hence is a moveable feast.

—Angela Carter

Finding affordable and suitable housing can be a daunting task. You may be tempted to rush this process, but take time to reflect on all the needs you want to address by the seemingly straightforward task of obtaining housing. Are you concerned with safety, convenience to the university, proximity to good elementary schools, or availability of public transportation? Do you prefer to have a roommate? Do you want to keep a pet? What values and meanings are embedded in your selection of a home (Fiffer & Fiffer, 1995)?

Much like writing a research paper, finding housing requires that you first frame your question and then collect data to answer it. In this case, the data collection includes finding listings from local and university newspapers, the university housing office, other students, or real estate agents. You may find that taking this step is an opportunity to become acquainted with helpful resources at the university and the surrounding community.

Most universities have a housing office that typically provides rental information, housing guides, bus schedules, and student directories. Similar to a chamber of commerce, the housing office may be able to assist you with other aspects of settling in the area, such as finding grocery stores and places for recreation. Find out if the office can help you with potential housing problems, such as lease difficulties, landlord conflicts, parking limitations, and transportation needs. Many universities also have separate housing available for graduate students. Although living in graduate-student housing offers some conveniences, you may want to explore other possibilities.

For example, Jocelyn and Michael used information from the off-campus housing office and advertisements in the local newspaper to find an apartment that was not "a stack of red bricks that looked like one big red brick." Unfortunately, they discovered that the typical landlord's view of students was very negative. They began to feel like second-class citizens. Their predicament was further complicated by their commitment to find a place that would accept them and their three cats. As Jocelyn said, "Evidently, adding a third cat puts you in the crazy-cat-person category." For Jocelyn and Michael, however, their pets helped them keep a sense of balance in their academic lives.

Other potential sources of housing information may be your program advisor, peer mentor, and fellow students. They can help you become settled by answering your questions about housing as well as about the university and the surrounding community in general. They can provide support, encouragement, and some very helpful tips about how to create your base of operations.

After you have collected enough data, you are off to the field to conduct the applied portion of your research project—finding the location. Once again, equifinality can be useful to keep in mind because many paths can lead to the same end. The following story illustrates a somewhat open-minded approach to finding a new home.

▲▲▲

Adventures in
Subsidized Housing Land
Chris' Story

LIKE MOST beginning grad students, I needed to visit my school's community well before classes started to find a place to live. This was not so easy because I knew nothing about the town. I didn't know about the shortcuts to school, where the grocery stores and fast-food joints were, or where to get a Slurpee at 3:00 a.m.

I had very specific requirements for the apartment itself: four walls, a floor, and, if at all possible, a ceiling. In other words, I wasn't choosy. I figured I'd be spending a lot of time at school, so my housing only needed to be comfortable enough for me. So it all came down to cash. I took the cheapest place.

Taking the cheapest place wasn't a bad idea—it's just that there were certain tradeoffs. One was the uninvited "roommates"—hundreds and probably thousands of little six-legged tenants. Although I have lived in some rundown places, and I'm okay with that, armies of marauding roaches were a new experience for me.

Fortunately, the other apartment dwellers (the human ones) were wonderfully diverse—ethnically, racially, and linguistically. Being a member of just about every privileged majority there is, I found myself in an interesting position. Here I was, pursuing an advanced degree, while living among marginalized folks who were struggling just to get by.

▼▼▼

By living where he did, Chris discovered the striking and vast inequalities in the everyday lives of his neighbors—an essential lesson for a student of human strivings, challenges, and resilience.

As you make your own decisions about housing, consider what needs your home may help satisfy. Bowlby's attachment theory (1979) emphasizes the importance of having a "secure base" from which to explore. That secure base refers to having an established relationship with someone who is emotionally available and responsive to your needs. Initially Bowlby based his theory on the need infants have for a secure attachment to their caregivers; he has since extended the construct to cross the life span. The protective influence of having a secure base is now considered a prominent factor, similar to the importance of Maslow's needs, for people of all ages.

A primary benefit of such a relationship—your home base—is that it helps you successfully explore your surroundings. It is natural to feel both apprehensive and excited when you are in a new setting and among unfamiliar people. You may cope with the anxiety by using a combination of defenses—withdrawing into isolation, retreating to your secure base, or "overexploring" your new environment.

Freshmen in college sometimes resort to these defenses. For example, some may have attended classes, but then they seemed to evaporate into thin air. Other students were homesick and scurried home whenever possible. And then there were those who were always zipping frantically around campus.

These defensive strategies, however, are neither satisfying, nor, in the long run, helpful in fulfilling your needs for safety or belonging. Instead, you should make time to deliberately connect with people who can provide you with a base for emotional security. By maintaining a firm foundation in those relationships, you will better be able to explore and keep your bearings as you investigate and build your new community.

Jocelyn and Michael helped incorporate their established secure base into their new surroundings in a number of ways. For example, they regularly E-mailed friends and relatives with news about their discoveries, mishaps, and adventures in adjustment. They also relied on generous doses of humor. As transplants from the East Coast to the Midwest, Jocelyn once commented to Michael about driving: "Today, I used my turn signal and someone actually made an opening in traffic so I could get over! Isn't that a sign of weakness where we come from?" They found a farmer's market and made a ritual of going there every Saturday morning and of always frequenting the same little coffee shop.

By taking similar steps to preserve your secure base and build your new community, you are more likely to create a comfortable place—both physically and psychologically—for yourself in graduate school. Give yourself some time to relish your new surroundings and reflect on the changes.

▲▲▲

Giving Up City Life to Fit into a Small Town
Dara's Story

M Y CAR's license plate is the only reminder of the city life that I left behind to do my doctoral training in a small community, where everyone's paths cross every day. My faculty advisor's office is next door to mine. One of my student colleagues is seeing the same therapist that I am. People's lives overlap so much here that I keep wondering, "What ever happened to the idea of *six degrees of separation?*"

In L.A., where I grew up, being able to drive across town in less than 10 minutes would have been considered a miracle, but it's an everyday experience here—and that's with what the locals call "traffic." It would have been extraordinary if all your L.A. friends knew what you did last night—before you even woke up in the morning. Yet it's commonplace for everything to be everybody's business in this town. And nobody in L.A. would ever ask, "Why did you ever move to *this* place?" But I get that question all the time in my new community, where Cracker Barrel is considered an elegant restaurant and chipped beef an exotic food. My Jewish heritage feels so out of place—the bakery here sells only two challahs a week.

As a transplant from a large city, I have discovered that it really helps to receive care packages of familiar foods. In my apartment, I have hung pictures of my favorite city scenes as comforting reminders. My computer's screen saver even shows different L.A. landmarks. I stay connected to my friends back at home. Regularly, I make excursions several hours away from here for a dose of big-city life. And finally, I share my culture— my favorite dishes, music and movies—with the new friends I have made here.

▼▼▼

■ ■ ■

EXERCISE 4.4 It Takes a Community
An Exercise in Imagination

You've heard the African proverb, "It takes a village to raise a child." Well, it also takes a community to support a thriving graduate student. Because your needs do not remain static during graduate school, it's helpful to spend some time periodically envisioning the ideal community setting for you to continue your development.

Build an imaginary community that would fulfill your needs. Where would you be living? In a house or an apartment? With or without a roommate? Who and what else would be in your neighborhood? What cultures would be represented? What family configurations would be present? Would there be a place of worship? A park, woods, or playground? A vegetarian restaurant? Is the setting urban or rural?

List these essential elements or draw a picture of this ideal community. What characteristics of your make-believe community exist already for you? If they do not exist wholly, are there parts you recognize? How can you build you community in reality? Who will you ask to help?

■ ■ ■

Financial Assistance

Spare no expense to save money on this one.

—Samuel Goldwyn

Lack of money is no obstacle. Lack of an idea is
an obstacle.

—Ken Hakuta

According to Finkle (1999), the most common reason why students
abandon their dream of graduate education is the enormous financial
burden of tuition, fees, living expenses, and supplies. No matter how
much financial assistance you are able to manage, you probably need
to prepare yourself for an austere lifestyle. As Hoskins (2000) urged,
"Ask yourself, how much macaroni and cheese do I want to eat for
the next three to five years?" (p. 32). The financial support available
from work, family, savings, university assistance, or government programs may be a significant factor in your decision to enter graduate
training. As you explore your financial needs and resources, reflect on
both the emotional and the fiscal costs and benefits of assistance.
If a government loan would be helpful, then, besides computing the
monthly payments and the years needed to repay the loan, consider
the implications receiving such a loan has for you, your spouse, and
your family.

How you address your financial needs can have an impact on your
progress through the program. Are you planning to work while you
attend graduate school? How will working affect your available study
time or commitment to the training? Are you considering borrowing or
using funds from family members? How will this arrangement affect
your relationships within your family?

About half of all doctoral students and a third of master's students
receive financial aid (Finkle, 1999). Financial aid is typically available
through a government-sponsored program or through your university.
Private organizations, businesses, and industry groups may also offer
some funding.

Financial aid for graduate school is usually based on financial need,
and most aid is in the form of student loans. Keep in mind that funds
sometimes go to members of particular groups, such as students with
disabilities, minorities, or international students. If you are a member of
a group that is underrepresented in higher education or the helping professions, funding may be available for you (Leider & Leider, 2006).

Graduate schools also disburse funds on the basis of merit to attract candidates with special talent or knowledge. Typically, merit-based funding support comes in the form of assistantships or scholarship awards.

Assistantships Assistantships usually cover tuition and a stipend. You receive this financial assistance in exchange for working about 15 to 20 hours a week during the academic year. To be eligible for an assistantship, you must carry a specific number of credit hours and be enrolled in a degree program. Assistantships are generally available in your department, as well as in other academic programs and services across the campus.

The responsibilities of graduate assistantships are varied and can range from conducting library research and providing laboratory support to photocopying and filing. You may qualify for a teaching or clinical assistantship if you meet specific qualifications. With a teaching assistantship, you may be responsible for teaching an undergraduate class or helping a faculty member with specific course responsibilities. With a clinical assistantship, you may be providing supervision, assessment, and counseling services at a university-based mental health center.

If you are seeking an assistantship, contact your university's financial aid office or the office manager of your department. Most assistantships are one-year appointments, so you will probably need to re-apply each year for this form of financial assistance. If you did not receive an assistantship your first year, don't give up! You may be more qualified for one as an advanced student.

Competition for assistantships is often keen, so you have no guarantees of being offered one. Graduate school offices report receiving three applications for every available assistantship, depending on funding. Even so, there are some steps you can take to tip the odds in your favor:

- **Take care of the basics.** As in any competition, you have to play to win. The sooner you complete (and return!) the application form, the better your chances. Also, always make copies of the paperwork you submit, noting dates and to whom it was submitted. You will want to be able to construct a paper trail to ensure that your application has not been delayed anywhere.

- **Know how the system works.** Each university has its own administrative network for conferring assistantships. Some universities have a single clearinghouse; others have more decentralized operations, in which programs operate as separate fiefdoms, with dramatically different application procedures for assistantships. Take care to learn the system and play by its rules.

- **Let people know.** Make certain that your program director, faculty advisor, and student mentor know of your interest in obtaining an assistantship. Ask for their advice and suggestions. While you're at it, give them your E-mail address so they can easily contact you if they hear of an opportunity.

- **Highlight your skills.** The application forms for assistantships typically ask you to list your skills. Keep in mind that computer, research, and people skills are in demand, especially for nonacademic departments.

- **Remember that neatness does count.** Yes, your elementary-school teachers were right, so be careful when filling out the application materials. People will assume that the care you show on these documents indicates the care that you would take with job assignments.

- **Be persistent.** Faculty and staff members are busy people, so it is important for you to be persistent and to ask questions about graduate assistantships.

Student Loans Financing graduate education with a student loan is the most used pathway for students in the helping professions. If you are considering this option, many resources are available to assist you in finding and evaluating potential loan sources (Leider & Leider, 2006). Again, your university's financial aid office is an excellent source of information about federal loans.

A major source of financial assistance is the Federal Stafford Loan, both subsidized and unsubsidized. You begin the application process by completing a Free Application for Federal Student Aid (FAFSA). To save time, submit your FAFSA application online at www.fafsa.ed.gov.

There are other time-saving suggestions you can follow: First, before you begin to complete the online form, gather the documents you need, such as your social security number, driver's license, income tax return, bank statements, and investment records. Next, print a hard copy of the FAFSA Web worksheet. You then can write down your answers before transferring the information to the online FAFSA form. Third, speed up the process by using a personal identification number (PIN) to sign your application electronically. If you have a valid E-mail address, you can apply for a PIN. It takes up to three days to get one electronically, but it could take ten days for a signature page to be processed through the mail. Fourth, check your eligibility for federal student aid. Carefully read the requirements and restrictions regarding assistance. Finally, apply as early as possible, by January 1 of each year.

After you have submitted, once the department of education receives your FAFSA electronically, it will process your application and send you a student aid report (SAR). Your school will also receive an electronic copy of your SAR. Review this report carefully, make any necessary corrections, and return it to the financial aid office as quickly as possible. The financial aid office staff reviews the SAR to determine your eligibility for aid and notifies you of its decision. The financial aid office calculates need using a hypothetical student budget for a year, minus any family contribution. If you qualify, you then receive the loan application form. You should complete the application and return it immediately.

If you are an incoming student or have taken a summer class at another school, you also can facilitate the process by arranging for your transcripts to be sent to the university's financial aid office, rather than waiting for the office to request the records. You will help speed up the process if you meet the deadlines for each stage.

One step that routinely slows down the process is verifying tax records. Applicants whose tax records are reviewed are usually chosen at random, and the financial aid office is then required to look at all their tax forms for the past year. If you are chosen for verification, simply provide the information requested. Typically, you are asked to present a signed tax form.

If your need is great enough, you may be offered a work-study job that you can choose to accept or decline. Other possible funding sources are graduate scholarships or fellowships.

Scholarships Scholarships, fellowships, and grants may be awarded according to need, merit, or membership in a specific group. These are the most preferred types of financial assistance because they do not have to be repaid. They are not, however, commonly available to graduate students, especially those who are planning to enter the helping professions.

You can be resourceful by looking for financial support from professional organizations and service organizations, such as the Kiwanis. The American Counseling Association, for example, offers a scholarship award to a graduate student who wins its annual essay competition. Assistance is sometimes available if you plan to work in particular areas of specialization, such as autism or death and dying.

Research has consistently identified the presence of a dedicated friend or determined advocate as a crucial contributor to an individual's resilience. Give yourself permission to rely on the help of others as you seek financial assistance, decipher directions on forms, and complete the process. Because financial assistance is an area that can change quickly, we urge you to use the Internet resources listed at the end of the chapter.

Wellness

I'm not into working out. My philosophy: No pain, no pain.

—Carol Leifer

Leisure time is that five or six hours when you sleep at night.

—George Allen

The dominant Western culture spends a great deal of time giving you messages about how to take better care of your body, how to eat healthier foods, and how to be more physically fit. Unfortunately, many of those messages are driven by the desire to promote corporate profits, not personal wellness. The emerging field of health psychology is reporting important findings about the relationship between your physical and mental well-being. Indeed, many of the results support a more traditionally Eastern concept of the wholeness of your self.

Let's face it: Like most of us, you probably know a lot more about healthy exercise and nutrition than you put into practice. Students in graduate counseling programs generally report high levels of wellness (Myers, Mobley, & Booth, 2003), but when you take on too many commitments in your training, you may find yourself abandoning some habits that promote physical well-being. Eating poorly, sleeping less, and rarely exercising can quickly become your lifestyle as a graduate student. As one student commented, "Sure, I drink plenty of water every day—if Dr. Pepper, Mountain Dew, and coffee count. And, yes, I also eat a well-balanced diet from the basic food groups—donuts from the round group, tortilla chips from the triangle group, and candy bars from the rectangle group."

As you consider your needs for good nutrition and regular activity, reflect on the meaning that eating well and exercising have for you. Here are a few questions to get you started. When you were growing up, what messages did you receive about food? In what ways was food part of family and community celebrations? Did you associate nurturance and comfort with food? Did you worry about not having enough food for everyone? Was finishing your plate an expectation? Why? What is the relationship between stress and eating for you? Is feeding other people a demonstration of your love?

What does fitness and activity mean to you? Who were the role models in your family for eating and exercising? Were messages about fitness gender-related? What messages do you believe about your self-esteem and your wellness? From your spiritual perspective, how do you view the human body? After you have reflected on these questions, you can come to a deeper appreciation of the regenerative power of eating well and the exhilaration of physical exertion.

The transtheoretical model of change (Prochaska, DiClemente, & Norcross, 1992) can offer another perspective. Counselors and therapists frequently examine the process of change that clients go through (for example, DiClemente, Schlundt, & Gemmell, 2004), but here, the focus is on *you*. The changes you will experience in your training and throughout your career are not time-limited events; they are ongoing and involve five important stages (Prochaska & DiClemente, 1983). *Precontemplation* is the first stage of change during which you do not intend to take any action. Of course, that may be due to a lack of information and feelings of futility, denial, or fear. As your consciousness is raised, you enter the second stage: *contemplation,* during which you begin to consider changing but are still feeling ambivalent about this new and threatening prospect. In fact, you may feel stuck, going over the pros and cons, procrastinating and delaying any real or meaningful action. *Preparation* is the third change. At this point, you have made a significant shift in your thinking. You have overcome the barriers of resistance and now truly believe that change is possible. Fourth, you engage in *action* by performing the specific, detailed, and overt modifications in your day-to-day lifestyle. *Maintenance,* the final stage, involves sustaining the new action and handling successfully the inevitable relapses that accompany any significant change. As you emerge from this change process, you have now entered into a new reality and have become a transformed self.

What does this model mean for you? Well, it's a great way to accelerate the momentum of the change process whenever you discover that your consciousness has been raised. For example, as you read and hear more about physical and psychological well-being, you may begin to contemplate a variety of lifestyle changes, such as better nutrition, more exercise, more fulfilling relationships, or more conscientious personal health care. Whatever alterations you consider, you can use this model to facilitate the change process. You can overcome your resistance by making plans, becoming energized, enlisting the help of others, and readying yourself for this transformation.

One counseling student, realizing that she was compromising her physical well-being, developed a plan. "I made an agreement with myself that I would get at least three hours of exercise a week to release stress, feel better about myself, and fit into my clothes again. My new schedule book would have that workout time in it" (Belcastro, 2000, p. 12). Another student, Martin, entered graduate school with many healthy practices already in place. He had attained a black belt in karate and carefully protected his practice time. After a while, his classmates learned to refrain from complaining about being tired in front of him, because they knew he would tell them, "You must not be exercising enough!" It was particularly irritating to hear his words because they knew he was right.

▲▲▲

Kicking and Sleeping
Martin's Story

EVEN THOUGH I would like to have maintained a more consistent exercise regimen than I have since entering the training program, I regularly do a Tae Bo routine, a kind of kickboxing-dance workout video. I make sure to do this whenever I feel stressed and have a need for physical activity. Also, in spite of my demanding schedule, I try to get at least eight hours of sleep a night. Getting a good amount of sleep replenishes my internal drive to tackle the demands and events of the upcoming day.

Finding and Creating Perspective

> Compared to what we ought to be, we are only
> half awake.
>
> —William James

Martin's observation is consistently supported in the research literature. If you take good care of meeting your physiological needs, you'll have more energy for other pursuits. You may heartily agree but believe that you just can't find the time for exercise. Covey (1989) offered a wonderful example to illustrate the fallacy of not making the time to satisfy your wellness needs. Imagine that, as you are taking a stroll in the woods, you encounter a person laboring frenetically to saw down a tree. The person, who's sweaty and haggard, is obviously worn out but has barely made a scratch in the tree after sawing for hours. Trying to be helpful, you suggest that if the person stopped and sharpened the saw, the work would go much quicker. But the person protests, "I don't have time to sharpen the saw. . . . I'm too busy sawing" (p. 287).

Covey's point is that we truly do *not* have the time to eat poorly and to avoid exercise. If we know these activities are important, why do we often systematically neglect them? He believes that we fool ourselves into thinking that neglecting wellness needs has neither immediate nor significant consequences. We know enough to do the right thing, but we need some help, as the Nike commercials say, to "just do it."

▲▲▲

The Road from Orange Crackers to Rice
Anne's Story

HAD LIMITED success in eating healthy meals as a graduate student. Nearly every day at lunch, for the better part of three years, I ate raspberry frozen yogurt ("You mean ice cream," a nutritionist finally told me) and those bright-orange cracker and peanut butter sandwiches. Fortunately, my body was in good enough health to somehow withstand this simultaneous neglect and assault. My weak defense was that the nearby grill did not have vegetarian entrees.

What finally helped me was to link my nutritional and exercise needs to my need for belonging. I now enjoy lunch with friends and make sure I eat a healthy meal. I take regular walks with my neighbor. Actually, I *talk* with my neighbor and we move while we do it. The other meaningful context is related to my role as a mother. It is important to me that my children develop good health habits. I know my children will be influenced by what they see me do in these areas, for better or worse.

▼▼▼

As you reflect on your needs and ponder their meaning for you, keep in mind that you are not alone. Linking with others to meet your needs can lead not only to good nutrition and exercise but also to good company. By addressing more than one area of need, you increase your thriving quotient (TQ) in ways that are both gratifying and enduring.

These "good habits" are similar to informal rituals observed in healthy families. Research informs us that having meaningful rituals in our lives provides a sense of cohesiveness and security (Driver, 1998; Imber-Black & Roberts, 1992). For example, a group of male graduate students decided to meet each Sunday to enjoy a meal together. First, the eating was paired with watching sports, a dominant interest for them in their pre-graduate-school lives. Over time, they regularly added a study component to their shared meal. Recently, their Sunday ritual has evolved into an informal men's support group—with good food.

EXERCISE 4.5 I'll Have the Combo
Meeting Multiple Needs

Think over Maslow's hierarchy of needs and jot down some activities that you want to do that correspond with the types of needs. Look for activities that might naturally combine to meet several needs simultaneously.

For example, to address your needs for safety and security, you may want to learn self-defense. You could enroll in a course that would teach you defensive skills, provide an excellent workout, and offer opportunities for developing new friendships. To meet the need to belong, you might find a camping or hiking club or a gourmet cooking club that could address both your wellness and friendship needs. In addressing self-esteem and self-actualization needs, you might use yoga, tai chi, or dance instruction for exercise.

Sometimes you hear another perspective and it immediately rings a bell. One student related that the most centering and helpful advice from her advisor was to picture the span of her entire life and then make a ratio of how much time she would actually spend in graduate school—an intense but relatively small part. That reminder helped this student put the challenges of school in the proper perspective. Like sitting in the dentist's chair, graduate school does not last forever—and reminding yourself that an ordeal is temporary can make it endurable. You can then focus on using this limited experience to forge a lifestyle of balance, beauty, and well-being.

Although you may focus more energy on satisfying safety and belonging needs at the start of graduate school, you'll find that these are ongoing needs throughout your training. For example, you may focus on financial aid more at the beginning, but you may find that additional support is available later for specific activities, such as funding designated for research or presentations at professional conferences. In the same manner, as you become more familiar with your community and make new friends, you may decide your belonging or safety needs will be better met by changing your living arrangements.

Five hundred years ago, Ficino (Moore, 1992) gave this good advice for staying well: "You should walk as often as possible among plants that have a wonderful aroma, spending a considerable amount of time every day among such things." Sounds good! Maybe you can even invite a friend to join you.

SUMMARY

In this chapter, we presented suggestions and guidelines for finding safe and affordable housing, obtaining educational loans, applying for assistantships and scholarships, taking care of your nutritional needs, and maintaining an active, healthy lifestyle. Meeting your needs in graduate school is not easy, but the experience can contribute to your thriving as a trainee. Through your struggles, you build an empathic bridge with the people you counsel. And in your successes, you gain an appreciation for your clients' personal strengths and social resources.

RESOURCES

Graduate School (Finkle, 1999) assembles an amazing variety of resources to help you research graduate programs, create successful applications, find financial assistance, and excel in your training. These resources include printed materials, Web sites, and on-line services.

Don't Miss Out (Leider & Leider, 2006), now in its thirtieth edition, is the undisputed leader in guides on financing your education. The authors describe the common myths about obtaining aid, how to complete federal forms, the role of the university, and employer-sponsored education. It includes information specific to women and persons of color. The book is comprehensive and has a terrific listing of suggestions and contacts.

Sage Publications Graduate Survival Skills series offers a comprehensive look at the graduate school experience, including how to apply and finance graduate school. The series has books that address the unique experiences and challenges that some students may confront in graduate school. For example, the series includes books geared toward women (Rittner & Trudeau, 1997) and African Americans (Isaac, 1998). The series is well written and provides detailed information on a wide range of topics, from studying and taking examinations to dealing with racism and clarifying goals.

Funding Education Beyond High School: The Guide to Federal Student Aid 2006–2007, published by the U.S. Department of Education and available at *http://studentaid.ed.gov/students/attachments/siteresources/StudentGuide.pdf,* is a comprehensive resource on student financial aid programs. Grants, loans, and work-study are the three major forms of aid available through the department's federal student aid office.

The Department of Education also publishes *Looking for Student Aid,* available at www.fafsa.ed.gov, which are guides that provide comprehensive information about applying for federal financial aid. You can also request print versions by calling the Federal Student Aid Information Center at 1-800-433-3243.

REFERENCES

Belcastro, A. L. (2000, February). Finding balance in school and life. *Counseling Today, 43,* 12.

Bowlby, J. (1979). *Separation.* New York: Basic Books.

Covey, S. (1989). *Seven habits of highly effective people.* New York: Simon & Schuster.

DiClemente, C. C., Schlundt, D., & Gemmell, L. (2004). Readiness and stages of change in addiction treatment. *American Journal of Addictions, 13,* 103–119.

Driver, T. F. (1998). *Liberating rites: Understanding the transformative power of ritual.* Boulder, CO: Westview.

Fiffer, S. S., & Fiffer, S. (1995). *Home: American writers remember rooms of their own.* New York: Vintage Books.

Finkle, J. (1999). *Graduate school.* Seattle, WA: Resource Pathways.

Hoskins, C. M. (2000, August). Get a life! Top 10 list for a first-year student. *Counseling Today, 43,* 32, 36.

Imber-Black, E., & Roberts, J. (1992). *Rituals for our times.* New York: HarperCollins.

Isaac, A. (1998). *The African American student's guide to surviving graduate school.* New York: Sage.

Leahey, T. H. (2000). *A history of psychology: Main currents in psychological thought.* Upper Saddle River, NJ: Prentice-Hall.

Leider, A., & Leider, R. (2006). *Don't miss out* (30th ed.). Alexandria, VA: Octameron Associates.

MacLaine, S. (2000). *The Camino: A journey of the spirit.* New York: Pocket Books.

Maslow, A. H. (1962). *Toward a psychology of being.* New York: Van Nostrand.

Maslow, A. H. (1970). *Motivation and personality* (2nd ed.). New York: Harper and Row.

Moore, T. (1992). *Care of the soul.* New York: HarperCollins.

Myers, J. E., Mobley, A. K., & Booth, C. S. (2003). Wellness of counseling students: Practicing what we preach. *Counselor Education and Supervision, 42,* 264–274.

Prochaska, J. O., & DiClemente, C. C. (1983). Stages and processes of self-change of smoking: Toward an integrative model of change. *Journal of Consulting and Clinical Psychology, 51,* 390–395.

Prochaska, J. O., DiClemente, C. C., & Norcross, J. C. (1992). In search of how people change: Applications to addictive behaviors. *American Psychologist, 47,* 1102–1114.

Rittner, B., & Trudeau, P. (1997). *The women's guide to surviving graduate school.* New York: Sage.

Answer to the Riddle The farmer first takes the chicken to the island, leaving the fox with the grain. The farmer then returns, picks up the fox, and ferries it to the island. Instead of leaving the fox alone with the chicken, the farmer brings the chicken back on the return voyage, drops off the chicken, and transports the grain to the island. Leaving the fox with the grain on the island, the farmer returns for the chicken once again to make the final transport.

CHAPTER 5

Enhancing Your Academic Skills

People get wisdom from thinking, not from learning.

—Laura Riding Jackson

Reason is, and ought only to be, the slave of the passions.

—David Hume

The Chinese character for listening combines not only the character for ears but also those for eyes, heart, and mind (Adler, Rosenfeld, & Towne, 1989). This wonderful fusion of symbols expresses the essence of successful counseling. As a counselor or therapist, you involve yourself totally—ears, eyes, heart, and mind—in a process of truly encountering your client in a helping relationship. Because counseling is a dynamic and complex process, you need to cultivate not only your observational competencies and emotional sensitivities but also your mental abilities. The purpose of your graduate curriculum is to prepare your mind, heart, eyes, and ears for the challenging work of counseling and therapy.

In this chapter, we discuss how to use the four basic academic skills—reading, researching, writing, and presenting—to enhance your training. Reading is the original virtual reality—it broadens and enriches your experiences by tapping into the observations, ideas, and discoveries of others. Research skills enable you to observe carefully, collect information systematically, and organize material into a coherent framework. Writing helps you give voice to your own experiences, makes your thoughts known, and helps clarify vague hunches. Finally, presentation skills enable you to communicate your observations and expertise with colleagues, clients, and the general public.

So how does improving those academic skills help you become a better counselor or therapist? These skills can help you stay current, think creatively, keep emotionally engaged, and approach your work mindfully, all of which can help you maintain your professional vitality and prevent burnout. These skills are not only essential during your training, but they are also indispensable throughout your professional career.

▲▲▲

More Than I Had Bargained For
Bonnie's Story

REMEMBER BEING the first person in the room the first time my course in my training to become a counselor met. That was a lot of "firsts"! There I sat, a forty-five-year-old woman, successful accountant, mother of two wonderful teenage girls, wife of nearly twenty years in a loving marriage, and now a brand-new counseling student. I had finally decided that if I really wanted to become a counselor, then it was now or never. Generally, I'm a pretty confident person but not right before my first class! Every other student entered the room as if he or she belonged there, and I couldn't help noticing how young they were. Some of them looked like they were still in college, and I must have been the oldest student by at least ten or fifteen years. I was even older than my professor! What, I wondered, was I doing here?

Sure, I had been a good student in college. Over the years, I had continued to read voraciously and to write newsletters for a volunteer organization for the mentally ill. I even helped my daughter with her calculus! But my days as a student were a long time ago. Even though I felt a calling to become a counselor, I was worried that I couldn't handle the demands of reading textbooks, writing term papers, and taking tests.

Of course, throughout that first semester of my training, I had to do a personal "crash course" on using the newer research services. I was so out of it that I thought Article Express must be a paper train and WorldCat sounded like a new super hero. Now,

I've become an old hand at using the PsycINFO database, and I've discovered I'm still a pretty good student.

My biggest surprise has been how emotionally charged and personally involved I am in the training. I've found that I cannot be a detached and disengaged spectator in my learning. Instead, I've watched my own life unfolding in the course on lifespan development. I've noticed all my own symptoms, as well as those of my relatives and friends, in the diagnostics class. And my counseling-skills class has stirred up all sorts of personal issues for me.

Early that first semester, we were watching a scene from a documentary, "The Farmer's Wife," which is a powerful account of a woman's courage in enduring the stresses of modern-day farming. I started crying because that could have been my mother on that screen. When it was time for the class to discuss the scene, I decided to share the memories and emotions that the scene had evoked in me. One student later thanked me for "enriching" her understanding of these issues. You know, this is more learning than I had originally bargained for, but I'm truly grateful that I'm able to take advantage of the opportunity.

▼▼▼

HEARTS AND MINDS

The heart has its reasons which reason knows not.

—Blaise Pascal

In his autobiography, Carl Jung (1965) described his journey to the American Southwest, where he encountered Ochwiay Biano (Mountain Lake), a Native American who was chief of the Taos Pueblo Tribe. Ochwiay Biano shared with Jung his concerns about "whites":

"We do not know what they want. We do not understand them. We think that they are mad."

I asked him why he thought the whites were all mad.

"They say that they think with their heads," he replied.

"Why of course. What do you think with?" I asked him in surprise.

"We think here," he said, indicating his heart (p. 248).

This account is more than just a "Jung at heart" story. In fact, research on emotional intelligence (Goleman, 1995) indicates that we think with *both* our heads and our hearts. According to Antonio Damasio (1994), a neuroscientist at the University of Iowa, Descartes made a huge mistake when he omitted emotions from the thinking process. Damasio's inno- vative research has revealed that emotions are actually essential to good thinking.

Many students who enter graduate programs in counseling may have been more of a "heart" person as undergraduates. When you first read a poem, you probably respond emotionally rather than critically. You become passionately involved in projects that captivate your attention. As you enter graduate school, you may view the academic courses in your training curriculum as merely ordeals that you must endure—the hoops you have to jump through—before you can qualify for the real learning experiences that take place in your clinical placements. If this description sounds like you, we invite you to examine carefully your academic skills. You can learn to study better, rather than harder, and make your academic work as personally rewarding and successful as the practice you'll do in your training.

On the other hand, you may be more of a "head" person in your learning style. You may have been a very competent undergraduate stu- dent, participating actively in your classes, carefully reading the assigned material, and completing assignments conscientiously. For you, emotions seem to get in the way of thinking objectively. Conse- quently, you may be less personally engaged and more emotionally detached in your approach to learning. If this description sounds more like you, you may find it challenging to explore yourself, your clients, and the counseling process in your graduate training.

Recalling your undergraduate education may seem like ancient his- tory to you. You may be one of the increasing number of "nontradi- tional" students returning to an academic setting after years of pursuing another career or raising a family. As a result, you may have only vague memories of those distant college days—and some strong apprehen- sions about re-entering the academic life. Whether you were passive and disengaged or active and involved during your undergraduate years may be irrelevant. After all, you're now at a different stage in your life. You've become more seasoned, mature, and thoughtful, all of which will be wonderful assets for you. But you probably have at least one major worry: that your academic skills may be too rusty.

In this chapter, we describe how you can develop critical reflection by enhancing the core academic skills of reading, research, writing, and presenting. "Isn't this stuff too basic for graduate training?" you may be wondering. "Aren't these just a variation of the three R's—reading, 'riting, and 'rithmetic?" Although these are basic skills, they'll be a little more complex and a lot more interesting in your graduate training. We share with you here some "tricks of the trade." But more important, we challenge you to commit both your heart and your head to becoming a lifelong learner and successful practitioner. After all, student and professional counselors who have higher levels of emotional intelligence are also more effective practitioners (Martin, Easton, Wilson, Takemoto, & Sullivan, 2004).

DEVELOPING CRITICAL REFLECTION SKILLS

The function of education is to teach one to think intensively and to think critically. Intelligence plus character—that is the goal of true education.

—Martin Luther King, Jr.

Simply put, critical reflection is the process of carefully and systemically examining ideas (Meltzoff, 1998). When you think, read, and respond mindfully, you challenge yourself to use higher-order thinking skills—to engage in critical reflection. Critical reflection is a requisite skill for becoming a successful counselor or therapist because you must ultimately rely on your own knowledge and judgment. Of course, you should never work without seeking supervision and consultation regularly from others. However, when you are alone dealing with a troubled client, responding to a suicidal caller, or even presenting a difficult case, you must rely on your own abilities. At these crucial times, you have to gather data, analyze complex information, synthesize different factors, present your ideas coherently, and then act on them mindfully.

To begin developing your critical reflection skills as a practitioner, you must have a thorough knowledge of theories, develop a repertoire of intervention skills, gain insight into your clients, recognize their cultural contexts, appreciate the intricacies of interpersonal dynamics, and become more aware of yourself. Mastering all this material is a daunting task, but it's only the beginning. Once you've gained some familiarity with these abilities, you need to play with the pieces to see where they fit and then arrange these elements into a complete picture. Ideally, the resulting mosaic will then serve as a working model for successful counseling and therapy.

One way you can facilitate the development of your own critical reflection ability is by striving to be mindful. Langer (1989, 1997) described mindfulness as being open to new information. Mindfulness is to thinking as flexibility is to athletics. Being mindful allows you to reach farther, notice connections, and discover parallels that you might otherwise miss.

Bloom and his associates (Bloom, Englehart, Furst, & Krathwohl, 1956) developed a hierarchy that may be helpful as you explore how you think. An anonymous cynic once insisted, "When it comes to thought, some people stop at nothing." But, according to Bloom, nearly everyone has at least some skills within the six levels of critical thinking. The first skill, *knowledge*, which involves mastering and memorizing, has probably served you well during multiple-choice or true-false tests. Similarly, *comprehension*, the second skill, is necessary to demonstrate your understanding of the basics and your ability to take them farther by interpreting and wondering about them.

Both of these skills are fundamental, but you'll find that graduate education challenges you to move up the hierarchy to other skills, such as application. *Application* requires that you use your comprehension to build new connections and, in some ways, "handle" the material. Application is at work when you try out your skills in your first peer-counseling experience.

The fourth skill, *analysis*, involves breaking down information to see how its components are related and connected. Your analytical skills are involved, for example, when you compare and contrast psychodynamic and cognitive behavioral approaches to counseling. Analysis is also essential in conceptualizing counseling cases.

Synthesis, the fifth skill, is the process of constructing new ways to integrate information. If your program requires you to describe your personal theory of counseling, chances are you'll use this higher-order thinking skill to put different pieces of information together to create a unified and comprehensive design. You may initially be shocked by the multitude of theoretical approaches in your beginning texts. Prochaska and Norcross (2007) place the most recent number of distinct theoretical approaches to counseling and psychotherapy at 400.

The final skill Bloom et al. identified is *evaluation,* which requires that you form a substantiated conclusion. "Hey, that's easy!," you may think. "I can tell right away if something is good or bad." Perhaps, but what are your criteria? To be truly mindful and stretch your critical-reflection muscles, you must establish and apply appropriate criteria so that you can make effective and consistent evaluations. Imagine, for instance, that a peer asks you to evaluate a recording of her counseling session. What will your criteria be? What are the bases for these criteria? How will you measure performance? Can you ensure that you'll evaluate this recording and another student's with some degree of consistency?

It's probably obvious that evaluation, as well as synthesis, analysis, application, and even comprehension and memorization, are complex skills. You can, however, make improvements in all these competencies if you practice. As Marilyn vos Savant once said, "My thoughts are like waffles—the first few don't look too good." If that's true for you, then keep cooking!

Stay mindful and stretch your intellectual muscles. Langer (1997) suggested that you can improve your mindfulness by asking good questions and looking for novel distinctions. You can practice this with your peers and your professors, while reading textbooks, and by yourself. As you do so, try to expand the ways in which you categorize the answers you get. For instance, rather than labeling a response as merely good or bad, search for a new evaluative description. At the same time, stay open to ideas or tasks that may at first seem unappealing or even boring. Approaching them mindfully by actively seeking novel aspects in them can actually increase your enjoyment of learning about a concept or performing an activity (Langer, 1997).

LEARNING BY HEART

> There is only one quality worse than hardness of heart and that is softness of head.
>
> —Theodore Roosevelt

The underlying assumption of most discussions about thinking is that it is much better to use your head than to follow your heart. Emotions, according to this orthodox view, only contaminate good thinking.

Therefore, the traditional goal of higher education has been to promote dispassionate thinking. The work of Damasio (1994) and Goleman (1995), however, have demonstrated that emotions play a vital role in performing academic tasks, engaging in effective problem solving, remaining open to new ideas, and thinking creatively.

In this section, we focus on three ways to use your emotions to strengthen your academic skills—riding the perturbation wave, finding "the zone," and using the Zeigarnik Effect.

Riding the Perturbation Wave

> The word "yes" may bring trouble; the word "no"
> leads nowhere.
>
> —Bantu proverb

In any significant learning experience, your mind is in a state of dialectical tension (Presbury, Echterling, & McKee, 2002). On the one hand, you are excited to discover new ways of thinking and to experiment with new ways of acting. On the other, you strive to have some sense of certainty and familiarity. This tension between chaos and order is the essence of learning. If your thoughts have been thrown into chaos, then you feel overwhelmed and confused; however, if you're not sufficiently challenged, you feel bored and stagnant.

The secret to getting the most out of any learning opportunity is to ride the wave of perturbation. Just as in surfing, you seek out the situations that make waves and create turbulence. You'll take a tumble now and then, but the adventure is well worth the risk. The learning tasks you encounter under these circumstances will be challenging and may even knock you off balance, but they are rarely overpowering. In contrast to surfing, the traditional ideal of disengaged, dispassionate thinking is like standing on the shore—you may never be in over your head, but neither will you experience the exhilaration of being carried away with an idea or totally caught up in performing a task.

Mihaly Csikszentmihalyi (1997) describes this invigorating process of immersing yourself completely in an activity as "flow." You are more likely to experience flow when several conditions are met. The first condition is that the situation requires specific actions to achieve explicit goals. When, for example, you are weaving, running, playing chess, or studying for a test, you are more likely to "become" that activity and achieve flow. Flow also requires that you receive immediate feedback on your efforts. You can see the pattern emerging as you weave, the route you are completing as you run, the new positions of your chess pieces as you move them, and your understanding enhanced as you continue studying. The final and most important condition is a manageable challenge. You can achieve flow if successfully completing a task requires that you make the most of your emerging skills. When the weaving pattern is particularly intricate, the running route especially demanding, the chess game unusually intriguing, and the subject matter extremely challenging, you have the opportunity to immerse yourself in the productive and satisfying experience of flow.

If you are a new student, you may not realize just how challenging your training experiences will be. Of course, in all graduate programs, the intellectual content of the curriculum will involve some difficulties and the workload will be heavy. But graduate training in counseling and therapy may seem much more manageable than other programs. Your textbooks, for example, may be more readable than those on physics, medicine, or law. Your counseling professors may seem nice—after all, they're also counselors—so you may initially assume that they won't be too demanding. However, you'll soon find that your professors, curriculum, readings, and learning experiences will all work together to consistently challenge you to deal with emotionally charged material, face your own personal issues, and learn painful lessons. Your training is more than hard work; it's *heart* work. The ride may turn out to be much more turbulent than you thought!

One of the common sources of turbulence you'll encounter as a counseling student is questioning your assumptions about yourself, people, and life in general. The assumptions that you have developed over the years are comfortable, like an old pair of shoes that you're reluctant to give up even though they've got holes in them. Particularly when you first begin to question your assumptions about cultures, gender, and values, you are likely to feel confused. As Milton Erickson pointed out (Erickson, Rossi, & Rossi, 1976), people have a powerful need to resolve confusion. Because you can't rely on automatic thinking anymore, you become attentive, focused, and mindful. At these times, you will embark on an intense search for new ways to view yourself, others, and the world. Embrace your confusion! Out of this chaos, you can create a deeper, richer sense of order and harmony.

Automatic thinking can cause you to see other people as stereotypes, whereas mindful thinking makes you aware of the unique qualities of those you encounter. Automatic thinking can also blind you to the often subtle forms of oppression that others endure every day.

▨ ▨ ▨

EXERCISE 5.1 The Birdcage:
Encountering Oppression

Frye (1995) offered a powerful metaphor to perturb our thinking about oppression. Take a couple of minutes to read the following fantasy.

Imagine that you are seeing a birdcage for the first time. But the birdcage is so close to your face that you can only focus on one of its bars. With the bar in front of your eyes, you can see its minute details—the gleam of light on its shiny surface, the texture of the paint, and its cylindrical shape—but not the other bars. If your conception of a birdcage was based only on this close examination, you could continue to examine it carefully and be incredulous to hear that a bird could not escape from it. Why couldn't a bird simply fly around this bar anytime it wanted? What's wrong with this bird? Lack of initiative? Some personal flaw? Or just plain laziness?

It's only when you have an opportunity to step back and gain a larger view of the birdcage that you can begin to appreciate how this systematic network of barriers works. Alone, each wire presents no obstacle to the bird's freedom, but together, these slender threads are just as effective as any prison made of solid stone.

Consider the meaning of this fantasy for you and describe your reflections below.

_____

_____

_____

_____

_____

▨ ▨ ▨

Finding "The Zone"

Life loves to be taken by the lapel and told: "I'm
with you kid. Let's go."

—Maya Angelou

Goleman (1995) found that a moderately elated or energized emotional
state is best for thinking flexibly and solving complex problems more
readily. The Yerkes-Dodson Law shows how your state of emotional
arousal affects your performance. You perform poorly when your emotions are at either extreme—disengaged or highly aroused (Martindale,
1981). At a moderate level of emotional arousal, you're at your best—
adrenaline pumping, memory enhanced, neurons firing, and attention
focused. When you're in "the zone," you can do your finest work.

One study discovered that first-year doctoral students in counseling
were plagued by concerns about the unknown and doubts about their
abilities to succeed (Hughes & Kleist, 2005). What helped those students
enter their productive zone was reminding themselves of their personal
strengths and previous successes. This emphatic belief in their capabilities, in spite of the uncertainties of these new challenges, was the essential
catalyst for engaging fully in the process of discovery and learning.

Most guides on academic success emphasize the importance of managing your time, but managing your emotional arousal is even more
crucial. If you led with your head as an undergraduate student, encourage yourself to follow your heart more in your graduate training.
Become a passionate scholar! Getting psyched can become part of your
preparatory ritual before you open a book, attend a class, or start an
assignment. You may want to remind yourself of the goals you are working to achieve, to visualize yourself as a successful counselor, or to ask
yourself important questions that your academic work can help you
answer. Get personal with the material. Explore, for example, how you
can use a particular concept to gain insight into yourself. How have you
experienced enmeshment in your relationships? When have you used
denial? How has modeling influenced you? Engaging with these concepts in such a personal way is like playing a sport—you're a participant
in the process, not a spectator.

If you've followed your heart throughout most of your previous
education, you may be more likely to hit the higher end of the Yerkes-
Dodson curve when you are facing important tasks in a counseling
graduate program. In that case, your routine for preparing for a
challenging assignment or test may include practicing relaxation and

focusing activities. When it comes to engaging your emotions in the learning process, you need to follow the "Goldilocks Principle"—not too hot and not too cold.

Using the Zeigarnik Effect

> The suspense is terrible. I hope it will last.
>
> —Oscar Wilde

Did you ever follow a television "soap opera"? No matter which one you may have watched, each episode would usually end with a cliffhanger. If soaps never interested you, perhaps you've read an adventure comic book that ended with the words, "to be continued," just when the hero was facing certain doom. Remember how badly you wanted to know how things were going to turn out? You may have replayed the events over and over in your mind, speculated about the possible consequences, and talked about the circumstances with friends. Until the program's next episode or the comic book's following issue, your curiosity continued to nag at you. At those times, you were experiencing the Zeigarnik Effect.

Hergenhahn (1992) described how Kurt Lewin, the famous Gestalt psychologist, hypothesized that a person who has not finished a task or achieved closure on a topic will remember the material better. Bluma Zeigarnik, a student of Lewin, tested this hypothesis in an experiment in which participants were permitted to finish only some tasks but not others. As predicted, she found that participants later remembered many more of the uncompleted tasks than the completed ones.

What the Zeigarnik Effect means for you is that if you want to "chew" on an idea, rather than forget it immediately, you should not rush to make up your mind about it. Similarly, because no graduate class ever resolves all the issues you will face in your counseling career, there is always naturally "unfinished business" in your personal and professional development. If you allow yourself to leave a classroom holding on to at least one suspenseful note, you are more likely to keep reflecting on it as you seek a richer and deeper understanding of the subject matter. In fact, we have a multitude of unresolved issues that face us in the counseling profession, unanswered questions that confront us in our personal lives, and vast, unexplored territories that beckon our psyches. Invoking the Zeigarnik Effect could be a great daily ritual to stay open, curious, and engrossed.

As you read the following material about basic academic skills, keep in mind that you can enhance your abilities in each of them by using your emotions to help you learn by heart.

THE CORE ACADEMIC SKILLS

Reading

Reading is a means of thinking with another
person's mind: It forces you to stretch your own.

—Charles Scribner, Jr.

Literacy is a fundamental skill for elementary school students, and the same is true for you in your graduate training. "Hey, reading is no big deal!" you may think. "I already read E-mails, newspapers, magazines, novels, and nonfiction books. I read all the time—what's so tough about the reading I'll do in a graduate training program?"

Well, the reading assignments in graduate school will differ significantly from the reading you've done so far. In addition to textbooks, you'll be expected to read seminal works in the field, as well as manuscripts written by your professors, drafts of collaborative papers by your fellow students, psychological assessments, client files, program evaluations, counseling protocols, and the most recently published professional literature. Some books and articles have become standards in the field and are often considered unofficial required reading for all counselors and therapists. Appendix A lists a few of these classics.

Although the content, style, and purpose of the material you read in graduate school will vary tremendously, it will have several common characteristics. First and foremost, the amount of reading will seem intimidating. You may not be able to prevent eyestrain, but many graduate students do invest in backpacks to manage heavy loads without straining their backs. Second, unlike a book you might read on the beach, this reading is not "fast food for the mind." The material is challenging in several ways; it may be difficult, complex, provocative, demanding, or even emotionally painful to read. This material requires your full attention. Otherwise, you are likely to miss subtle nuances and crucial details. You also need to read the material critically—with an inquiring mind. And afterward, you need to reflect on what you have read. This material is not something you can swallow in one quick gulp. You need to take the time to digest it.

Successfully handling both the breadth and depth of the reading material required in your graduate training is like baking a cake—you just have to combine a few basic ingredients.

The Place First, take some time to determine what environment is best for helping you engage in productive, intensive, and extensive reading.

Do you concentrate best in silence? With others around? With or without music?

Karen, a graduate student with two children, found that she did her best reading and reflection in a coffee shop near school. The smell of the coffee, the arrivals and departures of others, and the piped-in classical music were soothing to her. She could sit for hours, occasionally getting a refill of coffee or a biscotti, without being interrupted by family members. The others in the shop served as a welcome distraction when she needed to take a break, and she enjoyed getting to know the coffee shop employees, who occasionally inquired about her school work.

Rae, on the other hand, found that she was most able to read with depth and comprehension when she was at home, in total silence, sitting on a folding chair at a plain card table tucked in a small monastic-like alcove of her apartment—no coffee, no food, no distractions, and no visitors.

You may want to experiment to determine where and how you do your best reading. Once you've discovered what environment works for you, then find and claim it.

The Time Second, you need to set aside plenty of time. This suggestion, like the first, depends on your preferences. Many students find that when they begin graduate school, they have enough time to complete the assigned readings. As they become more involved in their classes and other activities, however, they find that the extra time has slipped away. They then struggle to keep pace, if not one step behind, with their reading assignments. After you've found your ideal place to read, figure out the best time to do it. Then claim this time as yours. Kelly, for example, found that the only way he was able to protect the time he had set aside was to schedule appointments with R.T.—Reading Time.

Yourself Of course, you have to put more than time into your reading—you have to put yourself into it, too. Read mindfully, asking questions of the material and of yourself. What does this information suggest to you? If you had to explain or perhaps defend the ideas to someone else, what would you say?

Whenever you read a text, consider yourself to be entering into a partnership with the author. Your role is to custom-design a personalized book based on the generic one that the author has written. As a collaborator, you will be jotting down comments in the margins, outlining the material in your own way, drawing visual representations of the ideas, critically evaluating the book's arguments, and even engaging in a dialogue with the author. In your own journal, you can also write at greater length about your own epiphanies—those "aha" experiences—that you experienced as you read the book. You'll find that this collaborative approach to reading is much more engaging than simply highlighting the text.

When the material is so challenging that you are having problems concentrating on it, you can use two strategies. First, remind yourself of the similarities between reading and counseling. Both involve an encounter between people through the medium of words. You certainly don't expect to completely understand a client in one session. You may at first have trouble reading your client's emotional state, deciphering the meaning of comments, or even comprehending important motives. Despite these difficulties, you can remain committed to working with your client because the payoff for a successful counseling experience makes it all worthwhile. You'll find that you're much more successful in your reading when you bring this same level of commitment to understanding what an author is saying. When you read, you don't have to fully comprehend a theory's every intricacy or articulate each nuance of an argument. Nevertheless, you can do your best to engage by mindfully attending to the words.

Another strategy to use when feeling overwhelmed by your readings is to remember that you are not alone in this endeavor. As one counseling student recommended, "Do not be afraid to ask for help or for what you need. No one gets through this on his or her own" (Hoskins, 2000, p. 36). You can ask a classmate to read or study with you. Together, you can support and encourage each other to read and reflect. When you're tackling particularly tough material, you can discuss it with your reading partner.

■ ■ ■

EXERCISE 5.2 What? So What? Now What?

The three W's, just like the three R's, can also serve you well. Choose a chapter in a textbook and take notes while you're reading it. First, pay attention to capturing the salient points of the content—the "What?" Then think about what you just read and figure out what it means—the "So what?" For example, you may want to jot down some of the idea's implications for counseling. Finally, after you understand this material, consider what you are going to do with it—the "Now what?" How are you going to apply it? How are you going to connect it to material from other courses? Write about this experience in your journal. Keep using the "What? So what? Now what?" approach with all your reading until it becomes second nature to you.

■ ■ ■

▲ ▲ ▲

I Learned How to Read All Over Again
Brian's Story

THIS WEEKEND, I learned how to read all over again. Last week I kept approaching my textbook with my highlighter in hand, trying to find the motivation to keep going. As I read, I realized that my book was almost glowing with all the yellow marks in it, but I couldn't recall a word. There seemed to be too much information, and I couldn't prioritize it, so I wasn't retaining anything. I'm new to this field, so I don't know enough yet to recognize the important concepts!

I finally asked my professor how to read this material. She told me to take my time, pay attention to the organization of each chapter, and then figure out what points the authors are trying to make and pay particular attention to anything that doesn't make sense to me. If I don't understand something, it's important that I note it and ask for clarification in class. I started taking notes when I read, and now I feel that I'm not only retaining more, but I'm starting to see the internal structure of the material. I'm starting to see how concepts relate to each other. Wow, I was really starting to feel worried for awhile that I couldn't do it.

▼ ▼ ▼

Researching

> Research is formalized curiosity. It is poking and prying with a purpose.
>
> —Zora Neale Hurston

The Need for Research Skills You may be wondering how research is relevant to becoming a competent helping professional. You came to a graduate training program to learn how to help people, not to crunch numbers—right? Well, there are several important reasons for integrating research into your training experience. First and foremost, if you're going to be a competent helping professional, you have to develop good research skills. To design successful interventions, you must be able to make careful observations, systematically collect relevant and comprehensive information, and organize this material into a coherent framework. Furthermore, research is not limited to the laboratory. When you gather background information on a school or community agency, review recent studies on a particular problem, and read up on new theoretical perspectives in therapy, you are doing important research. The knowledge you gain from these research activities is essential to being a capable professional who stays current in the field.

Second, research experience itself will hone your critical thinking skills. You are entering a complex, challenging, and ambiguous line of work. When you are confronted by troubled clients who are obviously in pain, it may be tempting to latch onto highly touted but untested techniques. But you need to maintain a healthy skepticism regarding fads, cure-alls, and biases in the field. Research experience reminds us softhearted helpers to be hard-nosed about the evidence needed to validate therapeutic effectiveness.

Third, throughout your training, you will be learning to plan, design, implement, and evaluate programs that meet the therapeutic needs of communities and schools. Once again, your research skills will help you assess people's needs accurately and evaluate programs carefully.

Another important reason for integrating research into your training is that it is one of the main ways that you can advance the profession. As an emerging professional in the counseling field, you have an obligation to contribute to the growing knowledge base through your scholarly activity.

Fifth and finally, an immediate and practical benefit of research is that it provides excellent opportunities for you to collaborate with faculty members and other students on important and stimulating projects. As you become more comfortable engaging in research activities, you'll be more likely to continue to collaborate with others on research studies. After you've graduated, you are likely to find that practicing as a counselor can feel at times isolating. You will most likely not always have a readily available peer group. Exploring areas of interest with colleagues is a great way to build and maintain a community of supportive professionals.

If you're still not sold on the importance of research, consider this scenario. You've graduated and have a position in a school, mental health center, community agency, or hospital. You begin to work with a client who has a problem that's more complex than those you've encountered previously. The situation may not necessarily demand that you refer the client to someone else, but you realize that if you're going to work effectively with this person, you'll need to find out more. The process of finding out more is essentially research. The more skilled you are at researching now, the more resourceful you'll be later when your client's well-being is on the line.

Learning Research Skills So how do you become skilled at research? This question may be especially pressing if you're nervous about or slightly afraid of research methods and statistics. Perhaps you're one of the many who read only the beginnings and ends of journal articles, skipping the methodology and analysis sections in the middle. Heppner and his colleagues (1999) stated that both the graduate school environment and the personality styles of the students themselves cause some trainees to struggle with research. The implication is that students who have investigative interests, are skilled in statistical analysis, or who are in research-oriented graduate programs may have an advantage over other students.

Certain activities in graduate school can, however, increase your comfort with research and improve the chances that you'll continue to engage in research efforts after graduation. Participating in research teams with other students can help you identify what aspects of research come more easily to you (yes, some things you will do quite well!) and which areas are more challenging. Then you and your colleagues can pool your expertise and help each other. In the process, you become not only more comfortable with research but also more critically reflective.

You can gain valuable research experience by joining faculty members' research teams or volunteering to work with a faculty member who is investigating an area that is interesting to you. Consider asking if you can assist, even if you'd primarily be doing literature reviews or library searches. If you're able to watch the research process from beginning to end—problem identification to manuscript completion—you'll likely improve your research abilities.

You may find that a literature search, which typically occurs early on in the research process, is an intimidating task. You may be overwhelmed by the amount and variety of information that is available on your topic. You may feel as if you're searching a hall of mirrors and doors. Which doors are real and offer you access to important information? Which doors are merely reflections? The following tips may help you choose wisely.

- Ideally, your undergraduate education provided you with training in library search skills. If so, then you'll feel fairly confident using the school library's search system or staying at home and searching the library online. (We'll talk more about online searching shortly; for now let's focus on general library searches.) If you feel rusty or underprepared, sign up for a workshop or ask a reference librarian for help. Most libraries use common databases, such as ERIC or PsycINFO, but ways of accessing those databases may vary. Don't hesitate to ask for help, and when you do, take notes! You'll find it easier to replicate a search on your own if you've made some notes to guide you. Similarly, don't limit yourself to one database. If you're truly stretching your thoughts and thinking critically, you may find that interesting connections exist between such fields as social work, biology, sociology, philosophy, anthropology, literature, medicine, and theology.

- Be organized. Even if you're not as a rule organized, take on some obsessive-compulsive traits when you work on your research. Keep your notepad with you so that you can keep track of your searches. You'll want to remember what keywords and databases you used to get your results. You may want to download, print out, or E-mail yourself search histories so that you won't have to start from scratch the next time you go to the library or sit down at your computer.

- As you find materials that relate to your topic, read the abstracts available on the databases and identify which articles you would like to read. Then find those articles. It'll help if you have your copy card (if your library uses these types of debit cards) or some money when you go to the library. You'll probably need to make copies of the most relevant articles. Since no library's collection is complete, you will also want to take advantage of interlibrary loan services.

- Learn how to use copiers, microfiche, and microfilm readers. Again, ask for help if you're not familiar with this equipment. Make sure that your copies are clear and complete before you leave the library.

- Save yourself lots of headaches by making sure you have complete citation information for each reference you may use.

- Keep copies of articles or chapters that interest you in a labeled folder or binder.
- Don't go to the library when you're exhausted, unless the idea of a couple of hours of searching is just what you need to wake yourself up!
- Take time to read what you have, and don't skip the middle section. This tip leads us to Exercise 5.3 below.

One advantage of doing research is that the process itself tends to use higher-order critical thinking skills. As you practice and gain experience with research, you may find that in general you are more mindful. Your knowledge base will broaden, and your ability to arrive at thoughtful conclusions will improve.

Remember that your research should be related to concepts and issues that you find truly intriguing. If you focus on what's captivating to you, you'll find that the process becomes easier if not genuinely exciting. Some students opt to choose one primary area of interest at the start of their program. They read about that area, investigate it, and focus on it whenever possible in course assignments. Those students generally go on to write theses or dissertations that build on their initial investigations. Other students find that they have several areas of interest. They may focus on play therapy when working with children in a practicum and then explore substance abuse issues when they take an addictions course. Advantages and disadvantages exist with both of these approaches, so don't worry that there's one right way to begin your research efforts. The key is just to begin!

▨ ▨ ▨

EXERCISE 5.3 Doing a Little Detective Work

Think about what interests you right now in the helping profession. What would you like to know about counselors or therapists? Clients? Problems? Processes? If you were to formulate one question you want to explore, what would it be? Remember that notepad you keep handy to jot down ideas and questions while you are reading? Use it now to write down your question. Now think about ways in which you may go about answering it.

At this point, imagine that you're a detective, either the sophisticated British variety or the tough American private eye. Whichever you choose, what would you want to know about your question (your subject)? Who would you ask? What would you ask? If you had to prove that there is a connection between two things, how would you do it?

Spend a little time thinking about this scenario. Don't worry right now about exact measurements, procedures, or instruments. Just try to expand your mind and become fully engaged and interested in your subject. After you've gotten to know your question, go to the library and do a literature search.

EXERCISE 5.4 Critiquing

Use your critical reflection skills to analyze the articles, chapters, and books you gathered in the Exercise 5.3. Maybe you have assumed that if research is published, it must be of good quality. We hate to disillusion you, but as blues singers often point out, "It ain't necessarily so."

Check this out by looking at how the articles are written, from beginning to end. How are research questions phrased? What hypotheses are presented? What information is gathered, and by what method? How does this information relate back to the hypothesis? If particular instruments are used, are these instruments reliable and valid? How are participants chosen? Are sampling procedures adequately described? Do you see any inherent complications in the sample or procedures? How are data analyzed? Look at your statistics textbook and see if the researchers' data match the assumptions of their analysis.

Writing

> Writing is not what the writer does after the
> thinking is done; writing is thinking.
>
> —D. Murray

The third core academic skill is writing. Writing is a little like eating raisins. People tend to love it, to dislike it intensely, or to enjoy it in small doses, as long as it's mixed into something good—like oatmeal cookies. If you belong to one of the last two groups, then the bad news is that you're going to have to write a great deal throughout your gradu-ate training, and do it well. The good news is that writing not only improves the more you do it, but you may even develop a taste for it—despite your feelings about raisins.

The Need for Writing Skills   At first, you might assume that whatever writing skills have brought you this far in your academic career will be sufficient to carry you through your program and professional career. After all, how frequently are people actually called on to write during their everyday activities? Actually, if you become a counselor, you'll be writing more than you think, especially if you plan to contribute to the field by sharing your research and clinical experiences.

Even if you decide against a career in academia, you'll be writing case notes, treatment summaries, reports, and correspondence on a regular basis. Your case notes must be clear and accurate in describing what occurred in the session. Likewise, your treatment summaries and reports must be thorough and complete, ensuring that others will be able to understand your words and use them to design an appropriate intervention strategy. Correspondence is another important way you will be representing yourself as a professional.

▲▲▲

Learning the Hard Way
Susan's Story

I N MY FIRST INTERNSHIP as a school counselor, I had the chance to present a guidance unit for students in the third grade. I decided, with the approval of my supervisor, that I would send a letter home to the students' parents introducing myself and explaining the purpose of the guidance unit. Like many interns, I was always busy, so I frantically wrote the letter late one evening, quickly showed it to my supervisor, and then sent the letter out to parents.

Within three days, the school had received two telephone calls complaining about the misspellings and grammatical errors in my letter. In addition, one parent returned the letter with each of the three mistakes circled in red, along with a written note admonishing me to review basic grammar rules and improve my writing skills before sending another letter on school stationery.

I felt humiliated! My supervisor was embarrassed, the principal was angry, and the parents were concerned about the quality of their children's education. I realized that I had made several foolish and serious mistakes here. First, I didn't take seriously my responsibility as a writer. Instead, I assumed that people would understand my meaning and give me the benefit of the doubt because I cared so much about the students. My second mistake was relying on my computer spell-check program to catch all the misspelled words. Finally, I had imposed myself on somebody else to carefully proofread my writing for me. As a result of my carelessness, my professional reputation suffered.

Fortunately, my story didn't end there. My internship instructor urged me to take that parent's advice and referred me to the campus writing lab. At first, I felt ashamed about going to the lab, especially because I was near the end of my school counseling training. Now I'm glad that I went. If I'm going to be a good counselor, I need to communicate effectively in writing, as well as in speaking.

(P.S.: One reason that I've written this story is to share with other students an important lesson that I learned the hard way. Another reason is to show you that I can write clearly and spell correctly!)

As a trainee and professional, you will be expected to express yourself clearly and to write in a style appropriate for your audience. Those conventions may feel stifling or rigid, but they are the minimum requirements for professional writing. When you write a term paper, research report, thesis, or dissertation, you'll want to have handy a copy of the *Publication Manual of the American Psychological Association* (American Psychological Association, 2001). Baird (2004) has written an excellent guide for writing effective case notes and summary reports.

"Oh, how boring!" you might think. "Where's the opportunity for me to express myself as a creative person?" Don't despair. You'll probably find that using the *APA Manual* will actually help you improve your ability to express yourself. Another helpful and much more entertaining guide is *The Elements of Style* (4th edition, Strunk & White, 2000). Writing well, in an engaging and clear manner is anything but boring.

Learning Writing Skills Earlier, we compared writing to eating raisins, so here's another comparison: Writing is also like playing a musical instrument. When you're learning to play an instrument, you have to focus on the mechanics and receive careful guidance from an instructor. You have to concentrate on where to put your fingers, how to hold the instrument, and how to read the music. But with regular instruction and diligent practice those mechanics will become second nature.

The same methods apply to writing. If you haven't mastered the basics of composition and grammar, seek instruction and begin practicing. As you practice, you'll find that you will no longer worry about the basics. A musician progresses from struggling to reach the high notes to improving his or her tone and phrasing. As a writer, you move from attempting to write transitional sentences to focusing on being more concise, vivid, and engaging. Along the way, you set higher expectations for yourself as a writer, and you probably find that writing becomes easier and more enjoyable.

If you haven't already done so, consider asking other students to join you in your writing exercises. Read each other's work and talk about it. As you read your classmates' writing, focus on what stands out as being particularly vivid, clear, and organized. Take risks with your attempts to express yourself, stretching yourself to engage fully in the process and reaching creatively for words that give voice to your experience.

You've probably guessed by now that this section on writing focuses primarily on practice. Of course, the practice can take a variety of forms. In Chapters 1 and 2, we recommended that you keep a journal to document your training journey. The habit of keeping a journal is not only a wonderful way for you to reflect on your experiences but also a great technique for practicing your writing skills. As the process of capturing your thoughts and expressing your feelings becomes a daily ritual, you can then read over your journal, watching the emergence of your own voice and recognizing when it's particularly authentic and clear. Those are the occasions that you'll want to pay attention to and build on as you work on improving your writing. The journal has the added benefit, by the way, of allowing you to make discoveries for yourself in your own time and place. Many students report that writing a journal, especially during their practicum and internship experiences, helped them see both important issues regarding their clients as well as vital information about themselves as counselors. If Chapters 1 and 2 didn't convince you to keep a journal, we hope that this chapter will.

Structuring So far, the writing exercises we've offered have been narratives or stories that take form as you're writing them. Now you're ready for a different type of skill. Exercise 5.5 will put some structure into your writing.

When you've finished that exercise, congratulate yourself. Organizing your material can be tough, but it's essential if you want others to understand what you've written. Even when you write case notes, you may find that your supervisor asks you to follow a specific organizational structure. The ability to organize, along with your understanding of the writing conventions mentioned earlier, will help you appropriately frame your writing.

Mindful writing—taking care to give voice to your experiences and ideas through the written word—is a skill that you can develop with practice and feedback. We think you'll find that it's well worth the effort because besides the improvements to your writing, you'll find that you also know yourself better, think more clearly, and have great trust in your creative hunches.

■ ■ ■

EXERCISE 5.5 Writing Twice-Told Stories

Take a few minutes to describe a story about yourself that you have often told others. For instance, you might have told others how you met your significant other, the way your family spends its vacations, or how you acquired your nickname. One friend's favorite story is how he was lost for several days in the Everglades! No matter what your story is, write it down. Write it out completely, imagining someone listening to the words as you write them, anticipating the questions a listener might ask, and providing enough detail so that the event or memory is captured as vividly as possible (Metzger, 1992).

In a couple of days, write down another story. Then, a couple of days later, write down another. As you practice, you'll find that writing comes more effortlessly. Expressing yourself through the written word, finding your own voice, and saying what you want to say will become second nature.

■ ■ ■

■ ■ ■

EXERCISE 5.6 **Reading**
A Writing Exercise

Read. Read novels. Read newspapers. Read journals. Read the backs of cereal boxes. Read. Now go back and improve one of the "Twice-Told Tales" that you wrote.

■ ■ ■

■ ■ ■

EXERCISE 5.7 **Structuring**
A Writing Exercise

Remember the topic that you investigated in the researching section of this chapter? Imagine that you will be writing a paper about it. The paper may be either expository or a research project. You choose. Then develop an outline for the paper. What are the most important areas to cover? How do those areas arrange themselves into headings and subheadings? Is there a natural or implied sequence in the headings and subheadings? Write down possible transition sentences you would use to connect the various components of the paper.

■ ■ ■

Presenting

> A speech is like an airplane engine. It may sound
> like hell, but you've got to go on.
>
> —William Thomas Piper

The Need for Presentation Skills The fourth core academic skill is presenting. "Presenting?" you may ask. "What do you mean? I want to be a professional helper—somebody whose career is listening and responding to clients." Although you may do most of your therapeutic work with individuals and small groups, sooner or later you'll be asked to share your expertise with others, and that process will often take the form of a presentation.

Many graduate courses require that you gain some experience in presenting your ideas to other students. As a matter of fact, one graduate program devotes the last two weeks of all courses to student presentations. Some cynical students claim that the instructors are simply tired of teaching. Although that interpretation may hold some truth, it's more likely that the instructors realize the importance of effective presentation skills.

If you're wondering why counselors and therapists need presentation skills, keep the following in mind. School counselors are regularly asked to present guidance units for classes, educational programs for parents and community members, and training sessions for school personnel. Family therapists are often asked to present educational programs to the public, psychoeducational programs to groups, and reports to boards, funding agencies, and local governments. In addition, many counselors and therapists find that giving presentations at state, regional, and national conferences enhances their own professional development while building a community of colleagues that can extend across the country. For counselors and therapists in private practice, offering mental health-oriented programs to community members is often an effective strategy for finding appropriate clients and referrals.

Learning Presentation Skills Presentation skills are undoubtedly essential for succeeding as a practitioner. Like many important skills, though, successful presenting is a craft that takes time to master. One obstacle to overcome is the common fear of public speaking. Another barrier is that you may not view yourself as a public speaker. If you don't have a dramatic flair or enjoy being the center of attention, you may assume that you're not cut out for public speaking. However, being a "good therapist" and a "good presenter" are not mutually exclusive. In fact, people who are successful in both roles have several important characteristics in common:

- **Focus.** They give an endeavor, whether it's counseling or presenting, their complete attention. In particular, they are adept at tuning into the emotional states of others and resonating with them.

- **Preparation.** They take the time beforehand to ensure that they know what they need to know. They also stay current and use appropriate resources and technologies to provide the best service.

- **Competence.** They may not always feel comfortable, but they believe in their own abilities.

- **Tolerance for ambiguity.** They understand that few things in life are concrete and that nothing is static. They allow themselves to trust the process and stay immediate.

The list could go on. Presenting, like other skills, requires that you practice and be open to feedback if you are to improve. The good news is that Heppner and his colleagues (1999) found that practicing increased students' self-efficacy ratings and thereby increased their confidence in presenting. Some students who participated in practice presentations also found that they felt more confident that they could contribute important information to the field. Furthermore, students evaluated practice presentation sessions as a useful educational tool. The researchers found that presentations not only were an effective way to learn public speaking but also promoted higher-order thinking skills. As you can see, these findings provide vindication for those instructors who require student presentations.

It's likely that there have been many times when you have been practicing your presentation skills without even realizing it. We're talking about being in class, being fully present, and participating in the learning process in as many ways as possible. Class participation (the two words that stir great dread in students who are a little shy) can help you read mindfully by improving your comprehension, keeping you focused, and helping you synthesize and build unique connections between concepts. Additionally, if you assume that you'll be participating in class, you're more likely to read the assignments carefully and systematically, preparing questions in advance.

Participation Anxiety   For you, the idea of class participation may be rather unpleasant. Deborah, for instance, found that when she started to share an idea or respond to a professor's question in class, she would immediately flash back to the time she threw up in front of her fourth-grade class. Of course, she knew that she was unlikely to repeat that scene, but even recalling her sense of profound embarrassment would make her recoil and flinch. By the time Deborah regained some composure, the opportunity for participating had passed. Over time, she simply quit trying to contribute her comments.

Similarly, in Chris's first graduate classes, he found that his heart would begin to race and his face would feel hot whenever he spoke in class. He began to fear that he was blushing, and although he couldn't identify what would make him feel so self-conscious, he decided to stop speaking in class.

Unfortunately, both Deborah and Chris taught themselves *not* to participate. In doing so, they deprived themselves of opportunities to connect more deeply with the course material and also created an additional stressor for themselves. Every class became stressful because they dreaded having to speak in class.

Certainly, some faculty members can be intimidating when they put on their "game faces" and challenge students. Keep in mind, however, that if you're having a problem with a particular professor, your first and best option is to make an appointment to discuss the issue directly with the person. If that doesn't help address your concerns, then by all means contact your advisor, another faculty member, or the program director.

In many cases, though, students who are worried about participating in class are apprehensive regardless of the instructor. If you're plagued by participation anxiety, consider that all these are forms of participation:

- asking questions
- summarizing to ensure comprehension
- reflecting critically while in class, either by taking notes or writing down questions to ask later.

The class experience is yours—you're entitled to it. You can do with it what you please. If you walk out of class confused about something because you didn't ask, you've made a choice to accept less than you deserve. You can also choose to push yourself to improve your class participation. For example, you can set a goal for your involvement. Maybe this week you'll ask one question. Next week you can make a connection between two different concepts. Another strategy is to ask your instructor for help. If you have an instructor with whom you feel relatively comfortable, ask her or him for some time to talk about class participation. The two of you can identify some ways to ease you into participation.

This worked for Adrian, who was very apprehensive about public speaking. She asked her statistics study group if they would listen to her presentation on human development and give her suggestions for improvement. The students not only listened and gave advice but also shared their own fears of public speaking. Soon, all the students in the group were sharing tips, encouraging each other, and providing general support. If you don't have a study group yet, ask your roommates or classmates to serve as an audience for you.

Improving Your Presentations When preparing for your presentations, remember that you want to challenge yourself and your audience. Ideally, you and the people to whom you're speaking will come together to share ideas and look at your topic in new ways. You can help your audience reflect critically on your topic by deciding what points you want to make and identifying the most effective ways to do so. People enjoy being challenged if you provide sufficient support.

Borrowing from Yoder (1999), we offer the following practical tips for improving your presentations.

- **Organize the presentation.** Decide how you want to impart the information (for example, lecture, discussion, group activities) and how much time you want to spend on the various points of your presentation. Some people follow the presentation rule, "Tell them what you're going to tell them. Tell them. Then tell them what you told them." You can use that rule if it helps. The "tell 'em, tell 'em, tell 'em" approach does tend to be systematic and can help you stay organized. If the idea of planning out minutes seems too rigid, then you may just want to plan approximately how much time you'd like to spend on each area.

- **Know the audience.** Does your audience consist of other students whose knowledge base on the topic is similar to yours? Or are they relative newcomers to your topic? You'll present differently based on the audience's needs. Similarly, if your audience is a class of third-grade students, you'll likely present differently (be more active, use different words and expressions, have a shorter time frame) than if your audience consists of national conference attendees.

- **Practice.** Practice more than once. If you can't find an audience with whom to practice, practice in front of the mirror. Go through the entire presentation more than once so that you develop a sense for timing, clarity, and organization.

- **Prepare for pitfalls.** You might expect 30 people to show up and find 5 in the room. Or 150! You might reserve the last ten minutes of your presentation for a question-and-answer period and find that not one person has a single question. You might plan to use a PowerPoint presentation only to discover that no equipment is available. What do you do in these situations? Try to anticipate problems and have a backup plan. Better yet, have several backup plans. A favorite professor used to always carry several case studies with him whenever he presented. He said:

  > If all else fails, no one talks, the electricity goes out, no one understands my points, or I forget everything I was going to say, I can pull out these case studies, pass them around, and say, "Okay. What do you all think?" I rest easier the night before the presentation knowing that I have that to fall back on.

- **Know your subject matter.** We recently attended a presentation in which the speaker consistently described her research findings incorrectly. The result was confusing and frustrating. Be sure to know what you're talking about, including understanding the meaning of figures and graphs that you use to supplement your talk. Similarly, have plenty of examples ready to help the audience understand your point.

- **Keep it lively.** Many people use technology (PowerPoint, videos) in their presentations so that they won't have to carry the ball alone in lecture format. Other options include role plays, group activities, panel presentations, and just about anything else you can imagine. Thinking creatively about how you can best communicate your ideas will likely improve your presentation and keep audience members interested. One caution: avoid being too cute. Some examples or metaphors can only be carried out so long before the audience starts to grow bored or (worse) groan.

- **Ask for feedback.** Receiving feedback on your presentation can be enormously valuable, but remember that you may be your own best evaluator. As Rogers (1961) wrote, "People can trust their own experiences; evaluation by others doesn't have to be our guide." In class, as well as conference presentations, the presenter typically receives some type of evaluation. Occasionally, especially at conferences, the evaluations will provide information that is not necessarily helpful. Some unhelpful comments include: "temperature was too cold," "room was too crowded," "I thought this was something else," "I work with the elderly, so this topic didn't really pertain to me." At times, though, an insightful participant will make a comment such as, "The section on unique characteristics was especially helpful. The part about the relationship could have been more thorough."

  Frequently, presenters will find that the evaluations are consistent with their own take on the presentation. They know, for instance, that they rushed the ending or lost their focus a little in the middle. The point is, then, to read the evaluations, but don't be crushed if one of your audience members didn't like your presentation. Pay attention to your own evaluation of your performance and set goals for next time.

- **Watch others' presentations.** Attend presentations whenever possible and critique them for yourself. What worked? What didn't? Learn from the successes (and mistakes) of others.

- **Use your emotional arousal.** Finally, and perhaps most important, use your emotional arousal by channeling that energy into productive preparation. Whenever you find yourself starting to tense up and worry, decide what particular task you can carry out to prepare for your presentation. Perhaps the task is to design your handout materials, develop your PowerPoint presentation, imagine yourself successfully articulating your major points, practice your delivery, or just enjoy a relaxing run. Whatever the specific task, you're transforming that worry and tension into positive and productive preparation—and the more prepared you are, the less anxiety you'll feel.

The tension related to public speaking can be unpleasant and distracting, but as you gain experience in using your arousal, you'll find that you're not just feeling more relaxed, you're also feeling more confident. One technique that we're certain will not work for you is avoidance. Unless you develop your presentation skills now, the anxiety will remain, lurking and waiting for the chance to emerge. Then, when you're called unexpectedly to present, you'll be less prepared to handle it.

Take time now to practice this essential skill, and remember, many of your peers are just as nervous as you are. You can be great resources for each other, so make the most of this time together and support each other as you try your hand at presenting.

EXERCISE 5.8 **Preparing and Practicing**

Take the topic you've been investigating as you've read through this chapter. You now have an outline for a paper, so use it to formulate a ten-minute presentation. Ask your study group if you can present it to them for their feedback on your presentation style.

EXERCISE 5.9 **Imagining Success**

Prior to giving a presentation in class, take time to imagine yourself as successful. Find a quiet, private place and sit or lie comfortably. Close your eyes and imagine that you're in the classroom and that it's time for you to go to the front of the class. You have all your materials ready, your name is called, you pick up your materials and walk confidently to the front of the room. You feel just excited enough to be sharp and energetic. You know your material. You're confident in your ability to present it effectively. Continue to go through your presentation, anticipating questions and feedback, and see yourself as you plan to be. Don't stop the imagery until you have finished the presentation, received applause or acknowledgement, and returned (triumphantly!) to your seat.

EXERCISE 5.10 **Breathing**

Lie on your back with your hands on your stomach. Breathe in and out, paying attention to how your stomach rises and falls every time you inhale and exhale. Do this for several minutes until you have a sense of what this feels like. Now sit up and continue to breathe in the same manner. Breathing from your diaphragm will help ease your tension and slow you down. It will also improve the tone of your voice!

SUMMARY

Being a successful counselor relies to some degree on your ability to think mindfully about the helping process, your clients, and yourself. Through reading, researching, writing, and presenting, you can savor the pleasures of pursuing knowledge, refining your skills, and gaining personal awareness. Honed academic skills do much more than help you earn good grades—they help you succeed as a counselor.

RESOURCES

The American Psychological Association of Graduate Students publishes *gradPSYCH* quarterly. Each issue includes articles with tips on succeeding in graduate school, interesting profiles of students, and advice on specific challenges, such as co-authoring with faculty, writing the discussion section of a dissertation, and pursuing an internship.

American Counseling Association's monthly publication, *Counseling Today*, offers a "Student Focus" column in each issue. Graduate students author these pieces, which cover such important topics as preparing for the comprehensive examination, coping with a personal health crisis, and maintaining professional boundaries. As you progress through your training, you may want to consider adding your voice to this forum by submitting your own column.

The Company Therapist, at www.thetherapist.com, is a Web-based drama about the fictional world of a therapist at a computer company. The story is written by the audience. This site is an entertaining way to improve your writing skills.

Study Skills Self-Help Information, at *www.ucc.vt.edu/stdysk/stdyhlp. html*, provides online study skills workshops and information on developing good study habits. It covers skills in scheduling time, setting priorities, and taking notes and has many other helpful study guides for students.

REFERENCES

Adler, R., Rosenfeld, L., & Towne, N. (1989). *Interplay: The process of interpersonal communication.* New York: Holt, Rinehart & Winston.

American Psychological Association (2001). *Publication manual of the American Psychological Association* (5th ed.). Washington, DC: Author.

Baird, B. N. (2004). *The internship, practicum, and field placement handbook* (4th ed.). Upper Saddle River, NJ: Prentice-Hall.

Bloom, B. S., Englehart, M. D., Furst, E. J., & Krathwohl, D. R. (1956). *Taxonomy of educational objectives: Cognitive domain.* New York: McKay.

Csikszentmihalyi, M. (1997). *Finding flow: The psychology of engagement with everyday life.* New York: Basic Books.

Damasio, A. (1994). *Descartes' error: Emotion, reason, and the human brain.* New York: Putnam.

Erickson, M. H., Rossi, E. L., & Rossi, S. I. (1976). *Hypnotic realities.* New York: Wiley.

Frye, M. (1995). Oppression. In M. L. Andersen & P. H. Collins (Eds.), *Race, class and gender: An anthology* (2nd ed., pp. 37–41). Belmont, CA: Wadsworth.

Goleman, D. (1995). *Emotional intelligence.* New York: Bantam Books.

Heppner, P. P., Rooney, S. C., Flores, L. Y., Tarrant, J. M., Howard, J. K., Mulholland, A. M., Thye, R., Turner, S. L., Hanson, K. M., & Lilly, R. L. (1999). Salient effects of practice poster sessions on counselor development: Implications for research training and professional identification. *Counselor Education and Supervision, 38,* 205–217.

Hergenhahn, B. R. (1992). *Introduction to the history of psychology.* Belmont, CA: Wadsworth.

Hoskins, C. M. (2000, August). Get a life! Top 10 list for a first-year student. *Counseling Today, 43,* 32, 36.

Hughes, F. R., & Kleist, D. M. (2005). First-semester experiences of counselor education doctoral students. *Counselor Education and Supervision, 45,* 97–108.

Jung, C. G. (1965). *Memories, dreams, reflections.* New York: Vintage Books.

Langer, E. (1989). *Mindfulness.* Reading, MA: Addison-Wesley.

Langer, E. (1997). *The power of mindful learning.* Reading, MA: Addison-Wesley.

Martin, W. E., Easton, C., Wilson, S., Takemoto, M., & Sullivan, S. (2004). Salience of emotional intelligence as a core characteristic of being a counselor. *Counselor Education and Supervision, 44,* 17–30.

Martindale, C. (1981). *Cognition and consciousness.* Homewood, IL: Dorsey Press.

Meltzoff, J. (1998). *Critical thinking about research: Psychology and related fields.* Washington, DC: American Psychological Association.

Metzger, D. (1992). *Writing for your life: A guide and companion to the inner worlds.* San Francisco: HarperCollins.

Presbury, J., Echterling, L. G., & McKee, J. E. (2002). *Ideas and tools for brief counseling*. New York: Merrill/Prentice Hall.

Prochaska, J. O., & Norcross, J. C. (2007). *Systems of psychotherapy: A transtheoretical analysis* (6th ed.). Belmont, CA: Thomson Higher Education.

Rogers, C. (1961). *On becoming a person: A therapist's view of psychotherapy*. Boston: Houghton Mifflin.

Strunk, W., & White, E. B. (2000). *The elements of style* (4th ed.). New York: Allyn & Bacon.

Yoder, B. R. (1999, September). How to survive a presentation and be successful. *Counseling Today, 42,* 22.

CHAPTER 6

Exploring Yourself

One of the most profound ways in which I can change myself is to change the story I tell myself about myself.

—Jerome Levin

If you don't stand for something, you'll fall for anything.

—country song

MAKE PERSONAL GROWTH YOUR GOAL

As you make your training journey, you need time alone to check your bearings, process your experiences, and reflect on the discoveries you are making. Like a photographer in a darkroom, you have been developing a more vivid picture of who you are. And like a novelist, you have been constructing a life story with yourself as the protagonist. Your self-concept, identity, and personal beliefs about the world and about other people are beginning to emerge. The "who I am," "where I stand," and "what I stand for" make up the person you have so far come to know as yourself.

Your training experiences will challenge many of your developing ideas about yourself. You might react by hunkering down and defending your self-image and your beliefs. But we invite you to consider remaining open to new possibilities and ideas. The one certainty about your journey is that you *will* be changed by it. In fact, a personal transformation is essential to becoming a successful professional helper.

In this chapter, we offer some guidelines for coping with the dramatic changes that you will experience during your training. Even when you're making positive changes, you'll find that they can feel uncomfortable, unfamiliar, and strange. You may even fear that you're turning into someone you won't recognize. At these times, remind yourself that you can become a new person while also preserving your basic integrity. Though you may be altering your beliefs, trying out new ways of interacting, and challenging how you experience yourself, you can trust that this change process is part of your fundamental identity. Your essential being is always becoming. Making personal growth your goal is the best way to stay vital, both in your training as well as in your career (Dearing, Maddux, & Tangney, 2005).

Whether or not you realize it, you are changing all the time. This change is the unfolding story of your life. But during your graduate training program, the change will be enormous—similar to the growth spurt you may have had as a child. You'll find yourself rewriting your life story as fast as you can. You are in training to become a helping professional, and you will find it an exciting process. At your center, you already have the basic ingredients to become who you wish to be. But you need to go through a metamorphosis to fulfill this potential. Such change is always stressful, but you have chosen to undergo this process. Welcome the change! Enjoy the journey!

▲▲▲

Thanksgiving Leftovers
Edna's Story

THANKSGIVING, I recently discovered, can involve other kinds of leftovers besides turkey, dressing, and pumpkin pie. This year, I was really looking forward to Thanksgiving because it was my first visit home since entering a program to become a therapist. I desperately needed a break and was excited about going home again. It was weird, though—it didn't seem like home anymore. I felt like a stranger in a familiar place. As an undergrad, I had gone to a nearby college and was home nearly every weekend—you know, so Mom could do my laundry and I could talk my parents out of a little more money for the upcoming week. So you might say that I was really never away from home before.

I've recently been finding that playing the role of my parent's little daughter is getting harder for me to carry off. I'm just not that girl any more. As we sat at the table on Thanksgiving, I was hassled to "eat up," my uncle was getting drunk, and my father told a racist joke. When I refused to laugh, he accused me of being "politically correct," and later, when I tried to tell people about what I was learning in school, they dismissed it as "psychobabble."

My mother scurried around like a servant and was up and down from the table so many times, filling people's glasses and offering second helpings, that she hardly ate a bite. She claimed not to be hungry because she had sampled so much while cooking the meal.

My cousins talked incessantly to each other as we ate and seemed to ignore me. We had been so close when we were younger, but we don't seem to have much in common. Then there was my best friend Jeannie, who's going to Tech and studying computer science. She kept talking about how much money she's going to make when she graduates. Dad said, "You see, Edna? You could be making the big bucks if you changed programs. You'll never get rich as a therapist."

I sat there watching these people with whom I had always been so close, and after a while all I could hear was "blah, blah, blah." "Who are these people?" I asked myself. When I was a small child, I thought that when I finally got to sit at the big table on Thanksgiving, I would officially be a successful grownup. But somehow, I felt as if I was still at the kids' table. Then it hit me, "I don't know who *I* am! I've been changing so much; I seem to have lost *me* in the process." I realized that I have a lot of leftovers here!

Why is it that understanding and keeping track of yourself is one of the most difficult tasks to do? Perhaps it's because a "self" is not a thing that you can observe and contemplate. Your sense of self is so close and yet so far. As Levin (1992) put it, "The self to which we think we are so close eludes definition and, indeed becomes more elusive as we attempt to grasp it" (p. 1).

Because your self is not a static substance, but rather a dynamic essence that is constantly with you, it may seem like an illusion. Part of your self is pure feeling or sensation. When you are "on top of the world," this feeling is vivid, but when you are ill or sleepy, the feeling is vague. Another part of your self is your self-concept—your identity.

In large part, this self-concept is an active determiner of your behavior and your feelings (Rogers, 1942, 1951). In addition, who you consider yourself to be is shaped by cultural influences. Your family, your gender, your race, and your location on the planet have all contributed to your conception of self. You have entered a training program for helping professionals in which you are asked to be authentic—to be the self you really are. But, at the same time, you are being asked to change. It can all be pretty confusing.

Concepts that can help you gain insight into this paradox come from Linehan's (1993) dialectical behavior therapy. Although her work has focused on clients diagnosed with borderline personality disorder, the dialectical issue of self-acceptance and change applies to all of us. How do we resolve our need, on the one hand, to accept ourselves as we are now and our fundamental impulse, on the other hand, to constantly change and grow?

Your willingness to embark on a journey of personal transformation may be sabotaged by worries about possible abandonment. At some deep level, you may wonder if your friends and family will accept and love the new you. Nevertheless, you can learn to be comfortable with—and even welcome—change in yourself, others, and the world around you. One strategy that Linehan recommended is the Zen practice of mindfulness. In Chapter 5, you learned how mindfulness can help you academically, but it is also an excellent way to deal with the sense of engulfment that you may experience during especially troubled and distressing times, when emotions seem to overwhelm and control you. When you practice mindful acceptance and validation of your emotional turmoil, you discover that the negative feelings actually decrease.

Your identity is really the story you tell yourself about yourself. You update your identity as new experiences alter your beliefs, your values, and your worldview (Sadler-Gerhardt, 2005). Usually this process is slow and difficult to notice. But now, with your entry into graduate school, you have been thrown into chaos, and you are developing your new identity more rapidly than ever before. It is your goal to become the best counselor or therapist possible. Such goals become part of your self-concept and then act like magnets. Drawing you toward your future and helping you focus your energies and activities. However, your current self is different from the self you hope to become as a counselor. This disparity is probably somewhat distressing because you're feeling as if you are a page or two behind in your story.

▦ ▦ ▦

EXERCISE 6.1 "I Am . . . " *versus* "A Counselor Is . . . "

On a piece of paper, write "I am . . . " at the top. Then take a little time to consider the qualities and characteristics that define who you are, what you believe, and what you can do. Finish the statement by writing twelve words or phrases that best describe you.

Then, on a separate sheet, write "A counselor is . . . " at the top. Reflect on the traits and qualities that characterize a successful counselor. Write a dozen words or phrases that describe the person you are training to become.

Finally, rate yourself on the number of attributes of a successful counselor you have now, using a scale of one to ten, with one indicating no attributes and ten being all the traits needed to be a successful counselor.

Obviously, you would not give yourself a one. If you had thought you didn't have any characteristics of a counselor, you would not have entered a training program. You already have many of the attributes you will need to be successful as a helping professional. On the other hand, you are not a 10 either. If you thought you had already arrived, you would not have embarked on this training journey.

Whatever number you chose to show where you are now, ask yourself this question: "What changes will I notice in myself that will let me know I am on the way to the next higher number?" Instead of immediately getting to ten, you'll be taking this process one step at a time. So what do you need to do to get to that next higher number? As soon as you answer that question, you'll have begun your journey.

▦ ▦ ▦

Ontological Security

> You really have to spend time with yourself to
> know who you are.
>
> —Bernice Johnson Reagon

In his classic work, *The Divided Self,* R. D. Laing (1969) created a vivid picture of what it means to have a secure base in life by contrasting this security with an uncertain experience of the world. According to Laing, "an *ontologically* secure person will encounter all the hazards of life . . . from a centrally firm sense of [one's] own and other people's reality"

(p. 39). If someone does not achieve this secure base, then the person grows up ontologically insecure, and everyday life seems threatening. Such an individual "cannot take the realness, aliveness, autonomy, and identity of . . . self and others for granted . . . [and] has to become absorbed in contriving ways of trying to be real" (pp. 42–43).

You may believe that to become a successful helping professional, you must first attain complete ontological security. But most of us have only achieved an ontological security that is "good enough," and we usually can recognize a small glimmer of our insecurity in the dark corners and recesses of ourselves. Furthermore, when we are in circumstances that put our self-esteem on the line, we feel this insecurity intensely. Your training program will require you to practice your skills in front of other students, on video, or while being observed through a one-way mirror. At these times, you're likely to feel insecure. You may find yourself so focused on what you are going to say next that you can hardly listen to what your client is saying.

You may find it reassuring to know that mistakes are unavoidable in such training situations. At first, you may attempt to preserve your self-esteem by acting as though you know what you are doing. After a while, as you begin to truly listen to what the other person is saying, you will get into the "flow" we described in Chapter 5. In flow, you lose yourself and become absorbed in what is happening. The paradox here is that when you get to the point at which you are really listening, rather than waiting for your turn to talk, you will lose your self-consciousness, but you also will be more ontologically secure.

"I" and "Me"

Your self-system is inherently divided between the core of your self (the "I" awareness) and the contents of your self (the "me" and those experiences that seem to happen to "me"). William James (1890) has been credited with making this distinction between the "I" and the "me." Deikman (1996) said that the "I" is what gives us our subjective sense of existence.

> [S]elf-image, the body, passions, fears, social category . . . are aspects of our persona that we usually refer to when we speak of the self, but they do not refer to the core of our conscious being . . . the "I" is identical to awareness. (pp. 350–351)

The "I" is the center of your existence, whereas the "me" is the object of your perception—the part of yourself you can observe. Erikson (1968) articulated the concept of "identity," or that observed part of us. There is some evidence that we do not begin to form an identity until we are about eighteen months of age and that we do not consolidate our identity until we are in our twenties. If you are recently out of undergraduate school, then you may still be in the process of putting yourself together. On the other hand, if you are a nontraditional learner—someone who has returned to school after years of establishing your identity—then you will be opening up your view of yourself to make room for the new you. In either case, there will be times when your sense of yourself will be less vivid and you will be experiencing ontological insecurity. At other times, you will be observing aspects of yourself that may be surprising and that must be incorporated into your identity. This experience will be what Erikson called "self-uncertainty." You will find that these experiences are way stations on your journey. They mean that you are on course to stabilizing your "I" and consolidating your "me."

THE NEED FOR PERSONAL GROWTH

The battles that count aren't the ones for gold medals. The struggles within yourself—the invisible, inevitable battles inside all of us—that's where it's at.

—Jesse Owens

Being a "Do-Gooder"

You are in a training program for helping professionals because you wish to prepare yourself to relieve the suffering of others. You are altruistic. Perhaps some of your more cynical acquaintances regularly accuse you of being a "touchy-feely type," a "bleeding heart," or a "do-gooder." By these terms, they mean that you are too softhearted for your own good. In an age in which it seems that self-interest and competition are essential to survival, someone with altruistic feelings for others may appear to be unnatural or naïve.

Jeffery Kottler (2000) investigated why animals and humans "do good," and he discovered that besides being natural it is essential to the survival of a species that individual members act altruistically for the good of others. Animals often do it to the point of self-sacrifice.

For example, Kottler found that birds will often sound alarms when predators are near. This behavior warns the other members of the flock but also calls attention to the bird giving the warning, placing that individual in danger (Trivers, 1971). Squirrels often give warning while risking their own safety (Sherman, 1980). Bees, termites, and ants have developed societies in which certain members sacrifice themselves to save the rest of the group from attack (Thomas, 1983). Higher-order species, such as monkeys and apes, engage in similar behaviors for the benefit of the troop (Gould & Marler, 1987). One adult member of a wolf pack forgoes mating and its own territory in order to help the alpha male and female raise their brood (Masson & McCarthy, 1995). So you see, there is nothing unnatural or rare about altruism.

Of course, we can never be absolutely certain about the meaning of such behavior among animals. However, you certainly have witnessed many instances of self-sacrifice among your fellow human beings. What is even more remarkable about the altruism of humans is that they consciously choose to perform these acts and obviously display tremendous empathy for the plight of others (Kottler, 2000). Charles Darwin considered empathy to be not only natural but also the very basis for an ethical society.

If you had chosen to be, say, an engineer, a physicist, or an accountant, you would expect your training to be centered largely on content and skills. You would be surprised if you were asked to work on who you are. But you have chosen to be a counselor, and the fact is that your success in this field will center largely on your personhood and the way you use who you are. In a classic study, Truax and Mitchell (1971) reviewed more than 100 studies of counselor effectiveness and found that counseling techniques are useful only when the counselor's personality is inherently helpful. Others (Perez, 1979; Seligman, 1995) found the counselor's personality to be the most important criterion for effectiveness with clients. Like members of the clergy who follow their vocation, successful helping professionals have somehow been called to their life's work and are ready to fully give themselves to it. The more willing you are to make such a commitment, the more likely you will be to experience joy and success in the work of helping others.

Having Empathy for Others The journey that has brought you to this training program has taken many years. It is likely that negative experiences in your life have sensitized you to the misfortune of others and stimulated in you the desire to be helpful. Henry (1977) found that, as children, counselors often had experienced illness, loneliness, or bereavement. Counselors were likely to have endured more traumatic events, and their families of origin were often in turmoil. Not surprisingly, counselors were likely to have been clients themselves before entering their training. Such findings have led to the "wounded healer theory" (Guggenbuhl-Craig, 1971; Rippere & Williams, 1985), which suggests that the healer's history of misfortune or trauma confers the power to heal.

Firsthand experiences of loss and suffering are certainly helpful in understanding what life might be like for clients. A counselor trainer of our acquaintance often says, "I wouldn't give you a nickel for a counselor who hasn't suffered." Such painful events in the counselor's life are, however, a two-edged sword. Although they may aid in the establishment of empathy, they could also result in the counselor overidentifying with the client's pain. One thing you will need to check in yourself is how strong your "rescue fantasy" might be. A rescue fantasy is the urgent need to fix the client's situation and then to be appreciated for the extraordinary intervention.

Handling Difficult Topics   You also need to explore your value system in order to become more aware of what "pushes your buttons" and what makes you uncomfortable. For example, you may have strong opinions regarding abortion, incest, infidelity, physical abuse, or alcohol and drug use. It's okay for you to have these opinions, but it is important that you work on respecting and accepting clients, even when their opinions or behavior are different from your own.

Often, your discomforts and prejudices may lie beyond your awareness. In such cases, you may communicate to your client, without realizing it, that talking about such subjects is out-of-bounds in the counseling relationship. For example, when he was a graduate student, Jack once had a meeting with an admired professor. In a horribly tragic turn of events, the professor committed suicide later that day. Although he retained feelings of guilt at having been the last person to see this man alive, Jack subsequently graduated and entered practice. Two years later, while discussing a particularly vexing case with a supervisor, Jack was asked if the client had talked of suicide. At that moment, Jack realized that none of his clients had ever spoken of suicide. Somehow, he had subliminally communicated to all his clients, "Don't talk about suicide—it makes me uncomfortable." After that epiphany, Jack's clients often spoke of suicide.

Like Jack, you may unconsciously hope that your clients do not bring up certain topics in counseling because they might make you feel threatened or helpless. Do you know what those topics are?

■ ■ ■

EXERCISE 6.2 Things I Hope My Clients Never Say
An Aversion Exercise

Listed below are some of the things clients have said to us. As you read them, imagine that the client is speaking directly to you. Try to identify the feelings you have as you read these quotes. Write your immediate reaction in the space below each quote, then think about what you could say that would be useful to the client:

1. "You look awfully young. I'm not sure you could understand a problem as deep and complicated as mine."

   _____

   _____

2. "I was raped last night."

   _____

   _____

3. " . . . and Goddammit! I'm so fucking pissed off at her that I just can't think about anything else!"

   _____

   _____

4. " . . . I don't know, they just told me I had to be here. I don't have a problem."

   _____

   _____

5. "I come in here week after week and spill my guts and all you do is listen. I don't think this is helping."

_____

6. "I've been to lots of counselors, but they were the pits! They had no idea how to help me. But I get the feeling that you are the one who can solve my problem."

_____

_____

7. "How about meeting me this evening at that bar down the street? I'd like to get to know you better."

_____

_____

8. "I've tried everything to get past this problem. I'm pretty discouraged. If you can't help me, I guess it's all over."

_____

_____

9. "You don't really care about me, you're just paid to listen—but you don't really care."

_____

_____

10. "There is something I have been wanting to tell you, but I am not sure you would understand . . . I'm gay."

_____

_____

11. "You remind me of someone I knew in college that I really hated."

_____

12. "I was sexually abused as a child."

_____

_____

As you read some quotes, you may have found yourself hoping that your clients will never say something like that to you. To which statements did you have greater confidence responding? How did you develop this self-assurance? Which quotes were most threatening to you? How will you go about developing the confidence to respond to these statements?

Consider Counseling for Yourself

> The key to understanding others is to understand oneself.
>
> —Helen Williams

The importance of counselor self-knowledge and self-awareness cannot be overstressed in the counseling relationship. You "must be able to differentiate between countertransference reactions that are triggered by client transference and those that are projections of unresolved personal conflicts" (McLeod, 1998, p. 364).

Although none of us will ever be problem free, it is our responsibility as counselors to always work to maintain "personal soundness." After reviewing the evidence, McLeod (1998) concluded that successful counselors "are people who exhibit higher levels of general emotional adjustment and a greater capacity for self-disclosure" (p. 351). Many counseling programs advocate personal counseling for their trainees. Besides being a great way of learning more about yourself and the therapeutic process, participating in counseling for yourself can be a powerful means to a more deeply empathic understanding of your clients. According to McLeod, there is also considerable evidence that participating in your own counseling can enhance your effectiveness. Personal counseling can give you "a reliable basis for the confident and appropriate 'use of self' in relationships with clients" (p. 351).

Of course, you don't have to be a paragon of mental health to be a successful counselor. All of us have our ups and downs, and counseling is useful for everyone. It helps you "clear the circuits" and stay in touch with yourself when the trials of everyday life make you begin to feel as though you have been "nibbled to death by ducks." Working with troubled clients expends a great deal of psychic energy and can result in a residual confusion and burnout unless you continually process your experiences. National surveys have suggested that at least three-fourths of all practicing counselors have received at least one sequence of counseling (Norcross, Strausser, & Faltus, 1988). Remember, you don't have to be sick to get better!

▲▲▲

It Feels Weird for a Counselor to Be a Client
Robert's Story

ENTER THE COUNSELING CENTER and take a seat in one of the empty chairs in the waiting room. People are coming and going, counselors are greeting their clients and then disappearing with them down the hall. The only sound following them is the squeak of the hinge as the door closes.

I know this feeling that is permeating my insides. I have had this reaction before, but not for some time. Because I am in my third year of counselor training, I thought I should be past this feeling by now. As I sit in the waiting room, the realization hits me that I have absolutely no doubt that this is what I needed to do and where I needed to be. This is a wonderful feeling! I am proud of myself for taking this step because it contradicts some very unconscious stereotypical masculine notions. By making the phone call and following through with my appointment, I was able to feel good about this decision and not let my internal "critic" voice its derogatory comments about my manhood.

Each of us has a personal story to tell and somehow I had lost or forgotten part of my story—what being a client was like. Books can convey a wealth of information and insight about counseling, but actual experience can be the door to true understanding. As my counselor appears in the waiting room, I realize that I have been so focused on learning how to be a counselor that I forgot how much was involved in being a client.

As soon as I sit down in the counselor's office, I am uncertain of my role. All at once, I feel entangled in a psychological web—confused as to whether I am a client or a counselor. I am immediately struck by my focus on the man sitting across from me. I am exploring every facial expression, scrutinizing each of his words, and making mental notes of his every move. I cannot help but compare and make judgments about what my counselor is doing and saying. "How dare you write down what I am saying? Where is the rapport-building? I was taught to be present with the client and taking notes was not encouraged. Where is the eye contact, the understanding head nod, and the empathic reflection? I have taken risks to be here and you are scribbling my history on a notepad. What's going on?"

I have learned to deal with a fair amount of ambiguity in my training program and have been challenged to think outside of traditional gender roles and cultural mindsets, but how to be a client again? I guess that if I expect my clients to make an honest self-assessment, I must be committed to this same quest for self-awareness. I think I am ready to do this.

▼▼▼

Allow Yourself to Mess Up

Life is very interesting if you make mistakes.

—Georges Carpentier

As a new counselor, you may tend to focus on the mistakes you are making with clients. You may even consider these mistakes as evidence that you have chosen the wrong career path. This is your crisis of faith. Be assured that such crises come with the territory. Counselors always make mistakes.

You are probably more sensitive to your mistakes because you really want to be good at this work, and you somehow have the idea that good counselors are infallible. In *The Imperfect Therapist: Learning from Failure in Therapeutic Practice*, Kottler and Blau (1989) suggest that it is not mistakes that cause us problems; it is our attempts to avoid acknowledging mistakes that can undermine our confidence and effectiveness. Therapeutic "failures" can lead to positive results because they can:

> . . . promote reflection, stimulate change, provide useful information, give feedback on the impact of action, encourage flexibility, teach humility, increase resolve, improve tolerance for frustration, and foster experimentation (Kottler & Blau, 1989, p. 163).

Maybe you have watched videos of master counselors who are modeling their approaches to counseling. You were probably in awe of some of them. You may have also felt overwhelmed by their abilities and doubted that you could ever do counseling with the skill level they display. Please remember that these people have been at this work for a long time. Besides, do you think you would ever see a video of them screwing up? No chance!

Explore Your Assets

When you decided that you had what it takes to be a counselor and applied to graduate school, you felt intuitively that aspects of your personality seemed to fit the role. Perhaps over the years, people regularly come to you with their problems, and you want to learn how to be more helpful. Hold that thought. You have obviously been able to establish warm and empathic relationships, and several studies have shown that the desire to be of help to others is perhaps the most indispensable aspect of a counselor's personality. You were correct to think that you had the right stuff.

However, if being a good listener is all that's needed for successful counseling, then you would already be an accomplished helper. Besides learning the theories and practicing techniques of counseling, you have to liberate "the authentic you" to use in a therapeutic relationship. As Parrott put it, "A counselor cannot fake authenticity; it is not something you do, but something you are" (1997, p. 28). Being authentic is not easy. We have all been taught to be less than forthright in our social relationships, often to

the point of feeling as though we have lost our way. The good news, however, is that under our social veneer, we are all authentic. Underneath is
who we really are. During your training, you will need to find your way
back to the authentic you. Socrates admonished us to "know thyself."
To do this, you sometimes need to uncover experiences that you have
sealed over or put out of your awareness. Socrates also said that the unex-
amined life is not worth living. Make a commitment to examine your life
and find the real you. Although this work is often exhausting, it is also
exhilarating. And it certainly will make you a better counselor.

Avoid the Groucho Paradox

The Groucho paradox comes from comedian Groucho Marx's explanation for canceling his membership in the Hollywood chapter of the
Friar's Club: "I just don't want to belong to any club that would have
me as a member" (Swann, 1996, p. 18). When we are in the midst of a
negative self-evaluation, it's difficult to accept positive feedback from
others. When something good happens to us that we feel may be unde-
served, our level of self-esteem can actually drop.

As you make this journey through your training program, at times
you will find yourself plagued with self-doubt (Hughes & Kleist, 2005).
Because you have such high standards for yourself, you will occasionally
feel vulnerable and incompetent, discouraged and confused (Egan,
2007). Your instructors expect this to happen, and they know that
because you are being asked to change in ways that no educational experience has previously demanded of you, there will be times when you
need to escape. Consult Chapter 3 on caring for yourself during the
training experience to keep balance in your life.

There is the story of a woman, blind from age six, who had her sight
miraculously restored by a new medical procedure. Prior to this surgery,
the woman had done well in school, obtaining a doctoral degree. She
married, had two teenage daughters, and held a responsible position
in a rehabilitation clinic. With her sight newly regained, she first felt
ecstatic, then ambivalent, then depressed. Her whole life, once happy
in spite of her disability, began to deteriorate. She alienated friends and
family, and her job performance suffered. On the face of it, something
wonderful had happened, but the results were feelings of confusion and
emptiness. She had undergone a profound change, and she just didn't
know how to "act sighted." She had to relearn all aspects of her behavior, and she felt as if she had lost something terribly important in her life
(Swann, 1996).

Such a positive change as suddenly being able to see should yield only good results. But think about your own situation: You've been accepted into a graduate program of your choice. The day you got the letter was probably a major milestone in your life. You initially felt great. You entered your professional training with positive expectations and a little nervousness. Then, because you were expected to change in so many ways, you began to have a crisis of faith: "Maybe I can't do this," "Maybe I was deluding myself to think I had what it takes," "Maybe they made a mistake when they accepted me," "Maybe I don't want to belong to a program that would have me as a member!" It's the Groucho paradox that's sometimes called the "impostor syndrome." You begin to feel as if you've fooled the admissions committee into believing that you'd be a good candidate for this work.

It is important for you to know that you can occasionally expect to have major misgivings about your career choice. It is part of your developmental process. Although you are finally preparing for the profession that has felt like your life's calling and that you are at last able to focus all your coursework on this goal, your feelings will not always be positive. You will question your decision about becoming a helping professional, and you will probably have times when you are really down in the dumps as a result of the changes you are going through. No matter how much you may desire to become the "new you," at times you will long for the "old you" and feel you have lost something very important. Gloria Steinem (quoted in Swann, 1996) put it this way:

> Change, no matter how much for the better, still feels cold and lonely at first . . . because it doesn't feel like home. Old patterns, no matter how negative and painful . . . have an incredible magnetic power—because they do feel like home. (p. 147)

BE A BEGINNER, NOT AN EXPERT

> When you forget the beginner's awe, you start decaying.
>
> —Nobuko Albery

As an undergraduate, you probably spent a great deal of time ingesting information that you later regurgitated on a test. You may have memorized definitions, names, dates, formulas, or scientific principles without truly being able to understand or apply them. You became expert in beating the system and making grades, often perhaps at the expense of truly learning. Now you are in a program that requires you to go beyond mere information and begin to apply concepts to guide your behavior. The test becomes whether you can actually do it, not whether you can talk or write about it.

Your problem may be that you have spent so many years going through the motions of learning that you have forgotten how to truly learn. You're finding that strategies that were once successful do not apply to these new situations. You are a rank beginner and are confused by this new environment. These circumstances certainly make you feel insecure, and you may attempt to cover your feelings of inadequacy by acting as though you know more than you do and by sticking to those areas of knowledge in which you consider yourself an expert.

Instead we suggest that you give yourself permission to know nothing—to be a beginner. The Zen philosopher Suzuzi (quoted in Kosko, 1993) said, "In the beginner's mind there are many possibilities. In the expert's mind there are few" (p. 44). The Zen master teaches students by confusing them, sometimes posing a koan, or riddle such as, "What is the sound of one hand clapping?" The Zen method of the koan is the way the master convinces students that expertise is precisely what keeps them from understanding fully the truth of a situation. A koan throws the student into ambiguity so that the problem at hand must be approached naïvely. Creative thinkers always approach a situation as a naïve beginner, never as an expert. Creative discovery requires a freshness and awe that, as Bruner (1973) has said, surprises and delights the onlooker, as well as the creator.

Experts know how to do things and how to think about things. Expert thinking often proceeds automatically as a convergent problem-solving process. On the other hand, novices approach each circumstance as a new experience and discover fresh ways of adapting to its demands. It is much harder work to stay fresh than to behave automatically. You have to burn a lot of calories dealing with something you have never encountered. Be careful about becoming an expert at helping people, because every person and every situation is a new experience.

Assimilation and Accommodation

Piaget (1970) stated that we develop our knowledge schemas using two major processes—assimilation and accommodation. You're *assimilating* when you apply new information to knowledge structures that you already have in place. This type of learning involves merely adding information or elaborating on previous knowledge. Assimilating new information that does not fit precisely within your existing schemas may tempt you to distort it. If you can't hammer the new data into some form that fits your knowledge structures, then you can either reject the information or accommodate it. You're *accommodating* when you actually change your own schemas and create new knowledge structures to take in and process new information.

Someone who assimilates but refuses to accommodate tends to deal with information in a rigid and narrow manner. Chances are you know people like this. They claim to be experts on everything, but they seem to be merely prejudiced and biased. They suffer from hardening of the categories. Believe it or not, some counselors are like this! You can avoid becoming an expert by remaining open to new information and being willing to accommodate—to change the way you see the world—as you encounter new experiences.

Clearly, you must be flexible to accommodate. If, however, you believe you are an expert on the new information, you are likely to consider accommodation unnecessary. As children grow up and develop what they consider to be a sufficient set of categories or cognitive schemas, they sometimes become refractory or resistant to much of the new information that challenges them to accommodate. After all, accommodation can feel uncomfortable. Everyone knows how insufferable adolescent experts can be and how at this stage parents suddenly lose at least 30 IQ points in their teenager's eyes. Adolescents who are striving for expertise are probably motivated by the feeling of security that comes from believing that they have everything under control and that no new disquieting mysteries are awaiting them. Adolescents become rigid in their beliefs as a defense against their rapidly changing world. Unfortunately, their bravado is transparent and pathetic.

Accommodating Information About Yourself

Certainly, you have enjoyed the "aha!" exhilaration of discovering an accommodation that offers new and exciting breakthroughs in your ways of thinking. This is not always the case, however, when it comes to accommodating new information about yourself. Sometimes when you're open to learning about yourself, the results are jarring and confusing. According to some historical accounts, the College of Cardinals refused Galileo's invitation to look through his telescope, which was pointed toward the heavens, because they were afraid they might see something that would contradict their beliefs. Similarly, when an instrument of clarification is pointed to an area within ourselves, all of us are reluctant to look too closely, fearing that we will discover that some of our own aspects, beliefs, or values are different from what we had always assumed was true. Like adolescents, we may prefer to think we know everything about ourselves that there is to know. Such assumptions provide a false sense of security so that we can continue to delude ourselves that we are completely in control of our behaviors and attitudes.

In your training program, you have the opportunity to discover who you are. You will realize that the ambiguity of the koan is rampant in your experiences. Many of your discoveries about yourself will make you feel uncomfortable, but that's only because you are human. Humans are not perfect. Karen Horney (1970) said that if we erect for ourselves an "ideal self" and attempt to maintain it, the result will be neuroticism. The only way to be mentally healthy is to accept yourself as you are. Take a beginner's approach to the challenge of knowing yourself, not that of an expert.

HOLD TO YOUR CENTER

> There comes a point when you really have to
> spend time with yourself to know who you are.
>
> —Bernice Johnson Reagon

Graduate school is, to say the least, a demanding venture, and you can easily feel overwhelmed by all you have to do. You certainly need to keep a calendar of your appointments, a daily to-do list of your assignments and chores, and maybe even a personal digital assistant, such as a Palm Pilot, to help you keep your life in order. Dealing conscientiously with each of the tasks you have scheduled is a fine idea, but take care to hold to your center through all the distractions of your days. It is easy to pay so much attention to the demands of your world and to focus so much on the expectations of others that you begin to disappear. You then become, like Lewis Carroll's Alice, unreal—a thing in the Red King's dream.

> "He's dreaming now," said Tweedledee, "and what do you think he's dreaming about?"
> Alice said, "Nobody can guess that."

"Why, about *you!*" Tweedledee exclaimed, clapping his hands triumphantly. "And if he left off dreaming about you, where do you suppose you'd be?"

"Where I am now of course," said Alice.

"Not you!" Tweedledee retorted contemptuously. "You'd be nowhere. Why, you're only a sort of thing in his dream!"

"If that there King was to wake," added Tweedledum, "you'd go out—bang—just like a candle! . . . You know very well you're not real"

Lewis Carroll, 1896/1991, pp. 173–174

The Demands of Others

Carroll's message to all of us is that we should take care not to allow others to define us or base our self-esteem on the approval of others. Carl Rogers (1961) called such perceptions "conditions of worth"—when we can only accept ourselves if we measure up to other people's standards. If we try too hard to become what others want us to be, we become existentially ill. Ironically, when we feel as if we are losing ourselves and becoming ontologically insecure, we often try harder to validate who we are by seeking the approval of others. We may also plunge into relentless activity as a distraction from our ill feelings. When we become so immersed in our activities that we lose contact with our center—our true self—we fear that the Red King may be waking and we will disappear.

In *The Roman Spring of Mrs. Stone,* Tennessee Williams (1958) described a character's ongoing pursuit of diversions as a futile attempt at self-distraction: ". . . the hairdressers at four o'clock, the photographer at 5:00, the Colony at 6:00, the theater at 7:30, Sardi's at midnight . . . she moved in the great empty circle. But she glanced inward from the periphery and saw the void" (as quoted in Gergen, 1971, p. 86).

Having an impossibly full appointment book and frantically attempting to run a marathon at top speed can quickly make you feel overwhelmed, but it can also keep you from looking at yourself. A demanding educational environment requires time management on your part and a more refined vigilance to the cues of professors. So go ahead and buy the personal digital assistant and make sure that you are fulfilling the requirements of your courses. But remember, when you find yourself feeling as if you are being hit from all sides by the expectations of others, don't just do something—*be* there. There is much wisdom in that old cliché about stopping to smell the roses.

▲▲▲

Learning from the Inside Out
Teresa's Story

A T THE END of my first year in the counseling program, I felt as if I was walking around inside out. I was certain when I started that I wanted to become a counselor, but I didn't know that this would involve such microscopic self-examination. In my classes, outside my classes, in conversations with my peers, I explored so many crevices, dark holes, files that had been shoved away—even those that wanted to remain hidden. It was a relentless process, and many days I came home feeling a mix of exhaustion and exhilaration from uncovering layers of meaning and emotion.

One of the most important discoveries that I made is that I have a great need for people to be happy with me, so much so that I lose myself and my needs in striving to be *all* for everyone. Because of the intensive focus on *my* thoughts, *my* feelings, *my* contributions, and *my* beliefs, I embarked on a slow process of change—of wanting to become my authentic self and to shed the self that I *thought* others wanted me to be. This process is not easy, and it felt, and still feels, strange—like I had entered into the Land of Fog, and everything in my life became murky. Nothing was clear until I accepted the strangeness and the realization that ambiguity is a state that can be traveled through.

As I muddle through my second year, this is by no means a met challenge, but I have learned how to read my own map. And, at least now, I am aware of what I am doing and can forge ahead in hopes that the result of this journey will be to emerge as the self that I am genuinely happy and comfortable being.

▼▼▼

Honor, But Modify, Your Style

Here's a news flash: no one's childhood was perfect. Even when parents have tried to do right by us, we all come into adulthood with unmet needs. To the extent that our needs were not satisfied, we developed strategies or styles to compensate for the anxiety of our unique situation (Teyber, 1997). Karen Horney (1970) has identified three prominent coping styles that people adopt. She calls them the "moving toward," the "moving against," and the "moving away" strategies. These coping styles serve to reduce anxiety from our unmet childhood needs. These strategies can, however, become a liability in adulthood because we tend to enact them over and over, even though modifying them would be much more productive.

The *moving-toward* style manifests itself as the need to please people. People who use this strategy are compliant and want others to see them as being unfailingly nice and good (Teyber, 1997). This style results in the need to be approved of by others and in the attempt to meet their needs in an almost servile way. Those with the moving-toward style "suffer under the self-imposed demands that they should be the perfect lover, teacher, spouse, and so forth" (p. 203).

Those who use a *moving-against* strategy respond aggressively or rebelliously to parental authority. In an attempt to protect themselves from feeling vulnerable, they try to control themselves and others. Such people are strongly assertive, sometimes to the point of being aggressive, and they expect themselves to quickly overcome all obstacles and difficulties. They try to use an act of will to control their feelings and to overcome their "bad moods."

People with a *moving-away* style physically withdraw from anxiety-producing situations, in an attempt to become self-sufficient. Those who use the moving-away strategy pay for this "by believing that they should be able to work tirelessly and always be productive. They demand that they should be able to endure anything without becoming ruffled or upset and that they should never need help or reassurance from anyone" (Teyber, 1997, p. 203).

■ ■ ■

EXERCISE 6.3 Toward, Against, or Away?
A Moving Exercise

Horney's three coping styles are obviously not mutually exclusive. Each can be used at different times. All of them serve to ward off feelings of anxiety. Because of this, you should respect your need to use these compensatory strategies in your life.

STEP 1

Look at the circles representing the three styles and think about which one you use most often. Put a "1" in that circle. Then put a "2" in the circle that represents your second most favored style, and a "3" in the remaining circle.

An Exercise in Self-Reflection

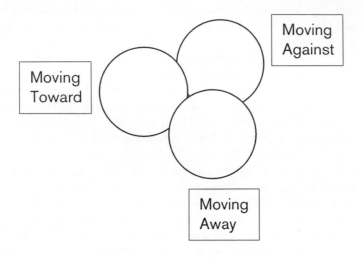

After you have completed this ranking, think about what purpose your dominant style serves in your life. How is it *helpful* to you? Reflect on recent stressful experiences in which your dominant style successfully dealt with the situation. Self-acceptance is a fundamental part of your personal growth. Just as you must honor resistance in your future clients, you must also honor it in yourself.

STEP 2

There is, however, an annoying paradox involved in these defense styles. They help you cope with anxiety-producing situations, but they also sometimes get in your way. The paradox is that, although you have adopted these styles to compensate for unmet childhood needs, they sometimes prevent your needs from being met as an adult. So the next step in this self-exploration exercise is to think about how this style *interferes* in your life, how it compels you to act in certain ways, and how your style may sometimes be off-putting to others.

STEP 3

The next stressful situation you are in will give you an opportunity to complete the final step of this exercise. Use that situation to deliberately refrain from using your favored style. For example, if moving toward is your dominant style, instead of immediately considering how to impress and please others, focus on your own needs and desires in this situation. Practicing a new style will seem strange and uncomfortable, but it will allow you to become more flexible in how you respond to challenges.

COUNTERTRANSFERENCE

It's déjà vu all over again.

—Yogi Berra

You inevitably have areas of emotional injury that may be too sensitive to fully explore, that are hidden and sequestered by protective layers of emotional shielding. Sometimes recent relationships with others uncover these unhealed injuries. Someone "touches a nerve," a sensitive issue that provokes a reaction that may seem out of proportion to the situation. Or perhaps you may find yourself responding negatively to someone, but you are unable to identify why you find that person to be so obnoxious. In other words, the ways in which you have been injured, frustrated, or disappointed in your past relations with others can affect how you perceive and respond to new relationships in the present.

This is particularly true if you have not yet fully explored and understood how past injuries or interpersonal problems influence you. Part of your journey of self-exploration includes becoming more aware of these areas of unresolved conflict. The less you are motivated by protective and defensive efforts to shield you from emotional pain, the more you will be able to engage others with full awareness of your authentic thoughts and feelings.

Playing out unresolved personal issues in new encounters with people is a response that Freud (1924) called "transference." In the therapeutic relationship, Freud observed that a client often acted as if the therapist were a sort of stand in for another important person in the client's life. The client may express emotions toward and assign motivations to the therapist that rightly belong to that patient's experience of someone else. Gaining insight into the origins and meaning of the client's transference constitutes one of the main goals of psychoanalytic therapy.

Although you're not in training to become a classic psychoanalyst, you will encounter transference in your clients. What's more, you will find that clients will evoke in you certain feelings and reactions that touch on your own personal conflicts and unresolved issues. Freud called the counselor's reaction in this situation "countertransference." He cautioned that it has the potential to derail a productive therapeutic relationship because the counselor's own unresolved feelings and conflicts get in the way of the client's self-expression. In other words, the therapist distorts the client's behavior to conform to the counselor's own expectations or biases.

Freud's concept is not a relic that is irrelevant to either counseling or interpersonal relationships. Most modern forms of counseling include some variant of the concepts of transference and countertransference. You can probably think of times that stand out as examples of your having had a strong transference reaction to someone. Of course, you will introduce your biases, distortions, and interpretive schemes in your subjective and unique fashion. The important point to remember is that self-awareness about how your past injuries become expressed in your interpersonal behavior is critically important to both your current personal relationships as well as to those you will foster with clients.

It is difficult to lift up bandages to look at old wounds and even more difficult to go poking around when they are not fully healed. But as you can see, the wounds that are still "alive" will influence your behavior toward others. Shoving painful life events down into a cellar of forgetting just makes you afraid to go down to the place in which your deepest, richest feelings may live. It is natural to want to "move on" from painful life experiences. How you choose to move is vital to whether you become an integrated and fully alive person or whether you insulate yourself in an attempt to forget your pain. As Freud observed, it is what we forget that we repeat.

GETTING CLEAR

> When one is a stranger to oneself then one is
> estranged from others too. If one is out of touch
> with oneself, then one cannot touch others.
>
> —Anne Morrow Lindbergh

What may be obvious to you by now is that becoming a successful counselor is more than simply veneering on a set of techniques and theories. A counselor is someone whose very personhood is therapeutic, and honesty is the counselor's most powerful asset. But to be honest with your clients, you must first be honest with yourself. As Carl Rogers said, the counselor must be authentic, congruent, and transparent in the counseling relationship.

Most people in everyday social situations cannot trust that they are receiving accurate feedback from others. As a result, most of us are uncertain about how others truly see us. This is why honesty is one of the characteristics that differentiates the counseling relationship from other relationships. One of the most refreshing and therapeutic aspects of the counseling relationship for clients is that they can rely on their counselor to be straight with them. Certain criteria must be met for such feedback to be effective. Clients must trust that your honesty is meant to be helpful and not to humiliating or self-aggrandizing. Your feedback must be timely and given in ways that clients can accept. But most of all, you must be clear as to your own motives for offering the feedback. Staying clear on your motives and values is a constant struggle that does not end with counselor training.

Trying to get a clear picture of your clients is like taking a photo with an old camera that uses glass plates. If the plate is clear, then the picture of your client will be reasonably accurate. On the other hand, if you have marred the surface of the plate, then it will be hard to tell which part of the picture belongs to the client and which to you. Striving to stay as clear as possible is a lifelong effort, and it requires that you are committed to continually work on yourself. As McConnaughy (1987) affirmed, the actual techniques you use as a counselor are not as important as your unique personhood. Moreover, "the more a therapist accepts and values himself or herself the more effective he or she will be in helping clients come to know and appreciate themselves" (McConnaughy, 1987, p. 304). The clearer you stay about yourself, the more room a client has to clearly understand his or her concerns.

Finding Your Roots

> Those of us who attempt to act and do things for others or for the world without deepening our own self-understanding, freedom, integrity, and capacity to love, will not have anything to give others.
>
> —Thomas Merton

Exploring or knowing yourself goes beyond trying to *understand* who you are. While this statement may seem confusing at first, there are really two parts to knowing yourself. Complete self-exploration also means developing an understanding of how other people regard you. Look at your reflection in the mirror. What do you see? The person that you see may not be the same person that others are responding to. How do you appear to others? They may see your ethnicity, gender, age, mannerisms, and many manifestations of your upbringing and values that are so much a part of you that you don't even notice them. Who you are to others creates an image that must also become part of your total self-understanding. Each time you encounter clients, they will be responding to an image of you that may or may not be in alignment with how you see yourself. Moment to moment you must attempt to view yourself through your clients' eyes and deal with their misgivings about whether you can be trusted, whether you care, and whether they feel safe in your company.

▲▲▲

I Need to Pay Attention to Who I Am
Michelle's Story

PRIOR TO MY FIRST practicum experience, I thought I knew myself pretty well. I had spent a good deal of time during my classes exploring my values and getting in touch with my beliefs. In one class we completed an exercise in which we imagined how it might be to counsel a pedophile, a substance abuser, or a wife batterer. I convinced myself that I would be able to transcend the "differences" of my clients and, as long as I treated each person with respect, my work as a counselor would be relevant and effective. Then I sat down with my first real client. The client seemed nervous, which helped me overcome my own anxiety and assume what I believed was a true helper role. I did my best to help the client feel at ease. After a few minutes of small talk and tentative "starts and stops," the client looked at me with a kind smile. "You know, I don't want to hurt your feelings, but I have to tell you I'm a little uncomfortable." No problem! I thought. I started to internally formulate a soothing reflective statement when my client continued. "I have a feeling you're probably Christian, and I really don't think I'll feel comfortable talking to a Christian counselor."

I can't begin to accurately express my reaction. All I can remember is a sinking feeling while I chanted to myself, "What do I do now? What do I do now?" I'll admit that in addition to feeling shocked, I was a little hurt that anyone would not want to talk to a Christian. What's wrong with Christians? I wanted to protest.

Later, after discussing this session with my supervisor and peers and experiencing a range of emotions, I discovered a few things about myself. During all my thinking about difference and what I can "tolerate" about other people, I never realized that the "different" one in the counseling session might be me. I also started to see that prior to that session I had never consciously explored my own ethnicity, religion, or socioeconomic status. As a person who sits squarely and comfortably in mainstream society (white, Anglo Saxon, Protestant, middle class), I've never had to think about these things. Unlike my peers who are Latina or African American, for instance, I've taken my identity and its implications for granted. Thanks to my sensitive client, I've begun an exploration of myself and my identity as white, female, Christian, and middle class. All of those identities mean something to me, and they obviously mean something to my clients. I need to pay attention to who I am.

Michelle could have responded in a variety of ways to her client's concerns. She could have acknowledged those concerns, addressed the religious differences, offered a referral, and so forth. In your training you will be developing skills to handle situations such as these, but our emphasis here is on your own self-understanding. As you can see, Michelle used this situation as a catalyst for her own growth, and she came away from the session with a much greater sense of who she was. Such awareness is much more useful to her than learning a new counseling technique.

Find the "I Am" Experience

Rollo May (1983) wrote about a client who had rediscovered what he called the "I AM" experience. When asked what this experience was like, the client said:

> [I]t feels like receiving the deed to my house. It is the experience of my own aliveness. . . . It is my saying to Descartes, "*I am, therefore I think, I feel, I do*" (p. 99, emphasis in original).

As you continue your training and discover the new you, you will find that you're also improving the old you. Somehow, your "I" and your "me" become united. Your self-confidence improves, and your self-trust becomes solid and more confident. This does not mean that you will never feel insecure about who you are. We all experience times when we lose touch with ourselves. But once you get hold of that "*I am*" feeling, you'll always have the deed to your house, and, contrary to what Thomas Wolfe said, you *can* go home again.

SUMMARY

In this chapter, we have hammered home the point that, in order to be an effective counselor, you must first be committed to your own "personal soundness." Being personally sound does not mean that you must be free of all wounds and troubles. In fact, the very program that you are going through will create new troubles for you and expose old wounds that must be dealt with. The main thing you must do is remain open to the changes that are happening in you. The Greek philosopher Heraclitus said that a person cannot step in the same river twice. But because the person cannot remain constant either, he might have gone on to state that the same person cannot step in the same river twice. You are always changing. You are different today than you were yesterday. As you make your journey through your training program, be sure to keep up with yourself!

RESOURCES

Two books are cited in this chapter that we think merit a thorough reading. They will be helpful to you as you explore yourself and navigate your own process of change. The writing style of both authors is quite readable and lively. Many of our students have reported that these books spoke to them and were personally reassuring during their "dark night of the soul."

The Discovery of Being, by Rollo May (1983), explains existential psychotherapy and its history. You may find this information interesting. But beyond gaining a better understanding of this way of working with clients, you will find that May has much to say about your "existential condition" as you become a helping professional. We especially recommend the chapter, "To Be and Not To Be."

Interpersonal Process in Psychotherapy, by Edward Teyber (2005), also describes a particular approach to working with clients and contains many useful examples of what to say in counseling sessions. The chapters that will be most helpful to you as you attempt to make sense of your own formative experiences are Chapter 6, "Familial and Developmental Factors," and Chapter 7, "Inflexible Interpersonal Coping Strategies."

Both these books will also be good resources as you develop your own counseling theory. Both are written in evenhanded and nondogmatic styles, and their ideas can be incorporated into many approaches to counseling.

We've also included two websites that you may find useful in the process of self-exploration.

PsychNet-UK

www.psychnet-uk.com

An interesting site based in the United Kingdom (U.K.) containing links to articles, jobs, chat rooms, games, MP3s, and "humour." You may find it interesting to see how the U.K. deals with issues of personal growth and psychology. This site also has a special section for students in the mental health professions.

Room 42

www.room42.com/store/health_center/selfgrow.shtml

This site is associated with Amazon.com. You can review video recordings, books, and software that you can order from Amazon. Each listing contains consumer ratings on the quality of the item. You can read what they have written and be better informed before you buy. Of course, you are not obligated to purchase anything from this site. By the way, we don't know why they call it "Room 42." You may recall that in *The Hitchhiker's Guide to the Galaxy*, "42" was the answer to the question about the meaning of life.

REFERENCES

Bruner, J. (1973). *Beyond the information given: Studies in the psychology of knowing*. New York: Norton.

Carroll, L. (1991). *The complete illustrated Lewis Carroll*. New York: Gallery Books. (Original work published 1896)

Dearing, R. L., Maddux, J. E., & Tangney, J. P. (2005). Predictors of psychological help seeking in clinical and counseling psychology graduate students. *Professional Psychology: Research and Practice, 36,* 323–329.

Deikman, A. J. (1996). "I" = awareness. *Journal of Consciousness Studies: Controversies in Science and the Humanities, 3*(4), 350–356.

Egan, G. (2007). *The skilled helper: A problem management and opportunity development approach to effective helping* (8th ed.). Belmont, CA: Brooks/Cole.

Erikson, E. (1968). *Identity: Youth and crisis.* New York: Norton.

Freud, S. (1924). *A general introduction to psychoanalysis.* New York: Washington Square Press.

Gergen, K. J. (1971). *The concept of self.* New York: Holt, Rinehart & Winston.

Gould, J. L., & Marler, P. (1987, January). Learning by instinct. *Scientific American,* 74–85.

Guggenbuhl-Craig, A. (1971). *Power in the helping professions.* Dallas, TX: Spring.

Henry, W. E. (1977). Personal and social identities of psychotherapists. In A. S. Gurman & A. M. Razin (Eds.), *Effective psychotherapy: A handbook of research.* Oxford, England: Pergamon Press.

Horney, K. (1970). *Neurosis and human growth.* New York: Norton.

Hughes, F. R., & Kleist, D. M. (2005). First-semester experiences of counselor education doctoral students. *Counselor Education and Supervision, 45,* 97–108.

James, W. (1890). *Principles of psychology.* New York: Holt, Rinehart & Winston.

Kosko, B. (1993). *Fuzzy thinking: The new science of fuzzy logic.* New York: Hyperion.

Kottler, J. A. (2000). *Doing good: Passion and commitment for helping others.* Philadelphia: Brunner-Routledge.

Kottler, J. A., & Blau, D. S. (1989). *The imperfect therapist: Learning from failure in therapeutic practice.* San Francisco: Jossey-Bass.

Laing, R. D. (1969). *The divided self.* New York: Pantheon Books.

Levin, J. D. (1992). *Theories of the self.* Washington, DC: Hemisphere.

Linehan, M. M. (1993). *Skills training manual for treating borderline personality disorder.* New York: Guilford.

Masson, J. M., & McCarthy, S. (1995). *When elephants weep.* New York: Delacorte.

May, R. (1983). *The discovery of being: Writings in existential psychology.* New York: Norton.

McConnaughy, E. A. (1987). The person of the therapist in therapeutic alliance. *Psychotherapy, 24,* 303–314.

McLeod, J. (1998). *An introduction to counseling* (2nd ed.). Buckingham, England: Open University Press.

Norcross, J. C., Strausser, D. J., & Faltus, F. J. (1988). The therapist's therapist. *American Journal of Psychotherapy, 42,* 53–66.

Parrott, L., III (1997). *Counseling and psychotherapy.* New York: McGraw-Hill.

Perez, J. F. (1979). *Family counseling: Theory and practice.* New York: Van Nostrand.

Piaget, J. (1970). Piaget's theory. In P. H. Mussen (Ed.), *Carmichael's manual of child psychology* (Vol. 1, 702–732). New York: Wiley.

Rippere, V., & Williams, R. (1985). *Wounded healers: Mental health workers' experiences of depression.* New York: Wiley.

Rogers, C. R. (1942). *Counseling and psychotherapy.* Boston: Houghton Mifflin.

Rogers, C. R. (1951). *Client-centered therapy.* Boston: Houghton Mifflin.

Rogers, C. R. (1961). *On becoming a person.* Boston: Houghton Mifflin.

Rogers, C. R. (1980). *A way of being.* Boston: Houghton Mifflin.

Sadler-Gerhardt, C. (2005, October). *Counseling Today, 47,* 7, 37.

Seligman, M. E. P. (1995). The effectiveness of psychotherapy: The *Consumer Reports* Study. *American Psychologist, 50,* 965–974.

Sherman, P. W. (1980). The meaning of nepotism. *American Naturalist, 116,* 604–606.

Swann, W. B. (1996). *Self-traps: The elusive quest for higher self-esteem.* New York: Freeman.

Teyber, E. (2005). *Interpersonal process in psychotherapy: An integrative model* (5th ed.). Pacific Grove, CA: Brooks/Cole.

Thomas, L. (1983). *Late night thoughts on listening to Mahler's ninth symphony.* New York: Viking Press.

Trivers, R. L. (1971). The evolution of reciprocal altruism. *Quarterly Review of Biology, 46,* 35–57.

Truax, C. B., & Mitchell, K. M. (1971). Research on certain therapist interpersonal skills in relation to process and outcome. In A. E. Bergin & S. Garfield (Eds.), *Handbook of psychotherapy and behavior change* (pp. 299–344). New York: Wiley.

Williams, T. (1958). *The Roman spring of Mrs. Stone.* New York: Atheneum.

CHAPTER 7

Being with Others

All real living is meeting.

—Martin Buber

It takes one kind of mind to absorb facts, and
another to absorb the presence of another human
being.

—Abraham Maslow

As you begin your training as a counselor, you'll soon realize that you are entering a whole new educational culture, one much different from your undergraduate experience. You are no longer among students with divergent courses of study, career goals, and professional aspirations; you and your fellow classmates all share the goal of becoming a counselor or therapist. There is a different feeling as you join with others to pursue not only training goals and a degree but also a new concept of who you are. Together, you are reaching for something that is not entirely known but that you sense has wonderful possibilities for your own growth and your relationships with others. You are suddenly part of a new community.

This chapter is about being in a community of peers, faculty, administrators, mentors, and supervisors. It is also about how changes in you—as you evolve as a person and forge a new identity as a counselor—influence the important people in your life. These people may be relatives, friends, romantic partners, and fellow students. One thing is sure: Because this journey will change your life, it will also change the lives of those closest to you. Your journey affects them all, and, in some measure, they are taking the trip with you.

You will inevitably change because you are entering a new, kind of milieu—one you have never experienced before. You notice that your new community calls on you to respond in fresh ways, take risks, collaborate with others, and be open and flexible to a degree that might be unfamiliar to you. You're expected to be "game" for new ventures, such as role-plays and experiential exercises. You become used to seeing yourself on videos, learning and practicing counseling skills. You also find that to really engage in a learning dialogue with others, you welcome critiques from supervisors and peers. Above all, being fully invested in forging an identity as a counselor requires you to be open, accessible, and collaborative with others, throwing your whole self into the experience.

Don't worry: Though you might feel that you don't know how to swim in these uncharted waters, you won't drown! Others will buoy you when you need it, and you will discover resources you never knew you had. At the same time, you find yourself learning new ways of relating to others that will serve you, not only with those who will one day seek your counseling but also with anyone whose life touches your own.

This chapter addresses not only the ways in which these new relational opportunities can test your ability to adapt, but also the ways they can provide memorable and joyful experiences. When you finally become a full-fledged member of the healing profession, you may look back on your training and say, "What a long, strange trip it's been!" But you will be grateful and alive with a new capacity for relating to others that is at the core of what it means to become a counselor. The question to ask yourself now is, "Am I open to this experience?"

▲ ▲ ▲

Being "Processed"
Rebecca's Story

CAN STILL RECALL how strange it felt sitting in a circle with my classmates, thinking, "Who *are* these people?" It was my first experience in a process group. I wasn't sure what that meant, but whatever it was, I sure was leery of being processed by this bunch. They were so different from what I had expected. Looking back,

I think I assumed that they would be more like me—you know, normal! Now, I can really appreciate the diversity in my classmates, but back then that beginning group felt like entering another world. I was disconcerted and a little scared. Later, I wondered how my previous world could have been so uniform. But at the beginning of that group, I felt out of place.

Apparently, "process" meant that we were supposed to share our thoughts and feelings about stuff that we were experiencing as new graduate students. Some students seemed fine with this and openly talked about their excitement as well as their frustrations. An older guy talked about being disoriented now that he's a student again. Somebody else talked about how her boyfriend felt threatened by her going to graduate school. One African American woman described how it felt to be the only person of color in the class, especially because she was from a "black" university. Her words about being in the minority stirred a guy to talk about his sexual orientation. Just when I was feeling like the most conventional person in the world, a young neohippy-looking guy, Robert, talked about "body-mind" stuff. He related how important yoga and meditation were to him. I thought to myself, "What a flake!"

I tend to be very private, so I kept wondering, "What am I doing here?" When it came to my turn to share my experiences, I mentioned a few things that were not particularly deep, but nobody seemed to mind. It creeped me out that some people in the group talked so freely, especially about personal stuff. I gravitated to Alicia, who was quiet like me and who was also nervous about being processed. We stuck together like we had been cast adrift and were clinging to the same life preserver.

Over time, though, I started to feel a little left out. I began becoming interested in the experiences my classmates shared and felt that I wanted them to know me better, too. I started to open up a little, and it wasn't so bad! This also kind of dragged Alicia along, and she began to loosen up around the others. By the time I was really feeling comfortable with everyone—well, almost everyone—we started our practicum.

This change set me back a little. It was hard because we had to show our work with clients and talk about our personal responses to client's issues. I was afraid of being criticized and felt exposed again. Strangely enough, Alicia, who had complained about all this personal disclosure, seemed to really like the process group for our casework, and eventually I enjoyed it too because it helped me develop my counseling skills. Now it's second nature to discuss my personal responses to client issues or how a particular experience affects me. I now realize that appreciating diversity is not just about ethnicity or race.

When I look back on how strange it had felt to be thrown in with people who are so different from me, I can't understand what I was nervous about. I am not as drawn to some of the people in the program, but I have been surprised that even they have something valuable to offer me. Sometimes it is the person who is most different from me that has helped me see things in a new way with my clients. That neohippy guy, Robert, has become one of my closest friends, and I've almost mastered the inverted swan position in my yoga repertoire!

▼▼▼

WHAT'S IN YOUR BACKPACK?

Remember that thriving principle about packing for the journey? Well, your counseling journey is the current leg of the larger journey that is your life. You already have things in your backpack, a lot of which influences how you relate to others. You may be fully aware of some of your pack's contents, and you pull it out all the time in your relationships. But you most likely forgot a lot that was in the backpack—or never realized what you had to begin with!

Like everyone else, you have a long history of interpersonal experiences that have helped contribute to who you are and how you relate to others. Discovering a quality or skill that helps you connect well with others is pleasantly surprising. The feeling is similar to an experience you possibly had as a child, heading off to camp on the bus. Just as you were starting to get hungry, you found that your mother had packed a peanut butter and jelly sandwich for you. Now, as a graduate student in a new program, you may discover you have the ability to take risks and have authentic encounters with people. Besides finding something nice, you may also realize that you've been carrying a bunch of rocks—dead weight from old relationships that prevents you from engaging with others in meaningful ways. You may wonder, "What is all this junk that I've been lugging around?"

SELF AND RELATIONSHIP

It takes two to know one.

—Gregory Bateson

You will continue to sort through that "junk" as you begin counseling, therapy, supervision, and other essential relationships that you will be establishing during your training. Even if you are skilled at forming new relationships, you will likely gain new perspectives as your counseling identity evolves. As you discover new insights, you will want to reevaluate your assumptions about how you interact with others.

Every profession has its own set of tools. In the helping professions, the most valuable tool is your ability to form a variety of interpersonal connections and relationships. Learning how your own experience manifests itself when communicating with others and becoming aware of the effect those communications have on them are major challenges in becoming a helping professional (Natterson & Friedman, 1995).

During the early phase of your graduate training, you use your interpersonal awareness and skills to develop relationships with your peers and professors. Later, awareness of how you structure your relations with others influences your interactions with your first clients. In your training, you learn new techniques, master new methods, and apply newfound knowledge to help your clients. It is important to understand, however, that all of these are secondary to the interpersonal context in which you practice these skills (Matthews, 2005). For this reason, your professors and supervisors encourage you to become more aware of how you encounter them as you work together. These relationships, as well as those with your new peers, are the laboratory in which you can discover your greatest counseling tool—yourself.

Exploring Your Relational Worldview

We are here to hand one another on.

—Walker Percy

You are the result, in part, of the unique psychological environment you and the people who have been important to you created. In that shared climate, especially with early caregivers, you forged a unique sense of self, as well as an awareness of how others respond to you. Your important early relationships, for instance, helped you learn to feel, regulate, and express emotion. The very structure of your emotional life took shape in a relational system (Stolorow, Brandchaft, & Atwood, 1987).

During that time, you learned to make sense of people's behaviors. You also discovered how your own actions, feelings, and expressions affected others (Stern, 1988). From myriad encounters that took place every single day of your young life, you developed a working model for structuring interpersonal relationships. More important, in the context of others you became yourself.

As you grew and developed, this formative matrix of relational experiences was the foundation you used to accommodate new interpersonal experiences, sharing a psychological environment with friends, relatives, peers, and intimate partners. That environment spawned your interpersonal style, which is the product of your early experiences, values, needs, traumas, motivations, and fears. All of those events are similar to pins on a map that show you where you have been and where you may be headed as you navigate new relationships.

Your unique itinerary records all the relational terrain you have traversed as you grew up. This map holds an enormously complex collection of interpretive categories that take shape from your unique interpersonal history, which informs every new relational event. These interpretive categories, with which you make sense of interpersonal encounters, are not often the focus of your conscious and deliberate examination (Stolorow & Atwood, 1992). Without even realizing it, you use these meaning-making templates all the time. You assume that they are accurate and reliable accounts of reality because you have a fundamental need to make sense of your interactions with others.

However, one reason for the success of your assumptions is that you develop relationships with people whose interpersonal assumptions are similar to your own. People with roughly similar sets of interpretive categories make you feel that they understand you. It feels like familiar territory, and because of that connection, a relationship is more likely to grow out of the encounter.

You did not select the members of your new learning community. Instead, you're thrown in among a wide assortment of people with whom you might not normally associate. Even though they may share a common commitment to a helping profession, your colleagues, professors, and supervisors most likely use vastly different organizing methods for interpersonal interaction. It is in this diverse and unfamiliar personality "salad bowl" that you are challenged to explore your own assumptions and expectations about others. In your class discussions, supervisory meetings, and counseling sessions, you will be stretching your capacity to accept alternate experiences of the same event. Like a single ray of light that is shed through a prism creates a spectrum of colors, a single, shared episode experienced by different people can have a spectrum of interpretations. In this psychological environment, you'll come to truly appreciate that others' subjective experiences of interpersonal events are as real for *them* as your experience is for you. By accepting and valuing these alternate perceptions, you can not only enrich and broaden your own perspective but also become a successful helping professional.

For example, facing the issues of racism and sexism can be very perturbing. White people, in particular, can be hesitant to bring up these concerns with people of color (Hayman, 2006). In your conversations, you may find yourself avoiding the topics of affirmative action, inequality, immigration, and race relations because you fear these will stir up strong emotions. One of the unfortunate results of this avoidance, however, is that you never become genuinely engaged in deep discussions about the pain inflicted by these social problems—and the ways of addressing them. Your training is an ideal time for you to explore yourself as a gendered, ethnic individual.

A central goal of your training is to gain a thorough understanding of how you structure your interpersonal experiences in the unique way that you do. In other words, as you make explicit your organizing frames of reference for understanding relationships, you become a more effective helper (Adams, 2006). As part of this process, you also discover how you respond to relational events. In your learning community, you can be open to revising your map, exploring your own relational assumptions, and becoming more aware of the impact you have on your fellow traveling companions.

EXERCISE 7.1 **Visitor from Another Planet**
A Guided Fantasy

For the next few minutes, imagine that you're from a planet where every member of the population looks exactly the same and has no distinguishing characteristics. Your spaceship lands in the United States and several government officials greet you. After determining that you pose no threat, the officials decide to familiarize you with U.S. culture. They suggest that you watch an evening of prime-time television programs and read popular magazines and newspapers. Imagine what you see and read. What is your impression of these men and women? What about

women who are racially or ethnically different from the majority of the
population? Or people whose ethnicity or sexual orientation seem different from the mainstream? What about people who have physical or emotional limitations? Take a few minutes to write your impressions.

_____

_____

_____

_____

_____

Now, imagine that the officials tell you that the United States is a
meritocracy in which people get what they work for and deserve and
that their country's government is based on the principle that all men
are created equal. What are your opinions now?

_____

_____

_____

_____

Reflect on the meaning this exercise has for you, consider the opinions and assumptions you have that you take for granted. What do your
findings imply about how different people may feel about their place in
society? How might this information apply to your clients?

_____

_____

_____

_____

_____

■ ■ ■

Growing in Relation

When we are listened to, it creates us, makes us
unfold and expand.

—Karl Menninger

Most students new to counseling programs are at first startled and later
excited by how much their programs focus not only on training but also
on personal growth, especially in relation to others. The experiences of
Alberta and Clare, both beginning graduate students in counseling,
typify what many undergo. Alberta, for example, was having trouble
with the emphasis placed on interpersonal self-awareness in her counseling program. Once she remarked with exasperation that her training
felt "more like personal therapy." Alberta was striving to deal with how
her interpersonal style, habits, and assumptions were being challenged
and made more explicit as she participated in forging new relationships
with peers and supervisors. These relationships were centered on the
cultivation of the person, as well as the skills, of the counselor.

Day after day, Alberta felt compelled to closely examine how her
interpersonal style affects others—much more so than if she had chosen
another profession. At the end of her program, however, Alberta shared
her feelings with her colleagues: "I thought that I could just come here
and learn what to do and not have to change myself. I guess I had this
idea that I would only 'do something to' others, rather than 'be someone with' others. Giving up that sense of control, and being open to
change and to all of you, was the hardest thing about the program."

One of the "rocks" in Alberta's "backpack" was the need she had to be
in control all the time to feel safe with others. It was difficult for her to
try new things or to be frank about her own thoughts and feelings
because she reserved trust only for lifelong friends. Being open to helpful
guidance, productive evaluation, collaboration, or mentoring was difficult because she felt threatened by not being the one directing the show.

Quite different relational issues may be more troublesome to you. Clare had always been the "star" in her academic pursuits. She proudly declared that she had a "high need for achievement." As her relationships with supervisors and peers developed, however, Clare began to realize that she actually harbored a strong and unrealistic desire for perfection. At first, she had a hard time trying new skills because of her fear of making a mistake—and of not being the star. As others watched her video recorded sessions, Clare felt overly sensitive to criticism. Her unrealistic aspirations hit a brick wall when her competitive desire to outshine her peers and win accolades began to disrupt her supervision group. Clare had difficulty accepting that her interpersonal style, rather than her external achievement, was fair game for discussion in this setting. However, as she began to understand how her interpersonal style affected her counseling effectiveness, Clare's desire to become a good counselor eventually enabled her to be open and receptive and to accommodate the feedback that others gave her. She discovered how her competitive behavior reduced, rather than elevated, the esteem with which others regarded her. Clare was also able to explore these interpersonal dynamics in terms of the family dynamics in which they had formed.

Like Alberta and Clare, you have a complex mixture of talents, fears, and interpersonal assumptions that serve as either peanut butter and jelly sandwiches or rocks in your backpack. Your expectations about relationships influence your defenses, fears, and hopes. Some of your habits of relating and communicating can work well, but some get in the way of being open, honest, and fulfilled in your relationships. Unlike the latest diet fad, which can offer you no guarantees, we offer you two assurances about your training experience. First, whatever your interpersonal style, you can discover its strengths and limitations as you continue on your journey. As you explore the baggage you bring to training, you can spread your backpack's contents on the ground so you can examine everything carefully before deciding what you want to keep carrying with you—and what you can discard. Our second guarantee is that, as you successfully make your way through training with a lighter load, you will relate to others in new and more fulfilling ways.

Mirrors

Your important relationships are like mirrors (Kohut, 1971). You see yourself in the experiences you have with others. Your professors, supervisors, peers, and clients form the relational laboratory in which you discover your professional identity. Undoubtedly, at times your reflection will be familiar and will confirm your assumptions. But it is just as likely that there will be times when you will think your reflection looks strange, unnerving, or disconcerting. As you ponder the many opportunities for growth that emerge out of these encounters, keep in mind that you are a work in progress and that the journey itself—not the destination—is most important.

▲▲▲

The Childlike Feeling of Possibility
Antoinette's Story

IT IS A BEAUTIFUL morning, so I decide to lie in the grassy arms of the campus quad. Sunlight speckles down on the noisy undergrads walking off the effects of last night's festivities. I am right next to the sidewalk. I wonder, "Is this somehow symbolic? In my life, do I dare not stray too far from safety?" I'm lying in a rare, unnatural pose of openness—bared arms, black skin shimmering in the fall sunshine, making me truly rainbow-like.

I feel the damp ground through my jeans. My black braids are long and soft. They comfort me as they sway in the breeze against the goose bumps on my skin. I sense the green, the wind, and the childlike feeling of possibility that I am often too scared to embrace.

I am almost 23, and I still fight the feeling of being alone. I can handle every day before I look in the mirror. No, I used to feel that way. But it still isn't a good idea to look for too long. Still, I see a life proposed again—one lived beyond mere survival. I am with these others, strangers and friends, different and the same. Now they are mirrors, too. I do not get the answers, but I ask the right questions, and I know there are options. I don't feel like I have to always question if I can live this life like some of the people I know. And I don't feel like I am left alone with the world balanced between teeth and tongue. I can't help but wonder how long today will last inside of me. But today . . . maybe today, I am strong and beautiful and confident enough to dare to say, "I belong."

▼▼▼

THE COUNSELING QUALITIES

Our fate is shared.

—Susan Griffin

Pondering the contents of your interpersonal backpack is good preparation for accepting traveling companions on your journey. To really get the most from your program, you need to join with others to help you navigate through the circuitous path of experiences that will foster your growth as a helping professional. These important persons are your professors, mentors, supervisors, clients, and fellow students. Some of your classmates will be farther along in the program and can help guide you when you feel disoriented and lost. With your new companions, you can discuss new ideas, practice your emerging skills, observe one another, and give feedback as you seek to apply what you are learning. You can practice therapy skills by watching videos of one another's role-plays and actual counseling sessions. You will become comfortable with giving and receiving constructive criticism and helpful observations. These activities can stretch your capacity for being "out there" and exposed to professors and fellow students in your learning process. If you open yourself to others, your companions can be there to encourage you when you need it—as well as challenge you to explore your potential to the fullest.

Two very important criteria are necessary for these relationships to truly have a profound impact on your growth as a counselor. First, you have to cultivate these relationships in an interpersonal climate of honesty and understanding. You need to really know and appreciate your traveling companions for you to fully trust and respect them. The good news is that your advisors, supervisors, and learning companions are very likely to value openness. However, you also have to let others truly get to know you, too.

The second criterion for successfully creating dynamic and profound relationships is that you must be a vital and engaged participant. Go out of your way to show the people who form your new learning community your animated interest, sincere curiosity, and unique perspective. By sharing your ideas and experiences, expressing your doubts and confusion, and communicating forthrightly, you help promote an environment that encourages discoveries and facilitates growth for everyone.

Many of the qualities that are essential to becoming a skilled helping professional are equally relevant to fostering meaningful relationships with your traveling companions. An attitude of respect and acceptance for persons different from yourself will enable you to reach outside your comfort zone and create connections with others whom you would not typically encounter.

Becoming open and accepting was particularly challenging to one woman at the start of her graduate program: Hannah grew up in a close-knit community of people who all shared her religious views. Until she learned to appreciate value systems different from her own, Hannah found it very difficult to create close and productive relationships with fellow students who were not of her faith. Her initial practicum experiences further challenged her to accept persons whose worldviews, values, sexual orientations, and religious beliefs were very different from her own. Hannah later acknowledged, "When I first started, I assumed that I would help people find answers to their problems. What I really assumed is that they would want *my* answers! It's still difficult for me sometimes to remember that my way of seeing things is not the only way."

Cultivating mutuality and interdependence means that you have to be open to give and take, to stand on an equal footing with others, and to be responsive to opportunities for engagement at a meaningful level. Many persons attracted to the helping professions enjoy the role of "helper" but have a hard time with mutual relationships that require reciprocal self-disclosure and trust. Such reciprocity implies a willingness to be vulnerable at times and to take a chance that others will accept you as you have accepted them. Another graduate student, Deaken, had savored how his peers celebrated him for his thoughtful and sensitive listening skills. Over time, however, his fellow students noticed that Deaken rarely revealed much of himself when it was his turn to participate in counseling exercises and role-plays. They also noticed, as friendships developed, that despite his supportive and caring attitude toward his fellow students in times of need, Deaken did not disclose his own struggles or feelings. When confronted about his one-sided relational style, Deaken acknowledged that he found it difficult to open up to others. His companions let him know that for mutual trust to develop, Deaken had to take the same risks that they did.

Mutuality means a willingness to be genuine with others, not pretending to show your real thoughts and feelings. For example, when his supervision group discussed his counseling video, Elias remarked that everyone complimented him on his strengths and commented on only what he was doing successfully. How could he improve his skills if everyone was merely being polite? Elias's candor and lack of defensiveness showed his peers that he was trying to grow and that they could respond forthrightly to him without creating ill will. When the other members pointed out where he had missed some important client expressions, Elias began to trust the integrity of the group process and to feel he was getting his peers' genuine reactions. You must do your part in helping to create a community of learners by sharing yourself, supporting and respecting others, and by being invested and engaged with all those whose lives are joined with yours in becoming helping professionals.

"TRUTH" WITH A CAPITAL "T"

Truth is always what a person believes privately and emotionally.

—Hergenhahn

Postmodernist thinking suggests that multiple truths exist. Therefore, you can truly encounter others only when you realize that your "truth" may not be someone else's. The bottom line is that to be both a successful and ethical helping professional, you must be able to accept others who are different from you.

Certainly, you have values that are sacred to you, but it's likely that you also consider yourself pretty understanding about different beliefs and lifestyles. It's also just as likely, however, that at times you react to certain differences with a "hard belly." Nothing about accepting that different perspective seems to penetrate—everything bounces right off. When you hear people talk about their life circumstances, it's as though you suddenly have "abs of steel." At that particular time, you are unable to absorb their experience. When do you have a hard-belly response? The best way to figure that out is to look at what purpose it serves.

Your hard belly is an example of distancing behaviors, those reactions and protests that may arise when you're faced with challenging ideas about diversity. Distancing behaviors include statements such as, "We don't have those kinds of problems around here," or "I don't see color," or "We've certainly come a long way in race relations/gender relations/accepting diversity." Although these statements may contain some element of truth, they're directly linked to the hard belly. These reactions protect you from feeling the intense emotions of others and genuinely connecting with their experiences. You may even recognize this pattern in yourself, but how do you move beyond that? Simple insight isn't enough.

The video, *The Color of Fear*, shows several men of different races and ethnicities who spend the weekend together discussing their experiences of themselves and others. One white man, David, consistently listened to the other men's stories with a hard-belly attitude. He rejected the legitimacy of the other's experiences, tried to convince them that racism isn't as bad as they think, and actually attempted to teach the others that being more like him would help them get along. Finally, Wah, a Chinese man who facilitated the group, quietly asked David what stops him from genuinely hearing the other men's experiences. David's reaction was startling. He began to cry, saying that if he believed the other men's stories, then he would have to face the fact that not everyone has the privileges that he has had as a white man.

As a future professional helper, you can learn from David's decision. These hard-belly behaviors do indeed protect you—not only from painful emotions but also from change and growth. You can make the commitment to engage with others authentically by being open to and respecting the reality of their experiences. The next time you feel yourself becoming rigid when encountering another person's experience, ask yourself, "What do I fear? What am I protecting myself from? What am I preventing myself from learning and experiencing?" This exploration is a vital part of your ability to be with others. In fact, it's a vital part of being an ethical practitioner. You are expected to know yourself and your own prejudices well enough to be able to practice effectively and refer appropriately.

■ ■ ■

EXERCISE 7.2 Your Hard-Belly Response
A Quiz

The American Psychological Association has adopted guidelines for therapy with lesbian, gay, and bisexual clients. You are expected to recognize how your own attitudes and knowledge about lesbian, gay, and bisexual issues influence your ability to assess and work with your clients. Let's test out your hard-belly response regarding this issue. If you are heterosexual, take the following quiz:

1. What do you think caused your heterosexuality?

2. When and how did you first decide you were a heterosexual?

3. Isn't it possible your heterosexuality is just a phase?

4. How does it feel to hear that heterosexuality doesn't offend me?

5. If you should choose to nurture children, would you want them to be heterosexual, knowing the problems they would face?

(e.g., sexism and inequality in intimate relationships; high rates of divorce)

6. Why must heterosexuals be so blatant, making a public spectacle of their heterosexuality?

7. Heterosexual marriage has total societal support, but why are there so few stable heterosexual marriages?

Did you feel the hard-belly response? If so, take time now to explore what you were protecting yourself from. What would you give up if you set aside this response?

GIVING AND RECEIVING FEEDBACK

If you don't risk anything, you risk even more.

—Erika Jong

Let's explore this idea of giving feedback to others a little further. As you can see, your psychological health and personal well-being depend greatly on the manner in which you conduct your interactions with others (Johnson, 1981). The ability to create and maintain cooperative and interdependent relationships is also fundamental to your success as a helping professional. Engaging in intimate communication with others is a personally nourishing experience, and such relationships help you become more self-aware. You can become more self-aware in two ways. The first is to listen to yourself and be sensitive to how you are feeling. The second is to seek feedback from others about how you are affecting them.

You are in a training program with other people who are very special. Like you, they recognize the value of authenticity in relationships, and they are also seeking to understand themselves better. You can help each other toward greater self-awareness—and thus greater psychological health—by engaging in truly honest discussions together. In such encounters, you not only disclose yourself to other people but you also give and receive honest and authentic feedback.

When you think about it, this may be the first time in your life when you have the opportunity to participate in such a special setting with colleagues who are acting in good faith to your benefit. Before, you may have been blind to the impressions and opinions others had of you. It is very hard to know how someone who says, "Thanks for shopping at Wal-Mart" or asks, "Do you want fries with that?" actually feels about you. Even worse, you've known people who have talked behind your back, withheld information from you, or deliberately tried to deceive you to serve their own ends. Even in some close relationships, there can be so many hidden agendas that you can't fully rely on what significant others say to you. They may not have wished to hurt your feelings, or they may have been afraid that you would stop loving them if they told you what they really thought.

So this is your chance. While you are with people who understand the value of straight talk, take advantage of the opportunity to receive honest feedback from them. It's a bit scary at first, but learning how other people see you is also quite exhilarating.

Giving Helpful Feedback

Given the right conditions, people can learn to trust that what others say to them can be accepted as given with good intentions. Such conditions need rules. Johnson (1981) suggested some guidelines for establishing a trusting environment in which feedback is helpful to you and others. We have modified these guidelines somewhat.

- Focus your feedback on the person's actions, not on his or her being.
- Describe the behavior, rather than label it. For example, if you say, "You talked a lot in today's group," rather than, "You've got diarrhea of the mouth today," the person will be less defensive, and you will still get your point across.
- Focus your feedback on descriptions rather than inferences. Instead of something like, "Just now I noticed that you were angry," you might say, "When Jane said that, your face got red and your lips narrowed." Leave the explanation of the behavior to the owner.
- Focus feedback on current happenings, rather than on history. If you say, "Last month when I said 'Hello' to you, you blew me off," the person may not remember the incident or may not be able to recall the mood of the moment. Keep your feedback as close to the "here and now" as possible.
- Share your perceptions, rather than give advice. Advice always comes across as a one-up–one-down relationship. "Shoulds," "oughts," and other admonitions always communicate that the

person is not doing it right. Advice also makes you come off as an expert on the other person's life.

- Make sure the other person is open to your feedback—don't force feedback on people. You might ask, "Would it be okay with you if I said something about that situation that has you upset?" Conversely, you don't have to take feedback from others if you don't want it at the moment. Just hold up your hand for them to stop if people are giving you more that you can process.

- Focus your feedback on something the person can change. Calling attention to the fact that someone blushes easily or that each of their eyes is a different color may be interesting to you, but it is probably not helpful. If the person does or says something that is bothersome to you, then it may be something the person can change.

- Make sure that the feedback you are giving is motivated by your desire to improve your relationship with that person rather than to "cut" the person down. Obviously, any feedback that is intentionally hurtful or vengeful is not in the proper spirit. Such feedback can destroy a trusting relationship.

- Feedback should never be given lightly. Timing is always important as well. "Excellent feedback presented at an inappropriate time may do more harm than good" (p. 25). When given in a respectful manner and received with an open mind, feedback can help each of us become more socially skillful, more self-aware, and more comfortable in the presence of others.

The Johari Window

Known Only to Self	Known to Others, Not to Self
Known to Nobody	Known to Everybody

The Johari Window, named after its originators, Joe Luft and Harry Ingham (Luft, 1969), is a way of looking at the four areas of the self.

"Known to Everybody" represents the "public self" that is known by others and ourselves. This area will be expanded as we disclose things about ourselves to others.

"Known to Others, Not to Self" is the so-called bad breath area that is unknown to us but is known by others. This area will be reduced as we encourage feedback from others, while the area of free activity in "Known to Everybody" would be increased.

"Known Only to Self" is the "avoided" or "hidden" area that we know but others do not. This area will be reduced by self-disclosure, and "Known to Everybody" will be expanded.

"Known to Nobody" is the area of "unknown activity," as it consists of material that is not known by ourselves and not known by others. According to Luft and Ingham, this area stays constant.

■ ■ ■

EXERCISE 7.3 Giving and Receiving Feedback

Briefly list four things that you would be comfortable disclosing in a training session with a colleague. These disclosures do not have to be deep, dark secrets but things about you (accomplishments, ideas you have, things about your family) that you usually would not share with anyone but a friend.

_____

_____

_____

_____

List four things that you have noticed about your training partner or significant other that you would be comfortable sharing with him or her as feedback. Even though this area is called the "bad breath" area, for the purposes of this exercise, we would like to have you offer observations that would fall into the "good breath" area, too. Remember to follow the guidelines for giving good feedback that appear earlier in the chapter and in subsequent sections.

_____

_____

_____

_____

Allow five minutes for one partner to give the other feedback. When you are finished, receivers describe what it was like for you to receive feedback in such a manner. Switch roles and repeat the exercise. Join the larger group and discuss if applicable.

■ ■ ■

AUTHENTICITY

> You don't have to be right. All you have to do is be candid.
>
> —Allen Ginsberg

All of the qualities we have been discussing are part of a concept that you will fully explore in your counseling studies—authenticity. The personal quality of authenticity is essential, not only to your relations with peers and professors but also ultimately to your work with clients as a helping professional. You probably know what authenticity means in everyday language, but as you delve deeper into your studies, you will discover that the word *authenticity* has a very specialized meaning in the helping professions.

Social Masks

To some degree, you wear a mask in your relations with others. You manage an impression of yourself that represents how you would like to be seen and that you hope others will find acceptable, likable, and appealing. Your social mask also helps you negotiate the complex demands of a variety of interpersonal encounters by making a "version" of yourself available to others. At the same time, you protect and preserve more intimate aspects of your own experience from others' view. Your social mask is very useful.

The problem with this mask is that sometimes it ends up getting stuck to you. Your mask, which should be removable for those with whom you wish to encounter closely and intimately, becomes a hindrance to deeper and more sustaining interpersonal connections. When your mask is stuck, you fail to show your authentic self to others. Carl Rogers (Kirschenbaum & Henderson, 1989) argued that to truly encounter another person means to demonstrate a sense of transparency. By transparency, he meant that you reveal your inner world of thoughts and immediate feelings.

Being and Seeming

The philosopher Martin Buber (1958) described these dimensions of interpersonal experience as the difference between "being" and "seeming." When you connect with another from the "being" dimension of yourself, your relations with others are characterized by all the qualities that we have been discussing. These qualities include immediacy, mutuality, acceptance, openness, and a willingness to access another person's inner world, while being anchored in one's own experience.

Buber believed that when persons have authentic encounters with each other, they can participate at the deepest levels of human experience. Buber described this interpersonal event as an "I-Thou" encounter during which something is created that is bigger than each of the persons. That is to say, in such a meeting, the whole is bigger than the sum of its parts. Something new and vital emerges that does not reside in either person but that exists *between* them. Buber said that this ability to "meet" another person authentically is really what defines us as human. Without it somewhere in our lives, we would live in an impoverished and shrunken interpersonal world. "All real living is meeting," Buber (1958, p. 93) said, as a testament to the importance of "I-Thou" connections with others. Carl Rogers (Kirschenbaum & Henderson, 1989) acknowledged his debt to Buber when he made a variation of this idea the cornerstone of his theoretical and therapeutic model.

In contrast to relationships grounded in "being" with others authentically, you may sometimes settle for "seeming," which is a poor substitute for a real connection. To protect you from encroachment or injury, you may develop a layer of protective shielding around your inner life. At the same time, however, your defenses also work against you by keeping you from being nourished and sustained by others at deep levels of engagement.

Of course, the needs you have for such nourishment and affiliation do not diminish just because you are unable to meet them in relationships. You still wish to be approved of, accepted by, and cared for by others. Instead of being authentic, you may seek connections by managing an impression, cultivating a "seeming" self that you present to others to gain favor and approval. Usually your "seeming" mask is successful, and you can elicit from others a response that looks accepting and approving. Unfortunately, even when you get the reaction that you are looking for, it fails to sustain or nourish you because it does not reach beyond the mask to touch your authentic self. "If Sara really knew me," you might say, "she wouldn't say such nice things about me." The self that needs that validating response is not the self that you show to others. Therefore the approval, acceptance, or praise merely bounces off the mask. Buber called this false and self-conscious presentation—the "I It" way of relating to others, because it is designed to objectify and deflect real encounters.

The greatest asset that you can bring to your studies in the helping professions is the ability to form real interpersonal relationships and connections with others. The degree to which your relationships are authentic is the degree to which you are likely to become a successful healer and helper. As you move through your program and become knowledgeable about different approaches to counseling, you will study these concepts in more depth. Do not simply learn them. Make them *come alive* for you. Examine your own assumptions, stretch your empathic abilities, celebrate diversity, and discover a new willingness to take some interpersonal risks. (What? Did you think it was just going to be multiple choice?)

IMPORTANT PEOPLE IN YOUR TRAINING

No matter what accomplishments you make,
somebody helps you.

—Althea Gibson

Always keep in mind that when you successfully complete your graduate program and launch your professional career, your professors and supervisors, as well as your fellow students and clients, go with you. Throughout your training, you will be internalizing the important and most significant others you encounter. You have already had experiences with others who have changed your life and have stayed with you through time. In fact, the constellations in your mythological sky are populated by the figures of those who have had the most profound influence on you. At this very moment, you can easily recall someone whose presence and interest in you made a difference in who you are today.

Mentors

Most myths involving journeys have the hero setting out on a quest that is a metaphor for self-discovery. The "hero cycle" goes something like this. The hero sets out with high hopes, full of confidence and courage. He or she has many adventures that test the hero's strength and determination. In the end, after many trials and tribulations, the hero prevails and discovers or achieves something of great value. Not content to selfishly possess the thing of great worth, the hero brings it back to share with the greater community (Campbell, 1973). But there is one important part to this hero cycle that we have not mentioned. That part, paradoxically, seems to be the most important, pivotal event. At some point between the idealistic outset and the return in wisdom and accomplishment, the hero gets hopelessly lost.

At this point in the story, the hero's weapons are broken, the food is gone, the horse is dead, and the reason for setting out in the first place is no longer clear. The hero is lost in an impenetrable forest, waterless desert, or endless night, or is washed up on a desolate shore. It seems as if the journey is a failure, and the hero is a goner.

But then something happens. Out of the deepest part of the forest, a person appears unexpectedly. This mysterious person never seems surprised at the arrival of the hero and possesses some knowledge or secret that is shared with the hero. Sometimes this wisdom helps the hero understand, in a new way, something the hero has always known. At other times, the guide gives the hero a new tool or weapon that the hero's courage and determination made him or her worthy to receive. The hero, fortified with new knowledge, self-understanding, and resources, eventually prevails, completing a journey that was perhaps less glamorous, but much more profound, than the one on which the hero had embarked.

Plenty of epic myths—both ancient and modern—feature mentors rescuing and guiding the lost heroes. Theseus, for example, went into the depths of the labyrinth, slew the Minotaur, and followed Ariadne's silver thread back into the light of day. Arthur had Merlin's magic to help and protect him. Luke Skywalker had crashed into a swamp, his spaceship—the horse equivalent—was nonfunctional, and he was out of options. It was then that Yoda appeared to guide his Jedi training. And when Dorothy crash-landed in Oz, she had the Good Witch to direct her to "follow the yellow brick road."

Believe it or not, your graduate school experience has a lot in common with those epic tales. You will have times of adventure, achievement, and clarity, as well as times of confusion, depletion, and indecision about which way to turn. In these bleak valleys, you may forget the reasons why you even began the journey. It's at those times that you especially need mentors and faculty members who can serve as guides for you. Of course, you can't just expect mentors to appear, as in the myths—you must cultivate relationships with them.

Seek out the help, guidance, and experience of a supervisor or professor whose values, personal qualities, research interests, or professional activities appeal to you. A mentor is someone who not only teaches you what you want to know but who is the embodiment of who you wish to become. Working closely with such a mentor who possesses the skills and knowledge you wish to acquire gives added meaning and dimension to your journey. These are lessons that you cannot learn from a book. Rather, by modeling yourself after persons who have gone before you on the adventure, you can discover the things of value that you wish to bring to your own community. When you near the end of your epic journey, you will have developed a professional identity and philosophical orientation that will represent and structure your work in the helping professions. In your undergraduate experience, you probably found that if you attended class, studied hard, and took your exams, you did pretty well. There was likely not as much opportunity—or demand—for you to become involved more directly with your professors. Fortunately, in most graduate programs, you can find faculty members who take a special interest in you. They can guide you to the kinds of experiences that stay with you long after you may have forgotten exactly the meaning of the Zeigarnik Effect (described in Chapter 5).

If you are wondering how you might connect with a faculty member whom you would like to have as a mentor, we'll let you in on a little secret. Professors, supervisors, and advisors love to work with sincerely committed, fully engaged, and curious trainees. Even mentors need to feel that what they do is meaningful and important; they like it when students want what they have to offer. Trainers of helping professionals are more than willing to really get to know you, to understand your needs and interests, and to mentor you in your journey—if you are responsive. It is enormously gratifying to professors and supervisors when they feel that their investment in and devotion to the helping professions are being passed on to their future peers. The strategy is simple—let your passion show!

Perhaps the faculty member you want to get to know seems busy, preoccupied with other projects, or simply hard to approach. That's okay. Just show how intrigued and fascinated you are by what your potential mentor is teaching, researching, or sharing. It is likely that he or she will make time for you. Then you can make the most of this opportunity to form a productive learning partnership—and a meaningful, lasting relationship.

As in the myth, someone in your graduate program is waiting for you to stumble into their forest. He or she will help you understand what it is you need to discover in yourself and to carry back with you as you continue your journey. Your mentor won't be wielding a light saber, like Obiwan Kenobi, or waving a magic wand, like the Good Witch. But your mentor, whoever he or she may be, will help you recognize and realize your unique potential.

Support Staff

We have been discussing your relationships with peers and professors. It is worth noting, however, that your program's support staff members are essential to having a successful training experience. They are often the first persons you speak with when you are in the application phase, and they help you with all the practical details of getting oriented. These staff members are typically underpaid and overworked but are truly devoted to making your experience a good one.

You would be wise to cultivate the goodwill of the program support staff. The kindness that you show them will be returned to you in many ways. Every seasoned graduate student knows that, in a practical sense, it is really the secretaries who know most about what is going on. They have the power to facilitate your progress—and to prevent it from becoming a living hell! These support persons can assist you in negotiating the various technical and bureaucratic hurdles that are an inevitable part of any training program.

As you progress through your training, regularly drop in on the program secretaries and offer them your thanks for their help and support. They are vital members of your learning community.

Significant Others

No one enters a graduate program alone. You have significant others in your life who are, in some small or large way, partners in your new undertaking. You may have been away from school for some time and have an established family or another career. If you are entering your graduate training with the support of someone important to you, the chances are that you have had many discussions about what this commitment means to your relationship. Perhaps you have to move to a new city, give up a good job, strain the family finances, or renegotiate family responsibilities. Perhaps your partner is concerned that you will not have enough time to spend on your relationship or nurturing other family members. Whatever your unique circumstances, you have had to take into account the needs, views, and feelings of important others in your life.

Graduate school often places new and unique stresses on intimate relationships. The amount of time and energy that you pour into your studies may reduce the personal resources you have to give other people in your life. How will your significant others feel about your being frequently absorbed and preoccupied with your projects? In the economics of your relationship, how will you redistribute your time, energy, and attention for your intimate connections to be preserved undamaged? Will you spend less time at the gym, with friends, or with the kids? How will you carve out a space in your life that is reserved exclusively for you and your partner to renew and nourish your love? Discuss these issues with your partner as you launch into your program. Once you begin your training, keep your "relationship antennae" up to stay sensitive to the shifts and changes in your partnership. Devise ways in which you can communicate with each other when things are getting out of whack.

Your intimate partner may not realize the degree to which he or she will be called on to adjust to and accommodate your graduate school commitments. In very real ways, your partner is taking the journey with you but may, for some time, receive less gratification from the experience than you do. After all, graduate school was probably your idea. If you are embarking on the hero's journey, your partner may be the unsung hero, the one standing in the background holding the reins of the horse while you take on the world—the Sancho Panza to your Don Quixote. Just remember—as you go tilting at windmills, you'll need your partner to celebrate your victory when it comes. Have discussions about some of the challenges you are likely to struggle with as you move into this demanding and time-consuming phase of your training.

Graduate school, especially in the helping professions, also introduces a more subtle challenge to your intimate relationships. If you truly throw yourself into the adventure of becoming a healer and a helper to others, you will also undoubtedly gain new insights into yourself and your relationships with others. These insights and experiences will dramatically change you. It's as if you have a new lens to view yourself and others. You'll look at your life differently and begin to question your values, assumptions, and motivations. As you gain understanding of individual development and family systems, you may reevaluate your own history in light of your new perspective. As you come to understand relational dynamics, you may find yourself realizing how certain themes play out in your own intimate relationships. You may begin to question your relationship's status quo and ask your partner to take into account your new perspective and feelings. You will be excited to share and apply what you are discovering with others in your life.

Without the benefit of the new lens on relationships that you have discovered, your partner will not automatically be able to share your newfound perspective. The changes you are experiencing may not be entirely welcomed by your loved ones because these changes may upset the homeostatic balance of your relationship. Your newly discovered insights may be disorienting or even threatening to your partner's sense of connection with you. The context of your program's culture that you take for granted and that makes certain interpersonal engagements possible may be unfamiliar to your family and friends. In your eagerness to share your new perspective on interpersonal dynamics, you may find yourself approaching your intimate others in the same way that you communicate with your classmates. For instance, one minute your partner may be quietly eating corn flakes and reading the paper, and the next, you're bringing up the passive-aggressive implications of hiding behind a newspaper every morning!

You want to make real what you are learning by applying new insights to your life and relationships, but this can be disruptive. People grow and change, and relationships must accommodate this change if they are to be vital and dynamic. Keep in mind, however, that one facet of empathy is to be sensitive to others' abilities to adapt to your new experiences. Your partner probably expected that you would go to graduate school, learn many new things, and later get a rewarding job. But, like it or not, that person has signed on to a program that influences you profoundly and has implications for your growth together.

We offer one last consideration for you to ponder regarding how your graduate school journey affects your intimate connections. Remember that you are gaining a new community of new friends with whom you are sharing very personal aspects of yourself and creating a new identity as a helping professional. You engage with others on a level that may have once been reserved only for your most significant others. Perhaps you're even fostering a sense of family with the people in your program and forming bonds that may last a lifetime. Although you may be including your partner in social activities outside of school, he or she may feel excluded from an area of your life that has become profoundly important to you. Your partner may have mixed feelings about your close bonds with others who are not in your usual circle of friends. Because your partner may not be involved in the helping professions, it may seem as if you are learning a foreign language and talking with others in a manner unfamiliar to your "normal" way of being with others. Remember that change is good but it can also be destabilizing. It is likely that you will need to make extra sure that you and your significant other find a new balance as your relationship seeks to keep up with the changes you experience as you become a helping professional.

SUMMARY

Have you ever had the experience of fondly remembering an event only to realize that your original experience of the event was very different from your current feelings? Our lives and the events in them involve multiple layers of meaning that are not revealed to us all at once. A sailor may battle a storm, cursing and fearing it, but later describe it almost with affection. The yarn the sailor tells is about the crashing waves, the tossing boat, the howling wind that drowns out everything else, and finally reaching calm water. Such a story is so exciting to tell and to hear because it describes a person in an extreme situation, mustering every resource to rise to the challenge. The sailor is never more fully alive, with all senses heightened, than when the challenge is the greatest.

Graduate school is a lot like surviving a storm at sea. It calls on all your talents and abilities. At times you may feel overwhelmed and challenged to the utmost. Perhaps you'll even wish that you had never left the safety of the harbor. Later, when you have reached calm water, you will recall things differently. People and events that were, at the time, simply part of the changing scene stand out as important. What you are most likely to remember are those times when you felt fully engaged, striving, connected, and open to the experience itself. At the center of this memory will be all of the traveling companions you had along the way. The most enduring, life-changing events always involve encounters with others—those who have shared some part of your life journey.

RESOURCES

Ohio State University and the American Counseling Association have a listserv for graduate-level counseling students. The Counseling Student Listserv, COUNSGRADS, is an active listserv for graduate students from across the country to communicate with one another. You can talk about classes, internships, papers, and ideas about the profession. Darcy Haag Granello, a counselor educator at Ohio State, is the list owner. Send questions about the listserv to her at *granello.1@osu.edu.* To sign up for the listserv, send an E-mail to *listserver@lists.acs.ohio-state.edu* with the following in the body of the message: subscribe counsgrads (your first name) (your last name).

The American Psychological Association of Graduate Students sponsors the Psychology Graduate Student Listserv, PSYCGRAD, a general discussion list for graduate students involved in any of the specialty areas of psychology. To subscribe to the listserv, send an E-mail to *listserv@lists.apa.org* with SUBSCRIBE PSYCGRAD (your first name) (your last name) in the body of the message. (Leave the subject line blank.)

REFERENCES

Adams, D. (2006, May). How I lost my voice and found it again. *Counseling Today, 48,* 12–13.

Buber, M. (1958). *I and thou* (R. G. Smith, Trans.). New York: Scribner's. (Original work published 1923)

Buber, M. (1988). *The knowledge of man: Selected essays.* Atlantic Highlands, NJ: Humanities Press International.

Campbell, J. (1973). *The hero with a thousand faces.* Princeton, NJ: Princeton University Press.

Hayman, J. W. (2006, April). Evolving from a racist worldview: A white woman's perspective. *Counseling Today, 48,* 41, 45.

Johnson, D. W. (1981). *Reaching out: Interpersonal effectiveness and self-actualization* (2nd ed.). Englewood Cliffs, NJ: Prentice-Hall.

Kirschenbaum, H., & Henderson, V. L. (1989). *Carl Rogers: Dialogues.* Boston: Houghton Mifflin.

Kohut, H. (1971). *The analysis of self.* New York: International Universities Press.

Luft, J. (1969). *Of human interaction.* Palo Alto, CA: National Press Books.

Matthews, M. (2005, December). Counselor know thyself: Education about intimate abuse. *Counseling Today, 47,* 7, 35.

Natterson, J., & Friedman, R. (1995). *A primer of clinical intersubjectivity.* Northvale, NJ: Aronson.

Stern, D. N. (1988). The dialectic between the "interpersonal" and the "intrapsychic": With particular emphasis on the role of memory and representation. *Psychoanalytic Inquiries, 8,* 241–250.

Stolorow, R. D., & Atwood, G. (1992). *Contexts of being: The intersubjective foundations of psychological life.* Hillsdale, NJ: Analytic Press.

Stolorow, R. D., Brandchaft, B., & Atwood, G. (1987). *Psychoanalytic treatment: An intersubjective approach.* Hillsdale, NJ: Analytic Press.

Wah, L. M. (Producer). (1994). *The color of fear* [Videorecording]. Berkeley, CA: Stir-Fry Productions.

CHAPTER 8

Thriving in Your Practicum and Internship

Until you are willing to be confused about what
you already know, what you know will never grow
bigger, better, or more useful.

—Milton Erickson

As any traveler knows, preparing for a trip and actually taking one are two very different experiences. Your coursework in counseling and therapy has prepared you well, and now you have the opportunity to put your skills into action with real clients. Your practicum and internship represent the next steps of your journey to become a full-fledged helping professional.

As you embark on these experiences, you may want to look into your training backpack again—just to double-check that you have all you need. At first, you may not see anything that appears useful. You may have overpacked with a lot of "just in case" items that now do not seem very helpful. Or you may feel as though you have left behind some important tools and valuable supplies. In either case, you will want to take time to reflect on your preparedness, review the knowledge and skills you bring to this experience, and take stock of your readiness.

When you are poised to begin counseling with actual clients, the responsibilities and complexities of clinical practice can seem overwhelming. In this chapter, we offer practical information and concrete suggestions for completing a practicum or internship. We also invite you to thrive in these settings by creating a secure base from which to venture out, take risks, and grow.

219

YOU ARE READY, ALTHOUGH
YOU MAY HAVE DOUBTS

We are the hurdles we leap.

—Michael McClure

During your practicum, you will face predicaments that challenge your sense of readiness. These dilemmas will come in a variety of shapes and sizes and will, in fact, continue to confront you throughout your internship. That's the point—these training experiences are demanding because you must be prepared to enter the challenging profession of counseling and therapy. Of course, your practicum and internship have other purposes. At these training sites, you will have plenty of opportunities to try out intervention approaches to see what fits your personal style and professional aspirations. While experimenting with different perspectives and techniques, however, you may be faced with issues of "fitting in" as a professional. And even though you will most likely be successful, you may sometimes feel as though you are playing a part or acting—rather than actually being yourself.

Along the way, it's also likely that you will encounter people— (besides yourself, of course!) who will question your abilities and decisions. For example, if you are a practicum student in school counseling, a parent may confront you with questions such as, "What do you know about children?" and "Are you a parent?" If you are a young intern, some client will be sure to ask, "How old are you?" If you are an intern at a substance abuse treatment center, clients may want to know if you're in recovery. Although no one looks forward to being questioned and confronted, you will quickly realize how exciting it can be to think on your feet and make some discoveries about yourself in the process.

You may think that because you are dealing with "real world" clients you should possess more skills and knowledge than you do. But give yourself a break. You have not been at this for very long. You are, after all, there to learn.

Someone has said that counselors and therapists—no matter how many years of experience they may have—are always guilty of not being good enough. This adage is even truer for your professors and supervisors. We must be willing to work constantly at improving ourselves and yet also be forgiving of ourselves for not being farther along than we are. Keep your expectations of yourself reasonable, and when someone implies that you should be older, wiser, or more skilled, don't feel as if you have been "found out."

▲▲▲

How Old Are You?
Grace's Story

THE FIRST CLIENT I ever saw during my master's program was a woman in her mid-thirties. I can still remember how nervous and excited I was to be actually working with a real live client! Although I felt relatively prepared for this first encounter, her first question for me threw me for a loop. After reciting my well-rehearsed informed-consent speech, I asked her if she had any questions before we started. Without hesitation, she asked, "How old are you?"

It was a simple question, and it would have been a simple answer if I had been anywhere but in my first counseling session with my first real client. I was flustered. I felt as though she saw right through me and wanted to expose my lack of experience. I tried to gain my composure and decided to fall back on the classic evasive maneuver that counselors resort to in a pinch.

I asked, "I find it interesting that you want to know how old I am. How is that important to you?" I hoped that would suffice! Surely this redirection would prove my professional competence. I was wrong. She was neither impressed nor satisfied with the reply and responded, "You just look so young!"

I somehow managed not to answer the question and steered her off the topic. Much to my surprise, the following week's session started off in an equally unsettling way. Though I hoped that she didn't have any more "bombs" to throw at me, when I asked her where she would like to begin, she said, "Since you never answered my question last week, I'll ask it again. How old are you?"

Off balance, without another counseling cliché, I meekly confessed, "Twenty-two." I felt as if I were raising a white flag in defeat.

After a pregnant pause—which I'm sure was not as long as it felt—she replied with an offhanded "Oh." She did not get up and leave. She did not laugh. She did not have a look of horror on her face. All along, I feared that she needed qualities that I did not possess. Much to my surprise, all she really wanted was honesty.

▼▼▼

Like Grace, you will find yourself making valuable discoveries about clients, the helping process, and yourself. You'll be developing a conceptual framework that makes sense to you, that works for you in helping relationships, and that allows you to be yourself. Your practicum and internship experiences are special times in your training when you can consolidate everything you learned in your classes—and everything you've learned about your own personhood. A theory is only as good as the person practicing it. Explore how you can bring your theory to life by making it your own.

YOUR PRACTICUM

> The great end of life is not knowledge but action.
>
> —T. H. Huxley

The practicum is your first hands-on learning opportunity to work with actual clients. The services you will be providing may include assessment, counseling, therapy, crisis intervention, consultation, education, and promotion of growth. Although the number of hours required for a practicum depends on your training program, you will likely be providing counseling and therapy services to individuals, groups, couples, and families. Your practicum is also your first hands-on experience working agency staff, supervisors, and administrators. Although most students have a generally positive experience at their practicum sites, a large minority have confronted serious misunderstandings and other problems. One survey of 321 students' practicum experiences found that 22% had much less supervision that they had expected and more than 34% had significantly less client contact than expected (Gross, 2005). Despite these problems, many students told no one about them, not even their friends and peers. Although such situations are unnerving and distressing, keep in mind that they give you invaluable opportunities to learn how to address these issues quickly, professionally, and productively.

Your practicum is the first bridge that connects the knowledge you've acquired in courses to the practical situations you'll face in the real world. At times, this bridge may seem long, high, and precarious. To cross it, you might avoid looking down, take a deep breath, and keep your eyes fixed on your destination ahead. You may even occasionally fear that if you venture a look to the left or to the right, you'll feel dizzy or off balance. In other words, you may fear trying new things or making mistakes. At these times, you can remind yourself that you're not alone. You have an instructor, supervisor, colleagues, and staff to guide, support, and help you along. Just remember, not only does this bridge help you reach your destination, but it also provides a terrific view!

Accommodating to Your Practicum

As you begin your practicum, you'll need to keep a couple of points in mind: First, most sites have a dual mission of serving clients and providing a training ground for those entering the helping professions. Therefore, you may need to make significant accommodations, especially at first, as you become oriented to the schedule and demands of the site. Clients, for example, may need to be seen at times that do not fit conveniently into your lifestyle.

The second point is that as a representative of your program, you will want to present yourself in a professionally appropriate manner. For instance, in your classes, you may have found that students, as well as faculty members, dress very casually. Your practicum site, on the other hand, is a different culture. You'll want to fit in and meet the site's expectations of how a professional should look and act. It's not that difficult to figure out. Ask questions, observe, and don't forget the old saying, "When in Rome, do as the Romans do."

▲▲▲

Pipe Dreams
Lennie's Story

EVEN THOUGH it was more than 30 years ago, I still remember vividly how insecure and unprepared my fellow students and I felt as we started our practicum course. To make matters worse, our professor looked like he had been chosen by central casting to play the role of the experienced and wise therapist. He was middle-aged, with distinguished graying hair, and was impeccably dressed in suit and tie, and, most importantly, he smoked a pipe. Now keep in mind that my training was back in the days when there were no restrictions on smoking in offices and classrooms. Many professors and graduate students smoked cigarettes during classes, meetings, and counseling sessions. A pipe, however, was considered a cultural icon of authority and wisdom.

One evening, when we were behind a one-way mirror watching our professor conduct a group session, I was entranced by how he used his pipe as a counseling tool. On one occasion, he pointed with his pipe stem to indicate the interpersonal dynamics between two members. Another time, while packing his pipe bowl with tobacco, he began a compelling commentary, "Well, the real issue that this group is struggling with is . . ." Then, when he had everyone's rapt attention, he paused dramatically to light his pipe and take a few puffs before finally finishing his pronouncement. I can't remember what he said, but it sounded really profound! The other male students in my practicum immediately took up smoking pipes. As a nonsmoker, I truly felt disadvantaged in my counseling because I couldn't use that talisman of insight and sagacity.

▼▼▼

Your practicum will challenge you in unexpected ways. At times, you may feel aggravated, insecure, and uncertain. Entering the subjective world of your clients and participating in this deep level of engagement will expose you to troubling events and disturbing circumstances. You may find it painful to deal with clients who are poor, drug addicted, or sexually abused. These encounters will provoke you emotionally and perhaps even disorient you at times.

Clients are not the only ones who will be stirring up your emotions. Staff members at your site may intimidate you because they seem so competent and knowledgeable. You may doubt that you'll ever reach their level of professionalism. At times, the staff may also appear to you as less than caring in how they deal with clients. And no matter how supportive your supervisor may be, your sessions with him or her will bring up issues that will be challenging and perturbing. Many of these encounters with clients, colleagues, and supervisors have the potential to leave you reeling and confused.

At some time during your practicum or internship, you may even wonder if you're cut out for this line of work. When you have these doubts, use your journal to explore your concerns and take time to reflect on their meaning. Talk to your supervisor and friends. What's important is not to ignore your doubts but to use them to seek deeper answers. After all, you will regularly face such "crises of faith" throughout your career. You'll be surprised how you can emerge from such an experience a stronger and more resilient counseling professional. In fact, graduate students with extensive practicum experiences have a much clearer idea of their vocational preference than those with no practicum training (Carless & Prodan, 2003).

Taking Pictures Along the Way

Many programs will use video recordings of your counseling and therapy sessions to help you refine your skills. If you are like most people, you may feel self-conscious and embarrassed watching yourself alone. However, watching these sessions with a supervisor, professor, or fellow student can produce real terror! Of course, you're not in the only one who feels this way. But over time, you will discover how valuable it can be to revisit your sessions, both by yourself and with others.

Videos are wonderful tools for exploring, discovering, and refining your skills. Because a practicum is so busy and hectic, you may be tempted to fast-forward through a session before you have mined the video for all its treasures. Baird (2004) recommended that you return to your video recordings several times to see them from different perspectives. Each time you review a session, you will notice elements that had not been apparent to you while you were participating in it. You can focus on the subtle nuances of phrases, emotional shadings, and minute gestures that offer a more textured and vivid understanding of the dynamics and themes of your therapeutic relationship.

With each encounter, ask yourself, "What do I experience now as I focus on this element of the interaction?" Also ask yourself, "If I could do this session over again, what would I do that would be different?" This question will help you think about how to conduct the next session with your client and will increase your general knowledge of how to make future sessions more productive. Involving yourself fully in the process can help you get the most from your experience.

▲▲▲

Sometimes the Therapist Learns More Than the Client
Jane's Story

MY FIRST practicum assignment in graduate school was in an inner-city agency that worked with low-income clients. I was really excited when I heard my first client was ready for me. But was I ready for my first client? My actual involvement with therapy was strictly what I had acquired in my own reading. I hadn't taken any formal therapy coursework prior to being thrown into the deep end of the pool. But I assumed that my supervisor knew what he was doing, so I reported at the scheduled time.

My client turned out to be a soft-spoken, moderately depressed young woman who complained about a conflictual, unsatisfying marriage. She detailed a fight she had with her husband about access to the only key to their house. We discussed some options that she might have to reduce the tension, including getting copies of the key made. She left my office feeling some optimism about ways to assert herself in their relationship.

In our next session, the client returned to my office covered with bruises and scrapes. What had once been only verbal abuse between them had turned into physical abuse. There was an ominous sense that something much worse was possible.

By the second therapy hour, I had already learned some very valuable lessons. Therapy is not advice. Human systems are complex; tinkering can produce unexpected results. Clients can be very forgiving. Sometimes the therapist learns more than the client does.

▼▼▼

INTERNSHIP

First to know, then to act, then to really know.

—Bishr al Hafifi

As we described in Chapter 2, during the final stage of your training, you participate in an internship that serves as a capstone of your training. During that time you undergo a major transformation. Your internship experience involves a change in your self-concept—you enter as a trainee and you leave as a professional.

One of our counseling colleagues, John, remembers the moment during his internship when his self-concept was suddenly reframed. After a particularly stressful day in the clinic where he was doing his internship, John went to a local restaurant for dinner. He struck up a conversation with a server who asked him, "What do you do?"

Without thinking, John replied, "I'm a counselor." Immediately, he felt a rush of pride and thought to himself, "I really *am* a counselor!"

John recalled how wonderful it was to consider himself in this new way—as a counselor. Almost imperceptibly, he had metamorphosed into a new person. As a result of your internship experience, you will also find yourself developing a new identity. You really will be a helping professional.

Choosing a Site

Internship sites include community mental health centers, counseling agencies, programs for survivors of sexual assault, university counseling centers, and elementary, middle, and high schools. The counseling services you will be offering within these settings might include assessment, as well as individual, group, family or couples counseling; emergency or crisis intervention; outreach, consultation, and education programs; and prevention activities.

Training programs use a variety of methods for making decisions about internship placements. In your program, you may be responsible for contacting sites and finding your own placement. In other programs, faculty members take responsibility for placing you while considering your interests, goals, and skills. In most situations, you have input into the placement decision (Simon, 1999).

When you explore your internship placement options, you'll want to consider the services offered at that agency, its client population, reputation, location, and, most important, the quality of supervision offered. According to Kiser (2000), the heart of your internship is the supervision you receive. Ask yourself this fundamental question about a possible supervisor: "Is this someone I think I can work with and who would be interested in helping me learn?" (Kiser, 2000, p. 5). Because selecting a field placement will be one of the more important training choices you must make, do not take the decision lightly.

EXERCISE 8.1 Refreshing Your Memory and Plotting Your Course
A Decision-Making Exercise

Gather all the materials you have from all the classes you have taken so far—handouts, textbooks, notes, counseling and therapy recordings, journals, and papers you have written. Mariners have used the stars to navigate their courses since ancient times, so as you revisit each class, put a star by an activity you really liked—a written passage you found particularly meaningful, a microcounseling segment in which you excelled. Be careful not to let any preconceived notions get in your way. Pretend you are lost and are searching for directions. Even if you think you have a pretty good idea of where you are headed, completing this activity will be a good test of your reckoning.

Now go back through everything, and see how your stars line up. Then converge on one or two clusters of common themes. You can use these clusters to chart your internship course.

Writing an Internship Agreement

Once you have located an internship site and have spoken with a helping professional who has agreed to supervise, you are now ready to formalize your relationship. Your training program will develop an agreement about what the internship is to include. Two types of agreements should be created before you begin an internship. The first is a written agreement between your academic institution and the internship site. Next, together with your program instructor and on-site supervisor, you should formulate an agreement that describes the specific details of your individual internship experience. Establishing such agreements in writing at the outset will help avoid any misunderstanding or confusion about what the internship site and supervisor expect of you and what you expect of them.

Because no two internships or academic programs are identical, there is no single model for institutional agreements. They do have, however, a number of common ingredients (Faiver, Eisengart, & Colonna, 2004). Gelman (1990) identified four types of training agreements. These can range from what he described as "friendly" agreements that are not legalistic to a more technical agreement that focuses on avoiding liability. Cooperative/joint agreements include the mutual benefits and responsibilities of the academic institution, student, and field placement.

Professional Liability Insurance

Being a student does not protect you from being sued. You need protection from the financial devastation that you could face in a lawsuit. Even if your program does not require it, we strongly advise you to obtain your own professional liability insurance. Both the American Psychological Association and the American Counseling Association have professional liability insurance for graduate students. You will need to join the organization as a student member, but the application process is simple, and the insurance rates are reasonable. In the "Resources" section at the end of this chapter, you will find contact information for both organizations.

Adhering to Ethics Codes

Competence The first and most important principle of most codes of ethics is to operate within one's level of competence. Pope and Brown (1996) pointed out that the work you will be doing requires both "intellectual" and "emotional" competence. Recall from Chapter 5 that you think with both your head and your heart. Intellectual competence refers to knowledge and skill, but emotional competence refers to your ability to manage the emotional challenges of working with clients.

No counselor is competent to work with every client or problem. You may find that certain clients "push your buttons" or overwhelm you. Don't try to fake it. Consult your supervisor and talk about those feelings. You will not be expected to work effectively with everyone. Furthermore, burnout, stress, family problems, and personal matters can impair your performance, regardless of your intellectual or technical ability. You can't take care of your clients unless you can take care of yourself.

Informed Consent Another important ethical principle is informed consent. Clients have a right to be informed about the treatment, assessment, or other services they will receive before they agree to them. To ensure informed consent, you must present the information in a manner and language that clients can comprehend. At a minimum, inform your clients about each of the following subjects (Harris, 1995):

- **Qualifications.** Clients should know that you are an intern and will be supervised. You should also explain your educational and training background.
- **Supervision.** Clients should be given the name and qualifications of your supervisor, should have an opportunity to meet with your supervisor if they desire to do so, and should know how they can contact your supervisor if they have any questions or concerns in the future. Your clients should understand the nature of your supervision, including the frequency of supervision and the activities involved (e.g., reviewing case notes, listening to tapes of sessions).
- **Services.** Your clients should be apprised of the nature of the counseling or assessment to be provided, including a brief description of the approach to treatment or the purpose of an assessment and the instruments that will be used. The frequency and duration of treatment sessions and a reasonable estimate of the typical number of sessions involved to address an issue should also be discussed.
- **Client responsibilities.** The client is expected to attend scheduled appointments, to notify you in advance to cancel or change an appointment, and to follow through with any therapeutic assignments.
- **Fees.** Information should include the costs for services and whether or not there are charges for missed sessions. Your client should understand how and when to make payments, as well as the procedures followed if payment is not made. Your discussion should also cover how insurance provider contacts will be managed and how this relationship affects confidentiality. If a client's insurance policy limits the number of sessions the insurance company will pay for, an agreement must be reached

about how to proceed if more sessions are needed and the
client is unable to pay without the assistance of the insurance.

- **Confidentiality.** The nature and limitations of confidentiality, including what is said in treatment, as well as what is contained in the client's records, should be included.
- **Questions.** You should encourage your client to ask questions at any time.

Confidentiality Confidentiality is the principle that clients have the right to determine who will have access to information about them and their treatment. In clinical settings, clients need to feel that the information they share will stay with you and not be released without their permission. Without this assurance, your clients are less likely to explore and express their thoughts and feelings freely. Such a situation might possibly make the client less willing to share certain information and may distort the treatment process (Nowell & Spruill, 1993). It is important to keep in mind the five situations in which absolute confidentiality does not hold and in which information must be shared. These exceptions are (1) dangerousness to self, (2) intent to harm others, (3) legal proceedings, (4) court orders, and (5) insurance company inquiries. Be sure to let your clients know the limits of confidentiality before they share personal information with you.

Putting It All Together

Most agencies and schools probably have photocopies of an informed-consent document that they give to their clients as soon as they walk in the door. Clients are supposed to read, sign, and date the document to indicate they completely understand everything they just read. Right!

When most of us are given a legal document that begins, "Whereas the party of the first part, heretofore known as the . . . ," our eyes glaze over as we search the page for some clue as to the meaning of what we are about to sign. Nevertheless, before they can enter into a therapeutic relationship, clients have to understand their rights and responsibilities. In most cases, the job of informing a client falls on the counselor.

Before each flight, every airplane pilot is required to perform a pre-flight check. A detailed list of "must do" procedures is performed and checked off before the aircraft enters the runway. Similarly, you need to be sure your client understands the essentials before the first session begins. Let's tune in as Eduardo, a counseling intern, is beginning the first session with his client.

Counselor: Before we get started, there are a few things I'd like to discuss with you. You've probably heard the term "informed consent" before, right?

Client: Yes, I think so.

Counselor: You have heard of it, good. As you know, "informed consent" means you have a right to know everything about the services you will receive here at the counseling center. We go through this procedure with everyone who comes to the center. It is the policy of the counseling center and our ethical responsibilities as service providers. Speaking of responsibilities, you and I also have responsibilities in our work together. I'll go over mine first, then yours, and then we can discuss anything you may have questions about. How does that sound?

Client: All right, I guess.

Counselor: There are quite a few things we have to cover, so I'll be using this checklist to make sure I don't leave anything out. First off, as you know, my name is Eduardo and I'm a graduate student in the school of psychology at the university. I have been working as a counseling intern since September, and I'll continue working here until summer. Because I'm still in training, I am being supervised by two licensed professional counselors. One is on the staff here at the counseling center and the other is my professor at the university. I meet with them both at least once a week, and I confer with them about my clients. Sometimes I show a recording of a counseling session. Both of my supervisors' phone numbers are on this sheet I'll give you so you can talk to them any time you want about any concerns you have about our work together. Okay so far?

Client: Okay, I guess

Counselor: Good. In addition to my two supervisors, two other graduate students will view the recordings and . . .

Client: Oh, great, that's all I need. Now everybody in town will think I'm a weirdo.

Counselor: Don't worry—they are mostly focusing on my counseling style and giving me feedback about my skills rather than sitting around analyzing every word you say. Plus, you are protected by confidentiality. I know you have heard that term also, but let's talk about it again, just to make sure. Essentially what confidentiality means is that you have a right to say anything you want to say in our sessions without having to worry about it being repeated.

What is said in this room stays in this room except for a couple of exceptions.

We have already discussed my supervisors and my classmates at the university watching recordings of sessions. In addition, if someone I'm counseling tells me that he or she plans to hurt himself or herself or someone else, I have to report that to my supervisors and to the proper authorities. Also, if I am subpoenaed by the courts or a client's insurance company, the confidentiality of our counseling relationship may no longer apply.

Client: So as long as I don't threaten to hurt myself or someone else, get in trouble with the law or with the insurance company, everything will be okay.

Counselor: Yes, that's right. We were told that it is standard practice pretty much all across the country.

Client: What else?

We aren't going to go through everything that needs to be covered in dialogue form, but we encourage you to develop your own "preflight checklist" for your site. Feel free to use what we've presented here as a guideline.

Taking the High Road

> In matters of style, swim with the current; in
> matters of principle, stand like a rock.
>
> —Thomas Jefferson

The Principles of Ethical Conduct As we discussed in Chapter 1, the sixth principle of thriving in your training is to always take the high road. To succeed as an intern, you need to practice the highest values every single day. Ethical conduct requires more than having good intentions and merely "following the rules." You will need to have a thorough understanding of the ethical standards that serve as the guiding principles for professional conduct (American Counseling Association [ACA], 2005); American Psychological Association [APA], 2002). Both the ACA and APA codes are included in the appendixes of this book. Accepted ethical standards help you structure the counseling relationship, place boundaries on its activities, and define aspects of its character that help you to promote client welfare.

Understanding your own values becomes especially important to your conduct as a professional when you confront ethical problems in an ambiguous situation that require you to interpret or apply ethical principles. Being ethical involves learning to make moral decisions based on criteria that emerge from the goals and context of the helping relationship. As you read through the ACA and APA ethical guidelines, you will notice that they constitute a body of regulations and rules that you are expected to apply in your work with clients. But they do not apply to all situations. You must become an ethical person who can make judgments that will benefit your clients and remain within the general ethical guidelines for counselors.

Dual Roles An important ethical consideration is avoiding a dual role with clients. This means that you should not provide professional services for someone with whom you have another, nontherapeutic relationship that might interfere with your ability to function effectively in a therapeutic situation. For example, according to the guidelines, it is unethical for you to provide counseling services to someone whom you employ. This employee may be your tax accountant or secretary or anyone with whom you have an ongoing relationship based on provision of goods or services. In relation to this person, you would assume a dual role because you interact with him or her in a specific context unrelated to the goals of your professional "helping" role. It is easy to see how this outside relationship, involving the exchange of money, the expectation of quality labor, the clear structure of power, and the difference in function of each of the persons involved can undermine the intent of a separate helping relationship.

Consider, however, a slightly different scenario that is not so clear-cut. Suppose you are one of only three mental-health professionals living in a small town. Your son's seventh-grade history teacher seeks your help with her problems with depression. You have expertise in this area, and she says she would feel comfortable with you as her therapist. In making a decision about whether to accept this client, you must evaluate the situation in light of the ethical guidelines on dual relationships but also take into account other relevant information in making a moral decision.

For instance, can you refer her to someone else who has similar expertise, or will she go without services otherwise? How acute is her need for intervention? How much contact are you likely to have with the teacher regarding your son? How might unforeseen events, such as after-hours emergencies or a hospitalization, influence whether the relationship is contained in the counseling sessions? What effect might these potential complications have on the teacher-parent relationship?

These are the kinds of questions that you need to consider when the ethical issue falls in the gray area of decision making. Therapists in very small towns frequently face these sorts of ethical dilemmas, and they quickly understand that ethical questions are often complicated and usually involve more than a "cut and dried" application of rules. As an aside, the good news about avoiding dual relationships is that, should your family and friends seek counseling from you because of your professional training, you can tell them that your ethics prevent you from being their counselor—and you are off the hook!

As you can see, to be an ethical practitioner, you cannot simply rely on "going by the book" without examining the values that influence how you apply accepted ethical standards. In the preceding scenario, it may be unethical *not* to accept the teacher as a client, at least temporarily, especially if she's depressed enough that serious harm may result in her not receiving services promptly. The application of ethics requires you to examine your own values. It is a vital part of knowing yourself as a person and a professional and understanding the process by which you interpret information in making moral decisions. A developed sense of moral reasoning, especially in ambiguous situations, is essential to becoming a truly ethical professional.

Handling Ethical Dilemmas Philosophers and thinkers who are working to understand how persons may distinguish between what is morally right and what is wrong have long since been interested in ethical theory. According to Aristotle, the ancient Greek philosopher, moral virtues are character states that pertain to rational control and direction of emotions (Cohen & Cohen, 1999). Recent discoveries in neuroscience have, however, suggested that good social judgment depends as much on emotion as on reason (Damasio, 1994). Sometimes you have to rely on your gut feelings in situations that pose ethical dilemmas. Ethics depend on both head and heart. Examine the situation carefully, explore your motives, and be aware of your emotions. Taking time to reflect on your choices and staying committed to developing your personal character can also help you form an ethical worldview.

Because of your desire to help others, you are way ahead of the game. Our greatest reference points are the principles that form the basis of the therapeutic relationship itself. When you choose actions that best honor and actualize the goals of the counseling relationship, then you remain faithful to an important set of organizing concepts that define ethical values. Thus your choices are based on values that reflect your use of your skills to foster growth and to communicate respect and acceptance of the person. Authenticity of expression, responsibility in actions, and courage to change become guiding principles when making ethical decisions. Fostering well-being and advancing the best

interests of clients become touchstones for structuring your interventions and making your decisions. Although your goals may be clear,
putting them into practice is often complex.

▲▲▲

Eric's Story

WHILE I WAS a practicum student, I counseled a man seeking
help for depression. In the course of treatment, the man
revealed that, though he was married with two children, he
engaged in unprotected heterosexual and homosexual activities
with many partners. This client learned that one of his frequent
homosexual partners had recently tested HIV-positive. The client
had not informed his wife of his secret life, nor of his own HIV
status. He continued to have unprotected sex with his wife. When
I encouraged him to get tested for HIV, he declined, saying he did
not want to know, though he felt guilty about his wife's potential
exposure. When asked whether he was willing to discuss these
issues with his wife, he protested, saying that she would leave him,
take his children away, and ruin him financially.

▼▼▼

Clearly, the ethical dilemma in this case is between maintaining
client confidentiality or invoking the principle that states that when a
client is a serious threat to him- or herself or others, confidentiality may
be breached. To keep client confidentiality may result in significant
harm to a third party. At the time, the legal precedents relevant to such
cases did not encourage informing a third party if a sexually transmitted
disease were the only identifiable indicator of harm. The case illustrates
that sometimes what is law and what is ethical may be in opposition.
Provisions by the ACA (2005) include a "Contagious Diseases, Life-
Threatening" clause that allows disclosure in some cases.

In this case, if the counselor had instantly broken confidentiality, the
client would have left therapy feeling betrayed, and the therapist's ability to influence the situation would have been lost. The client would
continue to have unprotected sex with other partners who would also
be at risk. On the other hand, even though the HIV status of the client

was undetermined, the counselor felt compelled to protect a third party from potential harm out of an ethical duty that transcended his relationship with the client.

Drawing on the principles discussed earlier, the counselor resolved to change the course of the therapy to address this central issue. First, the counselor secured an agreement from the client to cease sexual relations with his wife until the problem could be explored in therapy or until the client was tested. The client agreed to this provisional arrangement. The counselor concentrated on helping the client take responsibility for his choices, to be honest and authentic in his communications both inside and outside of the counseling room, and to rigorously examine the issues that led to such passive-aggressive behavior toward his wife and others. The frequency of sessions was increased, and within weeks of the initial discussion, with the strong support of the therapist, the client invited his wife to one of the sessions and disclosed the truth to her. He tested positive for HIV (his wife tested negative), and the couple divorced. The client continued to pursue therapy and to examine his sexual choices in regard to his HIV status, choosing to take more responsibility for protecting others. The client's wife was assisted in finding a counselor for herself as she sought to put her life back together.

Obviously, sometimes there are no happy endings, even when the counselor takes a proactive ethical stance. Cohen and Cohen (1999) provide a five-stage framework for conceptualizing and resolving ethical dilemmas. The following suggestions may be helpful to you as a template for resolving ambiguous situations.

- **Defining the moral problem.** The first stage involves identifying and defining the moral problem. How are the needs, interests, or welfare of the client or others threatened? The problem may be an intellectual one, such as "What should I think or believe?" The problem usually involves a practical question, such as "What should I do?" Defining these issues requires a developed moral sensitivity, insight, and awareness.

  In the preceding example, the counselor, rather than coercing the client, temporarily "stood in" for the client's lack of sensitivity by protecting the welfare of others. He emphasized the nature and scope of the moral problem by raising the central issue of responsibility for choices, a fundamental principle of the counseling relationship.

- **Identifying morally relevant facts.** The second stage focuses on identifying the morally relevant facts. How will the welfare of the client or others be affected by any decision? Morally relevant facts include such variables as the likelihood of suicide, test results from a medical examination, or history of violent behavior. In other words, what real factors impinge on the process of choosing a course of action?

- **Analyzing the issue.** This information gathering leads to the third stage, which is to analyze the issue philosophically in light of all the morally relevant facts. Facts by themselves are insufficient to reach an ethical outcome. The goal is to clarify key organizing moral principles. Examining values, reflecting on effects of choices, exploring frames of reference, and meaning-making help formulate an ethical principle. This principle should center on mitigating harm and promoting the welfare of all involved. As shown in the preceding vignette, the counselor's ethical action may have protected all parties from injury or pain.

- **Reaching a decision.** The fourth stage involves reaching a decision that is reasonable in light of the philosophical analysis. In that vignette, the client refused initially to seek medical testing or to address with his wife the issue of his hidden life. He was making a decision by not making a decision. If the counselor had gone along with the client's denial and procrastination, then the counselor would have colluded with the client in this avoidance behavior. The counselor reached a decision to address the moral issue through the therapeutic process only after securing from the client agreements that satisfied the counselor's imperative to protect the third party.

- **Acting ethically.** The fifth stage concerns putting the decision into action. For the counselor whose moral compass is responsive and accurate, implementation is often the hardest part of ethical functioning. For instance, most helping professionals eventually encounter a situation in which their client is at risk of harming himself or herself. The intensity and timing of intervention in such cases is often not clear. Deciding to break confidentiality or hospitalize clients for their own protection—and against their will—may severely or irreparably damage the therapeutic bond. Not to act in such instances, however, may also have harmful consequences.

Ethical conduct involves many other issues that are delineated in the codes. These principles include practicing within your scope of expertise, being sensitive to cultural differences, obtaining informed consent, and the nonsexual nature of the counselor-client relationship. The codes also address more practical matters, such as advertising, fees, bartering, and record keeping. Learn these ethical guidelines well. But remember that you must seek to implement them wisely, in consultation with your supervisor, keeping in mind the welfare of those who have sought your help and counsel.

Making Rest Stops Along the Way

In addition to performing your duties at your internship site, you will participate in weekly supervision sessions and may meet regularly with other interns. The internship class provides opportunities to share your experiences, explore the many opportunities for your professional development, look at your counseling work, learn from one another, clarify your professional goals, and help everyone to achieve those goals. It is also the time for support and encouragement among your peers—a designated time for you to "fill up your tank" so you can continue on the journey. Reflecting on the internship experience, students have commented that they "didn't feel so isolated and alone after talking with other interns." Others described the experience as a "support system that cheered" them on throughout the semester.

▲▲▲

Nathaniel's Story

WAS SEEING my first family in my practicum experience. In they trooped: father, mother, daughter. Then another woman came in who was introduced as an aunt. "What's she doing here?" I wondered. "Is this okay?" I was thinking about confidentiality and consent and trying to figure out what kind of family this was! Pretty soon, I found out. The mother was on "house arrest." She wore an ankle monitor and was allowed to leave her house only for work and counseling. The aunt was with us in the session because she had assumed primary caretaking responsibilities while the family was adjusting to Mom's situation. The father seemed stunned. He reported that he and his wife had been fighting frequently. The daughter was bright and hopeful, but I was uncomfortable with the banter and teasing that went on between her and her mother.

"These poor people," I thought with sympathy. "They have no money and this is their lifestyle. They probably don't know any better." As I listened to their stories, I judged every one of them. I remember vividly how I left the session shaking my head and telling my supervisor there was little potential for progress with this "family."

My supervisor seemed confused. What was the evidence for my gloomy prognosis? The entire family had come in, all expressing dissatisfaction with their current situation. Everyone present claimed a desire to work on the problem. What obstacles did I see to their progress and growth in counseling? I fumbled for words. "Well, you know, they're . . . Well, it seems limited." My supervisor looked at me inquisitively, patiently, and silently. Those were the longest few minutes of my life. It seemed as though my supervisor could see and hear every stereotype and prejudice that I had ever had. Furthermore, I started to suspect that I had been equally transparent to my clients.

My face began to feel as if it were on fire, and believe it or not, I started to get teary-eyed. I was so unprepared to face the ugly stuff that lies within me that I had avoided it until that moment. When it came, it came in a rush. I had always believed that prejudice was a given in our lives, and that I was in touch enough with my own "stuff" that it wouldn't interfere with my work. I was wrong. My supervision helped during that time, as did my own counseling. I've also come to appreciate the need to continually check on my own attitudes and beliefs and be responsible for my own growth. Even if prejudices are a given, that doesn't mean I have to be satisfied with my own.

▼▼▼

You may believe that you've effectively confronted your prejudices, only to be smacked in the face with a nasty reminder of old messages and beliefs that you learned as a child. Facing your prejudices and stereotypes can be painful and make you feel guilty. If you avoid doing so, however, you're bound to find yourself feeling like Nathaniel—ashamed and disappointed. Take time now, before you enter your practicum or internship, to again examine your own beliefs and attitudes about difference. Recognize that guilt is the great silencer, and don't let it stop you from being honest right now.

EXERCISE 8.2 **First Thoughts**
An Exploratory Exercise

Consider the following groups of people. Read through the list and write down the first thoughts that come to your head. Don't censor yourself. Just describe your thoughts. Now, imagine what might go through your mind if you were to counsel a member from each group.

Men

_____

_____

Sex abusers

_____

_____

Elderly

_____

_____

Athletes

_____

_____

Women

_____

_____

Whites

_____

_____

Alcoholics

_____

_____

African Americans

_____

_____

Disabled

_____

_____

Latinos

_____

_____

Rich

_____

_____

Asians

_____

_____

Of course, thinking of people as members of groups is always tricky. You run the risk of denying or ignoring individuality for the sake of categorization. Typically, however, you learn your prejudices and stereotypes about groups, not about individual people. That's why stereotypes are so specious—they erase your pictures of unique individuals worthy of respect and replace them with faceless images that create fear or contempt.

This exercise gives you a chance to explore how you really feel about yourself and others. Look over what you've written and work to identify your prejudices and stereotypes. Where did these messages originate? How have these beliefs affected you over time? After you've given some time and thought to this, talk with your supervisor and peers about how you approach and accept difference.

We offer one caveat regarding this exercise. You may find that you have to confront—at least in your mind—beloved family members. Your uncle Joey, for instance, who always took you sledding and gave you the most perfect birthday presents year after year, you may now realize is a first-class bigot. This realization need not be the end of your relationship with Uncle Joey. It may, however, cause you to evaluate your expectations of others and to consider how you want to handle differing opinions. Furthermore, attempting to understand where Joey got his ideas and what keeps him clinging to them might be a very illuminating exercise for you. Merely labeling him as a bigot and writing him off is contrary to the values in counseling and therapy. We try our best to understand how everyone sees the world. Good luck in your continued explorations.

Stages in the Journey

The real voyage of discovery lies not in seeking new landscapes but in having new eyes.

—Marcel Proust

Kiser (2000) suggested that internships progress through specific developmental stages that include preplacement, initiation, working, and termination.

Preplacement Stage During your preplacement, you'll be working with your professors to decide on internship locations. You'll also spend time carefully matching your needs, along with the program's expectations, to an appropriate site. Activities include writing a résumé or introductory letter to potential sites, visiting schools and community agencies, and interviewing. You may be discouraged if you are unable to find a perfect match. However, keep in mind that what you *want* in an internship may not necessarily be what you *need* in an internship. Keeping an open mind during this stage is essential.

Initiation Stage Once your internship is underway, you'll begin the initiation stage. During this stage, you meet new people and become familiar with the site's procedures. During this time you will begin to develop a trusting relationship with your site supervisor. You may at first "shadow" this person to help familiarize yourself with your surroundings. This stage is the "look" before the "leap" into counseling and therapy on your own. You may be asked to observe procedures, sit in on meetings, and take extensive notes. Remember, this stage does not last forever.

Working Stage At this stage, you are focusing your energy on reaching the goals that you developed during preplacement. You'll now begin to feel more settled and confident. A key element of this stage is taking advantage of learning opportunities that are available at your internship site. Kiser (2000) warned that you should not become too independent and urged that you continue seeking all the supervision, feedback, and teaching opportunities that are available.

During the working stage part of your journey, you may feel like turning on the "cruise control." When you feel confident about what you're doing, where you're headed, and the rate at which you are traveling, you can relax a little. This is not necessarily a bad thing—travelers cannot maintain a high level of stress and anxiety throughout such a long journey. But remember that you are still responsible for staying on track and heading in the right direction.

Final Stage The final stage of your internship is its termination. This stage includes saying good-bye to supervisors and colleagues and terminating with clients. Don't be surprised if you're feeling sad. Be sure to take time during this hectic period to review your internship, contemplating what you have learned, how you have changed, and what you have discovered. And give yourself permission to feel proud of your accomplishments!

Juggling

Once your internship is underway, you may feel overwhelmed at first. You may feel as if you've got one foot in the "student life" and the other foot in the "professional life." As classes start and supervisor's expectations become clear, you will begin to realize that this is an exciting time. You will be given opportunities to try things out while still receiving support and direction from your professors and peers. Once you begin to feel that you are standing on solid ground, take the time to explore. This is your time to ask questions, gather opinions, and formulate your professional identity. If the size of your internship class is small, take full advantage of the opportunity to use class time to share with your classmates. Although the start of your professional career is only a few months away, you may begin to wonder if you are ready for it, and you may begin to mourn the loss of the community that you established during your training program. Vow to stay in touch with your professors and your colleagues. They will want to know how you are doing, and they will be proud of your future accomplishments.

Making the Most of Your Internship

Remember to collect "postcards" along your journey. There are several different types of postcards you can gather to make the most of your internship. Your internship experience is a time to acquire as much information as possible from supervisors, peers, clients, professors, and other professionals. Besides being a time for putting theory into action, it is also a time for you to make the most of the resources around you.

One way to do this is to "pick the brains" of your colleagues at your site. If you are interning in a school, for example, make a point of scheduling meetings to learn from educational specialists, classroom teachers, principals, and students. Developing and maintaining a group of professional peers is important.

During your internship, also take the opportunity to attend as many workshops and conferences as possible. Use these events to see, hear, and talk about techniques, approaches, and interventions that are currently being tried in the field. Take advantage of the cheaper student membership fees and join professional organizations and affiliations.

Your internship is also a time to meet other professionals and to develop a networking system. Rather than loading your backpack with mementos from the journey, you can keep a journal of your personal reflections.

SUMMARY

Your practicum and internship experiences are unique opportunities to apply what you have learned. Each experience offers an opportunity to put your knowledge and skills into practice in a supervised setting. With careful planning and consideration, you can learn what it takes personally and professionally to thrive as a counselor. When you complete your internship, you will become a professional helper. Along with opportunities for employment will come many responsibilities. You will be well prepared for your new career, but remember that becoming a successful counselor or therapist is a lifetime pursuit. Make a commitment to yourself to realize your fullest potential.

RESOURCES

The Internship, Practicum, and Field Placement Handbook, (Baird, 2004) is one of the most helpful books for general questions about internships. The author includes such topics as preparing for an internship or field placement, getting started, and legal and ethical considerations. The book also provides many helpful lists and forms that will come in handy during your internship.

Getting the Most from Your Human Service Internship (Kiser, 2000) also provides another type of workbook for the counseling intern. It offers a variety of opportunities to reflect on your internship experiences. A list of "myths about internship" is included and is worth a look.

If you are concerned about paperwork, *Practicum and internship: Textbook and Resource Guide for Counseling and Psychotherapy* (Boylan, Malley, & Reilly, 1995) provides every possible document you will need for your internship and beyond. It is a great resource to have when you are starting out.

If you are interning in a school setting, you should take a look at *Developing Your School Counseling Program: A Handbook for Systemic Planning* (Van Zandt & Hayslip, 2001). Once your school counseling internship is underway, check out *The School Counselor's Book of Lists* (Blum, 1998). The author provides sample letters, activities, and definitions that are practical and useful.

Many practicum and internship supervisors require you to have personal liability insurance prior to working with clients. The American Counseling Association and the American Psychological Association both offer liability insurance at very reasonable rates for graduate students enrolled in training programs. The addresses are provided below:

American Counseling Association Insurance Trust
5999 Stevenson Avenue
Alexandria, VA 22304-3300
800-347-6647
www.acait.com

American Psychological Association Insurance Trust
111 Rockville Pike, Suite 900
Rockville, MD 20850
800-477-1200
www.apait.org

REFERENCES

Alle-Corliss, L. A., & Alle-Corliss, R. M. (2006). Human service agencies: An orientation to fieldwork (2nd ed.). Belmont, CA: Thomson Higher Education.

American Counseling Association. (2005). *Code of ethics and standards of practice.* Alexandria, VA: Author.

American Psychological Association. (2002). *Ethical principles of psychologists and code of conduct.* Washington, DC: Author.

Baird, B. N. (2004). *The internship, practicum, and field placement handbook* (4th ed.). Upper Saddle River, NJ: Prentice-Hall.

Blum, D. J. (1998). *The school counselor's book of lists.* West Nyack, NY: Center for Applied Research.

Boylan, J. C., Malley, P. B., & Reilly, E. P. (2001). *Practicum and internship: Textbook and resource guide for counseling and psychotherapy* (3rd ed.). New York. Brunner/Routledge.

Carless, S. A., & Prodan, O. (2003). The impact of practicum training on career and job search attitudes of postgraduate psychology students. *Australian Journal of Psychology, 55,* 89–94.

Cohen, E. D., & Cohen, S. P. (1999). *The virtuous therapist: Ethical practice of counseling and psychotherapy.* Belmont, CA: Brooks/Cole.

Damasio, A. (1994). *Decartes' error: Emotion, reason and the human brain.* New York: Putnam.

Faiver, C., Eisengart, S., & Colonna, R. (2004). *The counselor intern's handbook* (3rd ed.). Belmont, CA: Brooks/Cole.

Gelman, S. R. (1990). The crafting of fieldwork training agreements. *Journal of Social Work Education, 26,* 65–75.

Gross, S. M. (2005). Student perspectives on clinical and counseling psychology practica. *Professional Psychology: Research and Practice, 36,* 299–306.

Harris, E. A. (1995). The importance of risk management in a managed care environment. In M. B. Sussman (Ed.), *A perilous calling: The hazards of psychotherapy practice* (pp. 247–258). New York: Wiley.

Kiser, P. M. (2000). *Getting the most from your human service internship: Learning from experience.* Belmont, CA: Brooks/Cole.

Nowell, D., & Spruill, J. (1993). If it's not absolutely confidential, will information be disclosed? *Professional Psychology: Research and Practice, 24,* 367–369.

Pope, K. S., & Brown, L. S. (1996). *Recovered memories of abuse: Assessment, therapy, forensics.* Washington, DC: American Psychological Association.

Simon, E. (1999). Field practicum: Standards, criteria, supervision, and evaluation. In H. Harris & D. Maloney (Eds.), *Human services: Contemporary issues and trends* (pp. 79–96). Boston: Allyn & Bacon.

Van Zandt, Z., & Hayslip, J. (2001). *Developing your school counseling program : A handbook for systemic planning.* Belmont, CA: Brooks/Cole.

CHAPTER 9

Launching Your Career

To love what you do and feel that it matters—how could anything be more fun?

—Eileen Nelson

Several years ago, an advertisement page in an issue of *U.S. News and World Report* proclaimed, "Take this job and *love* it!" Why does this phrase capture our attention? Besides being a variation on the country music hit, "Take This Job and Shove It," it is the audacity of declaring your passion about your work!

A similar theme appeared in a newspaper comic strip a while ago. The first frame showed a man working at his desk with a sign hanging prominently behind him declaring, "Seize the Day!" The next frame showed the same man in the same place but with a different sign: "Survive the Day!" Beneath that frame, the caption stated, "Today's corporate philosophy." What a sad commentary on the current business world.

Why can't you both love your job *and* thrive each day at it? We believe you can. In this chapter, we discuss how you can forge a passionate and successful career in counseling and therapy. As you prepare to become a professional helper, you'll want to consider five specific goals: getting a job, becoming licensed or certified, involving yourself in a professional network, staying creative in your work, and continuing your personal and professional development. This chapter offers you guidelines for developing effective résumés, vigorous job-search strategies, and persuasive cover letters, and also for holding successful job interviews. You'll learn how to gather information about the different licensure and certification requirements across the United States and

explore some of the many opportunities for participation in professional organizations. You'll find out how to stimulate and keep your creativity fresh as a counselor or therapist. Finally, you'll explore ways to
maintain your professional vitality through a variety of continuing
training experiences.

Above all, you'll see that your career can be an exciting adventure,
another thrilling phase of your journey. You can make a difference
through your work—and one way to start is by being opportunistic.
Carpe diem! Seize this moment to make positive career choices that will
make a difference for you and for others.

▲▲▲

Around the Next Corner
Bill's Story

A T THE AGE of thirty-six, with three years of graduate school
and twelve years in one career, why would I now make a
change? I had a promising career that offered me financial stabil-
ity. Why would anyone in their right mind trade an annual
income of $64,000 for several years of financial worry and stress?
(Actually, during three of the five years of my doctoral program,
my average annual income was around $16,000.)

Most of my family and friends thought I was crazy! At times,
I thought I was too. But I wanted to be a counselor and make a
difference, and I needed more training and experience to get to
the place where I wanted to be. For years, I had been doing "counseling" and "crisis intervention" without the expertise, and I was
tired of pretending. I needed instruction, more experience, and a
sense of personal and professional integrity. So I studied for and
took the graduate record exams and then applied for and was
accepted into a Ph.D. program. I began the journey to become a
professional counselor.

Little did I know that, along the way, I would have the opportunity to teach counseling and discover my true life passion—
teaching! Now I have the best of all worlds. I am a lifelong learner
of the trade I teach, and I have the honor of teaching counseling
with some of the brightest minds in the field and the most caring
people in the world!

My best advice for you as you continue along your career journey is to be prepared for, and open to, the unexpected turns in the road, for around the next corner you may discover a surprising opportunity that may lead you toward discovering your life passion.

How do you discover your true passion in life? How can you make your work meaningful and successful? As you conclude your training and prepare to launch your career, perhaps you can identify with Laura Cornely (1999), who reflected on her own training journey:

> Look around and you will see that the road from student to professional is well traveled. Your peers, supervisors, and professors have each traveled the professional development road for various distances (p. 16).

Some of the signs that Cornely mentioned are what we want to call to your attention now.

EXERCISE 9.1 **Life-Span Time Line**

Think about all the career paths you have considered pursuing. As a child, you may have fantasized about becoming a professional actor, dancer, or athlete. As an adolescent, you may have seriously explored several career options. When you became a young adult, you probably experimented by taking a variety of jobs. Now you are at a point in your life where you are focusing on a few career options.

Describe your career fantasies, experiences, and plans at different points in the past, present, and future along the life-span time line below. Note the persons, places, or events that have influenced your decisions. Look for emerging themes, crucial turning points, and future aspirations. How do you move from the present to a successful future?

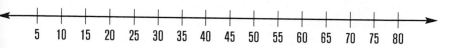

FROM STUDENT TO PROFESSIONAL

> It is good to have an end to journey towards; but it
> is the journey that matters in the end.
>
> —Ursula K. Le Guin

As you prepare to make the transition from student to professional, you'll begin to think more seriously about the specific career path you want to follow. New possibilities and opportunities are constantly developing in the fields of counseling and therapy. Before exploring your options, you should consider your values and family background, your unique interests and abilities, your personality traits, and the needs of others to whom you are committed. You will also want to know where to find the career opportunities that are best for you. You'll need to develop your résumé, prepare for interviews, and learn how to write effective cover letters and other correspondence that a job search requires of you. And finally, you'll want to ensure that your personal and professional journey continues to thrive through licensure, certification, and continuing education. Let's address these issues more specifically now.

Exploring Your Values

A great way to start your career development journey is by assessing your values—what you see as truly important—and the unique perspective you bring to life and work. As you gain insight about the role your values play in your career choices, you may feel greater confidence about the choices you are making. Here is an exercise to get you started.

■ ■ ■

EXERCISE 9.2 **Building a House**
A Values Exercise

All of us have values and beliefs that govern who we are and the decisions we make in life. Rarely, however, do we take the time to examine these values. For the next few minutes, think about the following questions, and then draw a symbolic representation of your answers in the form of a house. You don't need to be an artist to complete this exercise. Just go ahead and let yourself have some fun with it!

FOUNDATION

In Chapter 3, you wrote your training mission. Now take a much broader perspective and consider your *life* mission. What would be the motto for your life? What is the guiding principle that you live by every day? Draw the base of your house and write your answer inside the space you've drawn.

WALLS

Where do you get your support in life? Who or what provides the support you need? Draw some walls for your house, and write your answer on your walls.

ROOF

Certainly some storms come into every person's life. Who or what provides you with the protection you need when difficulties arise? Write your answer on the roof you've drawn.

CHIMNEY

How do you vent when life gets hard for you? What outlets do you have to use as a safe place to let off steam? Place your answer inside your chimney.

WINDOWS

What accomplishments or experiences are you most proud of, and what in your life are you most willing to let others see? Put your answers in the windows you have drawn.

DOOR

Who are the most significant and influential people who have entered your life? What have you learned from them? Write their initials on the door to your house.

TREES

What are you planting and nurturing that you hope will outlive you? Draw one or more trees to represent your legacy.

What have you learned about yourself and your values from this exercise? Share your drawing with a trusted colleague or mentor.

■ ■ ■

Exploring Your Roots

Sooner or later, thinking about where you want to go leads you to consider where you've been. As you try to make sense of your career choices, keep in mind that you can best be understood in a context and that your context includes the influences your family of origin has had on you. Family can be defined in a number of ways, so don't excuse yourself from this part of the chapter if your caretakers were grandparents, foster parents, or older siblings. You can define your family however you like. The important issue to consider is how your heritage affects your career and lifestyle decision making.

You can begin to answer this question in a number of ways. Think about what you learned from your family about work and career. Were certain jobs considered acceptable and others not? Did your family have different expectations for men than it had for women? Was higher education valued? How did your family balance love, work, and play? How are your current choices similar or different from those of your family? Finally, are you where you want to be?

Give yourself some time to ponder these questions. Your answers can be illuminating—and maybe even surprising.

▲▲▲

The Legacy of My Parents
Gabe's Story

I GREW UP in a blue-collar household and was the first member of my family to earn a college degree. As a matter of fact, my pursuit of a doctoral degree was primarily driven by my desire to prove that I could do it. I hadn't really given much thought to the type of lifestyle I would have after I graduated.

In my first job as an assistant professor in a counseling program, I couldn't believe how much my colleagues grumbled about their work. I kept thinking, "These whiners don't realize how lucky they have it!" I kept thinking about my mother and father and the hard physical work that they had done for years—and continue to do even now! I started to have doubts about my career choice, and I also felt distant from my colleagues.

At first, I felt like an impostor. Deep down, I didn't believe that it was okay for me to have a good-paying job that didn't physically exhaust me. Although I had earned my current position through my efforts in school, I felt guilty. I also didn't feel comfortable with aspects of my job that required administrative or committee work. I knew I could teach and do research, but the rest of the job seemed like uncharted territory to me. I chose not to participate in many university activities for fear of being rejected, labeled ignorant, or identified as an "outsider."

As I continued to think about my family, though, I began to realize a few things about myself. I came to understand that I do work very hard and that I can be proud of my accomplishments. One strength that I can now acknowledge is that I can easily empathize with first-generation college students in my classes. Although I still feel like an outsider at times, I'm working to make a place for me in my job while honoring the legacy of my parents.

A career genogram can help you identify your worldview, perceived barriers, role conflicts, intergenerational patterns, and beliefs about work and roles (Gysbers & Heppner, 1997). Constructing one and reflecting on what you find can be an important step for you at this stage of your journey.

Putting yourself in the context of your family, you can explore patterns and influences that have either helped or hindered your progress so far. You can then decide what to do with this information to make the most of your experiences.

EXERCISE 9.3 Career Genogram

Begin by constructing a genogram of three generations and include occupations for each person. (See *Genograms in Family Assessment* by Monica McGoldrick and Randy Gerson [1985] for information on constructing genograms.) Now spend some time responding to the questions below.

1. Who are you most like?
2. What were the dominant values in your family?
3. Did any family members have obvious vocational callings?
4. What roles did different family members play?
5. What values did you learn from your family about work?
6. How are love, work, and play balanced?
7. What do the vocational patterns that you see suggest to you?
8. What did you learn from your family about education?
9. If each person were to provide one word about work, what would it be?
10. As you notice any patterns, what do you want to do with that information?

USING THE CAMPUS CAREER CENTER

A good place to begin your career path is at your college or university career center. Most campuses have great resources available, with a professional staff ready and willing to assist you. Undergraduate students flock to these centers for help, but you may be surprised to discover that the center is available to graduate students, also.

The career counselors and advisors can assist you with résumé questions, interview preparation, job openings in your area, and contacts with alumni. Many colleges and universities have established wonderful career networks among alumni. Consider contacting graduates from your program through your college or university alumni network. Your career center may regularly sponsor a career fair and probably has many resources available for you to read. One such resource is the annual edition of *Planning Job Choices*. This magazine has excellent tips about the current job market, for writing outstanding résumés, interviewing successfully, and thriving in your first year of employment. The following is the "Top 10 Personal Characteristics Employers Seek in Job Candidates," taken from *Planning Job Choices* (National Association of Colleges and Employers, 1999) for information about what employers want most in job candidates.

Top 10 Personal Characteristics Employers Seek in Job Candidates

Honesty/integrity

Motivation/initiative

Communication skills

Self-confidence

Flexibility

Interpersonal skills

Strong work ethic

Teamwork skills

Leadership skills

Enthusiasm

Source: National Association of Colleges and Employers, 1999.

SEEKING CAREER COUNSELING

You may want to consider seeing a career counselor to explore the numerous areas of specialization in the counseling field. Bolles (2006) lists possible contacts from every state in his annual resource guide. Career counselors can help you sort through your concerns, and many offer testing and assessment services to further enable you to gain clarity about your career options. Possible career interest inventories include the Self-Directed Search (SDS), the Strong Interest Inventory (SII), and the Values Scale (VS). Personality instruments, such as the Sixteen Personality Factor Questionnaire (16PF), and cognitive scales, such as the Career Beliefs Inventory or the Career Decision Scale, may also be useful.

CAREER POSSIBILITIES BY DEGREE

Careers with a Master's or Ed.S.

With a master's or educational specialist degree in counseling, you can meet the coursework requirements for licensure and work in a variety of settings, including businesses, hospitals, schools, community mental health centers, and many other public and private institutions. However, these professional opportunities vary considerably and depend to a large extent on the type of training you receive. You may be involved in assessment, providing crisis intervention services, counseling, consultation, health promotion, vocational rehabilitation, or behavior management.

Licensing and Credentialing Licensed professional counselors may provide psychological services without supervision from other professionals. Currently, forty-eight states and the District of Columbia license professional counselors. Most of these states issue a general credential for a licensed professional counselor. All fifty states and the District of Columbia regulate school counseling through their state school boards.

Licensure and credential requirements vary from state to state. Typically, states have coursework, supervised experience, and examination requirements for licensure. The course requirements are generally based on the Council for Accreditation of Counseling and Related Educational Programs (CACREP) accreditation model for a counseling curriculum. The curriculum usually involves forty-eight to sixty semester hours of graduate study in the following areas: human growth and development, social and cultural foundations, helping relationships, group work, career and lifestyle development, appraisal, research and program evaluation, and professional orientation. The supervised experience requirement often involves up to 4,000 hours of work after the completion of your training. And the licensing exam requirement typically includes passing the National Counselors Examination. Also, the National Board of Certified Counselors nationally certifies CACREP graduates who successfully complete this examination.

For information on the licensing of professional counselors in your state, you can consult your telephone book's blue pages for the state regulation board's telephone number and address. For information about your state's regulations for credentialing for school counselors, contact your state's department of education. You can go to the American Counseling Association website (*www.counseling.org*) or call 1-800-347-6647, extension 222, and ask for the publication, *A Guide to State Laws and Regulations on Professional School Counseling.*

Other Helping Professions If you are seeking employment in school psychology, you probably hold an educational specialist degree, which usually requires at least sixty semester hours of graduate study. Most professionals in school psychology work primarily in the schools and are concerned with a variety of psychological and educational issues.

If you are seeking a general, research-oriented degree and you are not planning on pursuing further study at the doctoral level, you may find employment in teaching or research. Without a doctoral degree, however, you may find that your opportunities for employment or advancement in higher education are limited. You may discover that you are seldom able to provide services without supervision.

As a graduate of a professional master's degree program in industrial/ organizational psychology, you may find employment opportunities in private businesses and government organizations. You may devote much of your time to selecting and training employees. You may also focus on human resource development, employee assistance programs, and other programs related to personnel management and employee relations.

Careers with a Doctorate

Counselors and counseling psychologists with doctoral degrees assume many different occupational roles. You may work as a teacher, researcher, mental health service provider, administrator, or consultant. Doctoral-level counselors and counseling psychologists are employed in a variety of settings, including universities, elementary and secondary schools, hospitals, human service agencies, private business and industry, and government organizations. In addition, many helping professionals with doctorates maintain independent practices for the provision of counseling and psychological services. The doctoral degree offers you the most professional flexibility and leads to many career opportunities in counseling and psychology.

Obtaining a doctorate requires a deep commitment to academic training. The successful completion of a doctoral program entails at least four or five years of intensive graduate study. You must also pass a set of comprehensive examinations and write and defend a dissertation. If you wish to provide counseling and psychological services, you need to complete a year-long internship plus at least one additional year of supervised practice.

Admission to doctoral programs is highly competitive. The average acceptance rate for doctoral programs is approximately 11 percent; some programs in clinical psychology accept less than 2 percent of all applicants. Still, a doctorate in counseling or psychology is a very appealing option for students who are willing to make a substantial personal investment to achieve high academic and professional goals.

Counselor education is centered on the goal of training successful counselors who will be prepared to assume leadership roles in the field of counseling. A doctoral degree in counselor education is accredited by CACREP. CACREP emphasizes the training of professional counselor educators and counselors who will have competence in the core areas of counseling, teaching, research, and supervision. Counselor educators often fill multifaceted roles but are most often distinguished as helping professionals who work from a developmental and health perspective.

The majority of counselor educators and counselors who complete the doctoral degree will work in educational settings such as colleges, universities, public and private schools, technical schools, and a broad spectrum of human service agencies. Professional activities usually include counseling, assessment, diagnosis, casework, consultation, referral, and research.

PLANNING YOUR CAREER

Being Intentional

Selecting and pursuing your career goals are obviously important matters that will have a profound effect on your life. Explore your career options thoroughly, not only to improve your chances for eventual employment but also to choose paths that will lead to personal and professional satisfaction. Because of their extensive involvement in the field, faculty advisors and other helping professionals are in an excellent position to help you weigh your career alternatives. Rewarding professional experiences seldom happen by chance alone. You will need to carefully consider your options and to be intentional with your plans to achieve a happy, fulfilling career.

Where to Look for Jobs

The best way for you to discover an available employment opportunity is still the old-fashioned way—through other people. So it is still vital that you stay connected with your professors, fellow students, professional contacts in the field, and alumni of your program. In many, if not most, helping professions, job opportunities are found through personal contact—through someone you know or people who know you. So maintaining your personal contacts is essential. This does not mean that *what* you know is less important than *who* you know; however, counseling and other helping professions are less likely to advertise positions in more traditional ways, such as through newspapers or websites. You may discover a good job that way, yet we cannot tell you how often we have found our students receiving job opportunities through word of mouth or an E-mail. Keep this in mind.

Local newspapers are still a good resource for finding specific jobs in your geographic area. Most newspapers now have Internet sites available, allowing you access to almost any conceivable job market. Many websites are also maintained simply to provide employers with a means of reaching the largest possible audience of prospective employees. We have listed some of these popular websites at the end of this chapter. Thousands of jobs are posted on any given site. Some sites charge minimal fees for their services, and some are free to the public. Other services, such as résumé posting, are also available on many sites.

Professional organizations related to counseling, psychology, and other helping professions also advertise current position openings. The *APA Monitor* and *ACA Counseling Today* are outstanding resources in this regard. The *Chronicle of Higher Education* posts jobs in academic environments weekly. These professional newspapers also have websites with job listings, and these sites are included at the end of this chapter.

Remember to use your university's alumni office and career center. These centers often maintain binders with thousands of job opportunities that have been targeted for students about to graduate. Networking through professional organizations is also a great way to discover job leads.

■ ■ ■

EXERCISE 9.4 Interviewing Two Masters
A Journal Exercise

Schedule interviews with two professionals who are well established in the career field you hope to enter. Ask them their reasons for going into this profession and what keeps them in it. Ask what they like and dislike most about their jobs. You may even want to ask them what they would do differently if they had it to do all over again. Finally, you might ask what they see as future trends in their particular fields.

After each interview, write a reflective entry in your journal about the personal meaning and insight you gained. Sometimes it helps to compare or contrast your journey with those of others whom you deeply respect. This exercise may even emerge as the beginning point of a mentor/protégé relationship, as it has for many of our students.

Becoming Professionally Involved

As you consider your career options after graduation, you may be preparing to seek a position or to continue your education. Regardless of your current intentions, become involved in professional organizations. These organizations, such as the American Counseling Association, American Psychological Association, Association for Counselor Education and Supervision, and their regional, state, and local divisions, offer options limited only by your imagination and initiative. The student membership rates for professional organizations are much cheaper than they are for professional members, so take advantage of this opportunity while you can.

Through professional organization involvement, you can attend conferences, offer presentations, participate in workshops, serve on committees, find a mentor, lobby state and national politicians, keep abreast of current research, or simply meet and socialize with other professionals. Beginning this type of involvement now, while you're a student, will increase your network, perhaps enhance your capability to find an excellent job that matches your interests, and improve the likelihood that you'll stay connected and relevant in your own professional development.

When imagining such involvement, some students may immediately ask, "Yes, that sounds good, but how do I get involved?" You may feel intimidated by the idea of approaching strangers and asking if you can join a committee—especially if those strangers are well-known authors or researchers. Meeting a favorite author at a conference can feel like meeting a celebrity! One of the many advantages of being a student is that you can reasonably expect your professors to introduce you to "movers and shakers" in the field. In fact, you'll probably find that your professors and other mentors would love to "show you off."

As you meet people who are involved in professional organizations, ask them if there are ways that you can help. Most conference committees rely on graduate student assistance. Trainees who volunteer to work at national or international conferences usually receive compensation in the form of reduced or waived conference registration fees. They also enjoy the opportunity to see how professional organizations are administered and have the chance to meet colleagues from across the country.

Some of these interactions fall into the category of networking—a skill that may seem more appropriate for business and the corporate world. Actually, networking is essential for an active and successful professional in almost any field.

If you're trying to decide how to go about becoming more involved in professional organizations, consider the following tips (Huddock, Thompkins, & Enterline, 2000):

- Research organizations by visiting their websites and then consider joining as a student member.
- E-mail or telephone leaders to see if their committee needs your assistance. Don't be surprised to find that they do. Handle your shyness or nervousness by starting small. Contact local or regional divisions of professional organizations first. Ask a professor to introduce you to a committee chairperson via E-mail or telephone prior to making your first contact.
- Submit a proposal for a state, regional, or national conference. Ask a few peers to present with you. When you attend the conference, participate in the entire experience. Make the most of the opportunities that exist for you to meet people and become involved.
- Don't stop yourself with excuses. Just do it!

CONDUCTING YOUR SEARCH

Designing an Effective Résumé

As you begin the process of preparing your professional résumé, keep in mind the following basic tips. Choose high-quality paper, staying with basic colors such as white, beige, or gray. Use a font that is easy to read, such as Courier or Times New Roman, and a size that is legible, such as 11 or 12 points. Limit the length of your résumé to two or three pages.

Place your current personal data at the top of your résumé because this basic information is essential for the employer to contact you. Include your name, permanent and local addresses, telephone number, and E-mail address. Immediately below this personal information, offer a career objective statement that clearly reflects your interest in the position. Then list your undergraduate and graduate educational experience, highlighting specialized training, awards, and your grade-point average—if it's a good selling point!

Below the education section, present your employment experience, beginning with the most recent jobs. Don't forget to add your relevant volunteer, practicum, internship, and field placement experiences. You may also want to list any additional skills that seem relevant, such as website design, PowerPoint presentation, and word-processing skills. Following this section, include any professional presentations, publications, and research projects.

On a separate sheet, list the names of your references, along with the necessary contact information. Your references should be respected, responsible individuals who can describe in detail your personal qualities, work habits, and professional qualifications.

Be sure to ask someone to read and edit your résumé before sending it. Most colleges and universities offer this service to students through the career development office. Also many résumé writing services are available on-line. Choose this resource carefully, however, because some can be costly. Many websites will also post your completed résumé.

Writing Persuasive Correspondence

Carefully develop your résumé's cover letter to make it brief, yet informative. Again, use high-quality paper with a basic color scheme, rather than something flashy and gauche. Remember that basic color schemes will please almost everyone, but a unique paper may offend some personal tastes. It is best to stay conservative with paper choice, font style, and size.

Your cover letter should be brief—rarely longer than three paragraphs. In your introductory paragraph, write a clear, personal statement about your desire to apply for this particular position. In your middle paragraph, communicate succinctly several skills you possess that qualify you. Finally, express appreciation for being considered and respectfully request a personal interview.

Successful Job Interviewing

Before the Interview Find out all the information you can about your potential employer. Research the history and mission of the company, organization, or institution. These efforts not only demonstrate your personal initiative but also help you determine whether this position is a good match for you. Your research will enable you to speak with greater confidence and ask informed questions during your interview. It will be obvious to the employers that you've done your homework.

Practice a "mock interview" with a trusted peer or professor before you head out. Again, many campuses offer this service through the career development office.

At the Interview   Dress appropriately—wear only business or professional attire. Be prepared to offer several questions to the interview team. Remember that every interview involves finding the best match for a position, so seek out answers to your questions about this position, your potential colleagues, and the work environment.

You may want to bring along the portfolio that you have developed during your training. It can be a great way to showcase your experience, accomplishments, and developing areas of expertise.

Finally, make sure you remain energized and focused on the interview. Eliminate any possible distractions by turning off your cell phone or beeper. Above all, be yourself. You'll waste your energy and everyone's time by trying to be someone you are not. Trust who you are and the valuable experiences you've had.

After the Interview   Following an interview, write a personal note of appreciation to all key persons who participated in the process, especially those on the search committee. If you are offered the position, in addition to responding with a formal letter, write notes of appreciation once again—even if you decline the offer. These personal touches will go a long way toward establishing you as a thoughtful person determined to excel in all aspects of the position.

If you are offered the position, be prepared to negotiate salary and benefits. This is often the most difficult part of the hiring process, but it is essential that you prepare yourself for this crucial piece of the process. Research the salary range and benefits for this position. In other words, you must stay within the realm of possibility, but do not shortchange yourself, either. Remain confident in your abilities and experiences!

YOUR CAREER AND YOUR LIFE

Lifelong Learning

Be a lifelong learner. Even after you land your dream job, consider the importance of continuing your personal and professional growth journey. Take additional courses at a nearby university, participate in professional development workshops, and regularly attend conferences. If you are seeking licensure or certification, you will be required to receive additional training after you complete your degree. Enthusiastically embrace these opportunities as they come your way.

Fitting In and Standing Out

> Become aware of what is in you. Announce it,
> pronounce it, produce it, and give birth to it.
>
> —Meister Eckhart

So far, we have offered you advice on how to become a professional in your chosen field. Of course, to belong to any group or organization, you must behave in ways deemed appropriate to qualify you for membership. To the extent that you can do this successfully, you will be fitting in. But conforming to the standards and conventions of your field will also tend to make you ordinary—someone who is just like all the others.

Thriving as a counselor is much more than fitting in—it's standing out. Lefrançois (2000) asserted that just as not using your intelligence is being stupid, not using your creativity is being ordinary. So to become extraordinary in your profession, you must exercise your innate creativity. Being creative is simply seeing things in ways that others might miss and coming up with new ideas.

E. Paul Torrance conducted a longitudinal study over 22 years that focused on people in various professions who had been able to maintain their creativity (Millar, 1995). From this research, Torrance (1995) identified certain important factors and offered a seven-point "manifesto" to preserve your creativity.

- Fall in love with something and intensely pursue it. Staying fascinated with your work is only possible when you really love what you are doing. Of course, your interests will change, and if you are not paying attention to yourself, you may not even notice. As a result, you may go on doing something that you have long since "chewed the flavor out of" and, not surprisingly, finding that it bores you. Make sure that what you are doing continues to bring you joy. If it doesn't, do something else.

- Know, understand, take pride in, practice, develop, exploit, and enjoy your greatest strengths. Sometimes families seem to divide talents as if they were a scarce resource among the children. You've heard people comment about brothers that "John is the shy one, James is the confident one." Or they may contrast sisters by asserting, "Jane is the artistic one, Jill is the scholarly one." Or they simply slap on a label by saying that "Brad is athletic, Bob is bookish." Perhaps, because of this allocation-of-talent phenomenon in your own family, you believe that there are certain activities you can't do well or domains of endeavor you should avoid. Think again. Try your hand at everything that might interest you. You will be surprised at the many latent talents that you have.

- Learn to free yourself from the expectations of others. Free yourself to play your own game. All of us are raised under what Rogers (1961) called "conditions of worth." As children, we received the message that we would be lovable only if we behaved in ways that significant people endorsed. As a result, some of the ways in which you regard yourself are not truly you. Furthermore, you may harbor the belief that, to preserve your self-esteem, you must continue to please teachers, bosses, spouses, and all others who can withhold approval from you. Liberate yourself from the expectations of others. This does not mean that you must become an outlaw and ignore the wishes of people. It simply means that you can't please everyone, so you must first please yourself.

- Find a great teacher or mentor who will help you. Seek out someone who "knows the ropes" in your profession. Only veterans truly understand the many subtle dynamics of counseling that, as a novice, you are only beginning to grasp. In every setting, there are older people who are in the stage that Erikson (1975) called "generativity." They are eager to be helpful to fledgling professionals like you. Search carefully for such a person.

- Don't waste energy trying to be well rounded. Do what you love and can do well. Although you should explore everything that attracts your interest, don't feel that you must know and be able to do everything. In this era of information explosion, it is impossible for anyone to be a complete "renaissance person." Focus on those activities with which you have fallen in love, and refine your abilities in those areas.

- Learn the skills of interdependence. Remember that your professional development is not a journey that you have to take alone. Collaborate and cooperate. Share your talents and borrow talents from others. You will notice, for example, that this book was written by seven authors. We each contributed in the areas of our expertise, wrote the sections with which we were most familiar, and benefited from the contributions of our colleagues. Being a team player has many rewards. Give up the notion that you must be competitive to stand out. You will be more respected if you generously give of your creativity and seek the contributions of others in the work that you do.

Think You're Not Creative?

> There is a vitality, a life-force, an energy, a quickening that is translated through you into action and because there is only one of you translated in all time, this expression is unique.
>
> —Agnes de Mille

Perhaps you're thinking that you are not a creative person. If so, you are either confusing creativity with certain abilities, such as painting or playing music, or you have buried your creative spark somewhere along the way. When you were a child, you were constantly creating, inventing new games, allowing yourself to be enchanted by imaginary play, and proposing all sorts of fabulous ideas. But something happens to many children as they grow older and become formally educated. "Many people with the potential for creativity probably never realize it. They believe that creativity is a quality they could never have" (Sternberg & Lubart, 1995, p. vii).

What happens to these creative children? Why do they arrive at adulthood having misplaced their potential? What happened to you? In their book, *Defying the Crowd*, Sternberg and Lubart (1995) stated that creativity can be developed, but they suggested that one reason why all of us are not more creative is that creativity is generally undervalued and overlooked in our culture. Critics of our educational system, such as Gardner (1991) and Goleman (1995), view school as a place that values only certain kinds of learning. The traditional cognitive, convergent, and conforming biases of school make it difficult for students to develop their creative thinking.

Compulsive conformity is the antithesis of creative thinking. Imagination, a precondition for original thought, is often considered a liability early on. One study found that, in preschool children, the percentage of original responses on ideational fluency tasks was about 50 percent. However, that number dropped to 25 percent during elementary school. Whether you entered adolescence equipped to preserve your creative thinking depended on whether your home and school environments valued the thought processes that support creativity.

Along about the fourth grade, you began to face increasing expectations that your thinking should be free of emotion and concerned only with facts, not fantasy. Torrance (1967) identified what is called the "fourth-grade slump." At about this stage of education, an alarming number of children display a marked decline in their creative production. This is the stage at which male and female roles become important, peers become significant evaluators, children are expected to behave in more adultlike ways, and the school curriculum changes:

> Children, it is thought, need to learn that the world isn't all roses, that animals don't talk, that competition is keen, and that the rewards of life go to persons who are alert, practical and realistic. (Strom & Bernard, 1982, p. 309)

Torrance (1963) studied teachers from several countries, focusing on their attitudes toward creative behaviors in their students. He found that, of sixty-two student behaviors listed, conforming behaviors, such as being courteous and obedient, handing work in on time, and accepting the judgment of authorities, were most prized, but creative behaviors were consistently listed as least desirable. Teachers and parents complain that highly creative children don't pay attention and get off task.

Does any of this sound familiar to you? If you remember yourself being criticized for your daydreaming or off-task behavior, you were probably targeted as someone who needed to be less creative. But the good news is that your creative ability is still *there*, buried under layers of conventional behaviors, and you are past the fourth grade now. You are in a program in which you can once again exercise your creativity. Your professors will appreciate it, and you will feel the exhilaration of rediscovering a part of yourself that you had carefully packed away in elementary school.

Clock-Watchers and Workaholics

Some people work to live, and some live to work. Those who see their work only as a means to an end are the clock-watchers. They live for the time when they are no longer at work. Perceiving their jobs as boring and the time they spend at work as endless, clock-watchers are under-committed to the work they do.

On the other hand, people who seem to have no time for anything but work are workaholics. Their cell phones and briefcases are their constant companions. Instead of enjoying pleasant midday meals, workaholics "do working lunches." They regard vacations as merely interruptions to their jobs and are overcommitted to their work, experiencing time as fleeting and frantic.

Both of these extreme attitudes toward work pose dangers. Workaholics tend to burn out, whereas clock-watchers tend to rust out. The philosopher Aristotle preached the "golden mean" in all things and was among the first to say that you must find balance in your life. You want to enjoy work and also enjoy your free time. Unless you are independently wealthy, you must work to live, but don't be a clock-watcher. If you truly enjoy your work, you will live to work, but don't be a workaholic. Be careful to find the proper ratio of work to play for yourself. The only way to test whether you are achieving this balance is how you are feeling at the moment. Consult that inner voice.

By the way, if you are a clock-watcher during your counselor training program—marking time until you graduate—you are not getting the most out of your classes and practicum experiences. Conversely, if you are a workaholic who is trying to get better grades than anyone else in your program, you need to lighten up and have more fun. See if you can turn your work into play, so that it becomes a joy rather than a grind.

Leaving the Nest and Making Mistakes

> Do not fear mistakes. There are none.
>
> —Miles Davis

No matter whether your training has been a joy or a grind, as you near graduation, you may be surprised to find that you are approaching it with mixed emotions. You are excited about finally reaching your training goal, but you are also probably feeling some sadness about what you are leaving behind—and even some dread about what lies ahead. You now have to go out into the real world, leaving behind the safety and comfort of your learning community. Looking for just the right opportunity and interviewing for the "dream job" can lead to disappointment and rejection. But thinking creatively about this phase of your journey will give you a good start.

Of course, only being creative will not ensure your success. Creativity may be essential for thriving in your career, but other personal qualities, such as determination and perseverance, are also necessary. This little ditty below clearly makes that point:

> *Reflective on Creative*
> While I am very receptive
> To your urging convective,
> My experienced perspective
> Leaves me somewhat skeptive,
> 'Cause most of my inventive
> Is a little bit not productive.

John Irving, author of several critically acclaimed novels, including *The World According to Garp* and *The Cider House Rules*, described writing as "one-eighth talent and seven-eighths discipline"(Gussow, cited in Amabile, 2001). That claim brings to mind Thomas Edison, holder of more than a thousand patents and widely described as one of America's true geniuses, who said, "Genius is 1 percent inspiration and 99 percent perspiration."

Edison also showed an amazing passion and positive attitude. A reporter once asked him what it felt like to have failed 10,000 times in searching for the right material needed to make a light bulb. Edison replied, "I have not failed. I've just found 10,000 ways that won't work." He was also wonderfully opportunistic because some of his greatest inventions were accidental or resulted from failed experiments (McAuliffe, 1995). For example, when a large supply of chemicals was ruined in storage, Edison stopped all his experiments and used that calamity to invent new techniques for storing and combining chemicals.

No one in your graduate program requires you to write like John Irving or to be as inventive as Edison, but to make the most out of your professional career, we offer four clichéd but important reminders:

- Think outside the lines.
- Walk the extra mile.
- Accept your mistakes as "practice."
- Seek clues for success in your failures.

▦ ▦ ▦

EXERCISE 9.5 **Putting It All Together**
A Balancing Exercise

We are sure you have noticed the pictures of loved ones and vacation postcards that most professional people have sitting on their office desks or bookshelves. You have probably also observed that most people also have little mementos, souvenirs, and knickknacks sitting around in conspicuous places. Just as these photographs of friends and family serve as reminders, sources of inspiration, or metaphors, so may the knickknacks have more meaning than mere "conversation pieces."

One of our colleagues has this interesting structure (pictured in the figure) resting on his desk to remind him of how the important things in his life must remain in harmony. As you can see, six larger nails are balanced on one smaller nail, which is anchored to a solid foundation of oak. The structure is freestanding. That is, the nails are not magnetic and they are not held together with any type of adhesive, yet the figure remains intact, connected, and balanced.

The themes of becoming connected and maintaining balance in your personal and professional lives have been addressed throughout this book. As you prepare to launch your career, it can be valuable for you to

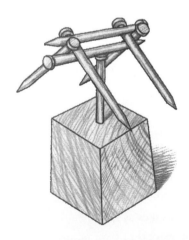

construct a personal reminder or symbol that you could take with you on the next part of your journey.

Make a list of things that would make up your foundation (the oak block), the fulcrum (the smaller nail) and six elements in your life (the six larger nails) you would like to remember from this book and from your training that must always be balanced and connected.

FOUNDATION POSSIBILITIES:

_____

_____

_____

FULCRUM POSSIBILITIES:

_____

_____

_____

POSSIBILITIES FOR SIX NAILS:

_____   _____

_____   _____

_____   _____

It's fun to construct one of these structures, but maybe you lack the time or inclination. If so, you have our permission to copy the picture and use it instead. Perhaps you would like to invent your own connecting and balancing structure. Let us know what you come up with!

SUMMARY

In this final chapter, we discussed how you can begin exploring strategies for finding employment, obtaining licensure or certification, becoming more involved in your professional life, and continuing your personal and professional development.

ONE FINAL POINT

Leap, and the net will appear.

—Julia Cameron

Remember the Zeigarnik Effect that we discussed in Chapter 5? It refers to your ability to remember and take with you those lessons that are ongoing and not fully resolved better than those that have been resolved. We therefore leave you with one final point. Your most important discovery about thriving in your training is an emerging insight, unfolding before you like a velvety, deep red rose on a spring day. You are discovering that thriving is . . .

_____

_____

_____

_____

_____

RESOURCES

The following books all provide a wealth of resources and current ideas, including exercises for self-discovery, questionnaires that provide insights into your work values, and tips to assist you with résumé writing and interview preparation:

What Color Is Your Parachute? (Bolles, 2006) *Career Focus: A Personal Job Search Guide* (Lamarre, 2006), *Life Skills: Taking Charge of Your Personal and Professional Growth* (Leider, 1994), and *The Search for Meaning in the Workplace* (Naylor, Willimon, & Osterberg, 1996).

The following resources and websites are great places to find job openings as well as career-related articles and other information.

American Counseling Association Career Center

www.counseling.org/CareerCenter

This is the official employment site of the American Counseling Association. In addition to position openings, you can also find answers to career-related questions and read suggestions for enhancing your career.

American Psychological Association Online Career Center

www.psyccareers.com

On this site, which is sponsored by the American Psychological Association, you can search for job opportunities for psychologists, read tips on successful interviews, and even post your résumé.

Career Magazine

www.careermag.com

Career Magazine is similar to Monster (described below), just a little less overwhelming. The site often has some wonderful articles as well as services similar to Monster's.

Chronicle of Higher Education Job Listings

jobs.chronicle.com

The Chronicle is the primary publication of higher education, so college and university jobs are posted here.

Monster Board

www.monster.com

Billed as the largest website for job hunters, Monster is a great place to find job openings, post your résumé, read career-related articles, research organizations you're interested in, or contact prospective employers. Monster often has nearly half a million job openings posted!

Occupational Outlook Handbook, 2006–2007 edition

www.bls.gov/oco

The *Occupational Outlook Handbook* is a nationally recognized source of career information, designed to provide valuable assistance to individuals making decisions about their future work lives. Revised every two years, the *Handbook* describes what workers do on the job, working conditions, the training and education needed, earnings, and expected job prospects in a wide range of occupations.

REFERENCES

Amabile, T. M. (2001). Beyond talent: John Irving and the passionate craft of creativity. *American Psychologist, 56,* 333–336.

Bolles, R. N. (2006). *What color is your parachute?* Berkeley, CA: Ten Speed Press.

Corona, J., & March, P. A. (2000, June). Into the real world: Moving from school to work. *Counseling Today, 43,* 31–32.

Cornely, L. (1999, October). Travels from student to professional: Signs along the road. *Counseling Today, 42,* 16.

Erikson, E. H. (1975). *Life history and the historical moment.* New York: Norton.

Gardner, H. (1991). *The unschooled mind.* New York: Basic Books.

Goleman, D. (1995). *Emotional intelligence.* New York: Bantam Books.

Gysbers, N. C., & Heppner, M. (1998). *Career counseling process, issues, and techniques.* Boston: Allyn & Bacon.

Huddock, T. J., Thompkins, C., & Enterline, C. (2000, May). Counseling students need to get involved in networking, conferences. *Counseling Today, 43,* 16, 23.

Lamarre, H. M. (2006). *Career focus: A personal job search guide* (3rd ed.). Upper Saddle River, NJ: Prentice-Hall.

Lefrançois, G. R. (2000). *Psychology for teaching* (10th ed.). Belmont, CA: Wadsworth.

Leider, R. J. (1994). *Life skills: Taking charge of your personal and professional growth.* San Diego, CA: Pfeiffer.

McAuliffe, K. (1995). The undiscovered world of Thomas Edison. *Atlantic Monthly, 276,* 80–93.

McGoldrick, M., & Gerson, R. (1985). *Genograms in family assessment*. New York: Norton.

Millar, G. W. (1995). *E. Paul Torrance: The creativity man. An authorized biography*. Norwood, NJ: Ablex.

Morrison, T. (Summer, 1998). Generate opportunities: The latest in résumé writing trends. *The Quill of Alpha Xi Delta*, 11–23.

Naylor, T. H., Willimon, W. H., & Osterberg, R. (1996). *The search for meaning in the workplace*. Nashville, TN: Abingdon Press.

National Association of Colleges and Employers (1999). *Planning job choices* (42nd ed.). Bethlehem, PA: Author.

Rogers, C. R. (1961). *On becoming a person*. Boston: Houghton Mifflin.

Sternberg, R. J., & Lubart, T. I. (1995). *Defying the crowd: Cultivating creativity in a culture of conformity*. New York: Free Press.

Strom, R. D., & Bernard, H. W. (1982). *Educational psychology*. Monterey, CA: Brooks/Cole.

Super, D. E., & Super, C. M. (1982). *Opportunities in psychology* (4th ed.). Skokie, IL: National Textbook.

Torrance, E. P. (1963). The creative personality and the ideal pupil. *Teachers College Record, 65*, 220–226.

Torrance, E. P. (1967). *Understanding the fourth-grade slump in creative thinking*. Washington, DC: U.S. Office of Education.

Torrance, E. P. (1995). *Why fly? A philosophy of creativity*. Norwood, NJ: Ablex.

American Counseling Association's *Code of Ethics and Standards of Practice 2005*

PREAMBLE

The American Counseling Association is an educational, scientific, and professional organization whose members work in a variety of settings and serve in multiple capacities. ACA members are dedicated to the enhancement of human development throughout the life span. Association members recognize diversity and embrace a cross-cultural approach in support of the worth, dignity, potential, and uniqueness of people within their social and cultural contexts. Professional values are an important way of living out an ethical commitment. Values inform principles. Inherently held values that guide our behaviors or exceed prescribed behaviors are deeply ingrained in the counselor and developed out of personal dedication, rather than the mandatory requirement of an external organization.

PURPOSE

The *ACA Code of Ethics* serves five main purposes:

1. The *Code* enables the association to clarify to current and future members, and to those served by members, the nature of the ethical responsibilities held in common by its members.

2. The *Code* helps support the mission of the association.

3. The *Code* establishes principles that define ethical behavior and best practices of association members.

4. The *Code* serves as an ethical guide designed to assist members in constructing a professional course of action that best serves those utilizing counseling services and best promotes the values of the counseling profession.

5. The *Code* serves as the basis for processing of ethical complaints and inquiries initiated against members of the association.

The *ACA Code of Ethics* contains eight main sections that address the following areas:

1. Section A: The Counseling Relationship

2. Section B: Confidentiality, Privileged Communication, and Privacy

3. Section C: Professional Responsibility

4. Section D: Relationships With Other Professionals

5. Section E: Evaluation, Assessment, and Interpretation

6. Section F: Supervision, Training, and Teaching

7. Section G: Research and Publication

8. Section H: Resolving Ethical Issues

Each section of the *ACA Code of Ethics* begins with an Introduction. The introductions to each section discuss what counselors should aspire to with regard to ethical behavior and responsibility. The Introduction helps set the tone for that particular section and provides a starting point that invites reflection on the ethical mandates contained in each part of the *ACA Code of Ethics*. When counselors are faced with ethical dilemmas that are difficult to resolve, they are expected to engage in a carefully considered ethical decision-making process. Reasonable differences of opinion can and do exist among counselors with respect to the ways in which values, ethical principles, and ethical standards would be applied when they conflict. While there is no specific ethical decision-making model that is most effective, counselors are expected to be familiar with a credible model of decision making that can bear public scrutiny and its application.

Through a chosen ethical decision-making process and evaluation of the context of the situation, counselors are empowered to make decisions that help expand the capacity of people to grow and develop.

A brief glossary is given to provide readers with a concise description of some of the terms used in the *ACA Code of Ethics.*

Section A: The Counseling Relationship

Introduction

Counselors encourage client growth and development in ways that foster the interest and welfare of clients and promote formation of healthy relationships. Counselors actively attempt to understand the diverse cultural backgrounds of the clients they serve. Counselors also explore their own cultural identities and how these affect their values and beliefs about the counseling process. Counselors are encouraged to contribute to society by devoting a portion of their professional activity to services for which there is little or no financial return (*pro bono publico*).

A.1. Welfare of Those Served by Counselors

a. *Primary Responsibility.* The primary responsibility of counselors is to respect the dignity and to promote the welfare of clients.

b. *Records.* Counselors maintain records necessary for rendering professional services to their clients and as required by laws, regulations, or agency or institution procedures. Counselors include sufficient and timely documentation in their client records to facilitate the delivery and continuity of needed services. Counselors take reasonable steps to ensure that documentation in records accurately reflects client progress and services provided. If errors are made in client records, counselors take steps to properly note the correction of such errors according to agency or institutional policies. *(See A.12.g.7., B.6., B.6.g., G.2.j.)*

c. *Counseling Plans.* Counselors and their clients work jointly in devising integrated counseling plans that offer reasonable promise of success and are consistent with abilities and circumstances of clients. Counselors and clients regularly review counseling plans to assess their continued viability and effectiveness, respecting the freedom of choice of clients. *(See A.2.a., A.2.d., A.12.g.)*

d. *Support Network Involvement.* Counselors recognize that support networks hold various meanings in the lives of clients and consider enlisting the support, understanding, and involvement of others.

e. *Employment Needs.* Counselors work with their clients considering employment in jobs that are consistent with the overall abilities, vocational limitations, physical restrictions, general temperament, interest and aptitude patterns, social skills, education, general qualifications, and other relevant characteristics and needs of clients. When appropriate, counselors appropriately trained in career development will assist in the placement of clients in positions that are consistent with the interest, culture, and the welfare of clients, employers, and/or the public.

A.2. Informed Consent in the Counseling Relationship

(See A.12.g., B.5., B.6.b., E.3., E.13.b., F.1.c., G.2.a.)

a. *Informed Consent.* Clients have the freedom to choose whether to enter into or remain in a counseling relationship and need adequate information about the counseling process and the counselor. Counselors have an obligation to review in writing and verbally with clients the rights and responsibilities of both the counselor and the client. Informed consent is an ongoing part of the counseling process, and counselors appropriately document discussions of informed consent throughout the counseling relationship.

b. *Types of Information Needed.* Counselors explicitly explain to clients the nature of all services provided. They inform clients about issues such as, but not limited to, the following: the purposes, goals, techniques, procedures, limitations, potential risks, and benefits of services; the counselor's qualifications, credentials, and relevant experience; continuation of services upon the incapacitation or death of a counselor; and other pertinent information. Counselors take steps to ensure that clients understand the implications of diagnosis, the intended use of tests and reports, fees, and billing arrangements. Clients have the right to confidentiality and to be provided with an explanation of its limitations (including how supervisors and/or treatment team professionals are involved); to obtain clear information about their records; to participate in the ongoing counseling plans; and to refuse any services or modality change and to be advised of the consequences of such refusal.

c. *Developmental and Cultural Sensitivity.* Counselors communicate information in ways that are both developmentally and culturally appropriate. Counselors use clear and understandable language when discussing issues related to informed consent. When clients have difficulty understanding the language used by counselors, they provide necessary services (e.g., arranging for a qualified interpreter or translator) to ensure comprehension by clients. In collaboration with clients, counselors consider cultural implications of informed consent procedures and, where possible, counselors adjust their practices accordingly.

d. *Inability to Give Consent.* When counseling minors or persons unable to give voluntary consent, counselors seek the assent of clients to services, and include them in decision making as appropriate. Counselors recognize the need to balance the ethical rights of clients to make choices, their capacity to give consent or assent to receive services, and parental or familial legal rights and responsibilities to protect these clients and make decisions on their behalf.

A.3. Clients Served by Others

When counselors learn that their clients are in a professional relationship with another mental health professional, they request release from clients to inform the other professionals and strive to establish positive and collaborative professional relationships.

A.4. Avoiding Harm and Imposing Values

a. *Avoiding Harm.* Counselors act to avoid harming their clients, trainees, and research participants and to minimize or to remedy unavoidable or unanticipated harm.

b. *Personal Values.* Counselors are aware of their own values, attitudes, beliefs, and behaviors and avoid imposing values that are inconsistent with counseling goals. Counselors respect the diversity of clients, trainees, and research participants.

A.5. Roles and Relationships with Clients
(See F.3., F.10., G.3.)

a. *Current Clients.* Sexual or romantic counselor-client interactions or relationships with current clients, their romantic partners, or their family members are prohibited.

b. *Former Clients.* Sexual or romantic counselor-client interactions or relationships with former clients, their romantic partners, or their family members are prohibited for a period of 5 years following the last professional contact. Counselors, before engaging in sexual or romantic interactions or relationships with clients, their romantic partners, or client family members after 5 years following the last professional contact, demonstrate forethought and document (in written form) whether the interactions or relationship can be viewed as exploitive in some way and/or whether there is still potential to harm the former client; in cases of potential exploitation and/or harm, the counselor avoids entering such an interaction or relationship.

c. *Nonprofessional Interactions or Relationships (other than sexual or romantic interactions or relationships).* Counselor-client nonprofessional relationships with clients, former clients, their romantic partners, or their family members should be avoided, except when the interaction is potentially beneficial to the client. *(See A.5.d.)*

d. *Potentially Beneficial Interactions.* When a counselor-client nonprofessional interaction with a client or former client may be potentially beneficial to the client or former client, the counselor must document in case records, prior to the interaction (when feasible), the rationale for such an interaction, the potential benefit, and anticipated consequences for the client or former client and other individuals significantly involved with the client or former client. Such interactions should be initiated with appropriate client consent. Where unintentional harm occurs to the client or former client, or to an individual significantly involved with the client or former client, due to the nonprofessional interaction, the counselor must show evidence of an attempt to remedy such harm. Examples of potentially beneficial interactions include, but are not limited to, attending a formal ceremony (e.g., a wedding/commitment ceremony or graduation); purchasing a service or product provided by a client or former client (excepting unrestricted bartering); hospital visits to an ill family member; mutual membership in a professional association, organization, or community. *(See A.5.c.)*

e. *Role Changes in the Professional Relationship* When a counselor changes a role from the original or most recent contracted relationship, he or she obtains informed consent from the client and explains the right of the client to refuse services related to the change. Examples of role changes include 1. changing from individual to relationship or family counseling, or vice versa; 2. changing from a nonforensic evaluative role to a therapeutic role, or vice versa; 3. changing from a counselor to a researcher role (i.e., enlisting clients as research participants), or vice versa; and 4. changing from a counselor to a mediator role, or vice versa. Clients must be fully informed of any anticipated consequences (e.g., financial, legal, personal, or therapeutic) of counselor role changes.

A.6. Roles and Relationships at Individual, Group, Institutional, and Societal Levels

a. *Advocacy.* When appropriate, counselors advocate at individual, group, institutional, and societal levels to examine potential barriers and obstacles that inhibit access and/or the growth and development of clients.

b. *Confidentiality and Advocacy.* Counselors obtain client consent prior to engaging in advocacy efforts on behalf of an identifiable client to improve the provision of services and to work toward removal of systemic barriers or obstacles that inhibit client access, growth, and development.

A.7. Multiple Clients

When a counselor agrees to provide counseling services to two or more persons who have a relationship, the counselor clarifies at the outset which person or persons are clients and the nature of the relationships the counselor will have with each involved person. If it becomes apparent that the counselor may be called upon to perform potentially conflicting roles, the counselor will clarify, adjust, or withdraw from roles appropriately. *(See A.8.a., B.4.)*

A.8. Group Work

(See B.4.a.)

a. *Screening.* Counselors screen prospective group counseling/therapy participants. To the extent possible, counselors select members whose needs and goals are compatible with goals of the group, who will not impede the group process, and whose well-being will not be jeopardized by the group experience.

b. *Protecting Clients.* In a group setting, counselors take reasonable precautions to protect clients from physical, emotional, or psychological trauma.

A.9. End-of-Life Care for Terminally Ill Clients

a. *Quality of Care.* Counselors strive to take measures that enable clients 1. to obtain high quality end-of-life care for their physical, emotional, social, and spiritual needs; 2. to exercise the highest degree of self-determination possible; 3. to be given every opportunity possible to engage in informed decision making regarding their end-of-life care; and 4. to receive complete and adequate assessment regarding their ability to make competent, rational decisions on their own behalf from a mental health professional who is experienced in end-of-life care practice.

b. *Counselor Competence, Choice, and Referral.* Recognizing the personal, moral, and competence issues related to end-of-life decisions, counselors may choose to work or not work with terminally ill clients who wish to explore their end-of-life options. Counselors provide appropriate referral information to ensure that clients receive the necessary help.

c. *Confidentiality.* Counselors who provide services to terminally ill individuals who are considering hastening their own deaths have the option of breaking or not breaking confidentiality, depending on applicable laws and the specific circumstances of the situation and after seeking consultation or supervision from appropriate professional and legal parties. *(See B.5.c., B.7.c.)*

A.10. Fees and Bartering

a. *Accepting Fees from Agency Clients.* Counselors refuse a private fee or other remuneration for rendering services to persons who are entitled to such services through the counselor's employing agency or institution.

The policies of a particular agency may make explicit provisions for agency clients to receive counseling services from members of its staff in private practice. In such instances, the clients must be informed of other options open to them should they seek private counseling services.

b. *Establishing Fees.* In establishing fees for professional counseling services, counselors consider the financial status of clients and locality. In the event that the established fee structure is inappropriate for a client, counselors assist clients in attempting to find comparable services of acceptable cost.

c. *Nonpayment of Fees.* If counselors intend to use collection agencies or take legal measures to collect fees from clients who do not pay for services as agreed upon, they first inform clients of intended actions and offer clients the opportunity to make payment.

d. *Bartering.* Counselors may barter only if the relationship is not exploitive or harmful and does not place the counselor in an unfair advantage, if the client requests it, and if such arrangements are an accepted practice among professionals in the community. Counselors consider the cultural implications of bartering and discuss relevant concerns with clients and document such agreements in a clear written contract.

e. *Receiving Gifts.* Counselors understand the challenges of accepting gifts from clients and recognize that in some cultures, small gifts are a token of respect and showing gratitude. When determining whether or not to accept a gift from clients, counselors take into account the therapeutic relationship, the monetary value of the gift, a client's motivation for giving the gift, and the counselor's motivation for wanting or declining the gift.

A.11. Termination and Referral

a. *Abandonment Prohibited.* Counselors do not abandon or neglect clients in counseling. Counselors assist in making appropriate arrangements for the continuation of treatment, when necessary, during interruptions such as vacations, illness, and following termination.

b. *Inability to Assist Clients.* If counselors determine an inability to be of professional assistance to clients, they avoid entering or continuing counseling relationships. Counselors are knowledgeable about culturally and clinically appropriate referral resources and suggest these alternatives. If clients decline the suggested referrals, counselors should discontinue the relationship.

c. *Appropriate Termination.* Counselors terminate a counseling relationship when it becomes reasonably apparent that the client no longer needs assistance, is not likely to benefit, or is being harmed by continued counseling. Counselors may terminate counseling when in jeopardy of harm by the client, or another person with whom the client has a relationship, or when clients do not pay fees as agreed upon. Counselors provide pretermination counseling and recommend other service providers when necessary.

d. *Appropriate Transfer of Services.* When counselors transfer or refer clients to other practitioners, they ensure that appropriate clinical and administrative processes are completed and open communication is maintained with both clients and practitioners.

A.12. Technology Applications

a. *Benefits and Limitation.* Counselors inform clients of the benefits and limitations of using information technology applications in the counseling process and in business/billing procedures. Such technologies include but are not limited to computer hardware and software, telephones, the World Wide Web, the Internet, online assessment instruments and other communication devices.

b. *Technology-Assisted Services.* When providing technology-assisted distance counseling services, counselors determine that clients are intellectually, emotionally, and physically capable of using the application and that the application is appropriate for the needs of clients.

c. *Inappropriate Services.* When technology-assisted distance counseling services are deemed inappropriate by the counselor or client, counselors consider delivering services face to face.

d. *Access.* Counselors provide reasonable access to computer applications when providing technology-assisted distance counseling services.

e. *Laws and Statutes.* Counselors ensure that the use of technology does not violate the laws of any local, state, national, or international entity and observe all relevant statutes.

f. *Assistance.* Counselors seek business, legal, and technical assistance when using technology applications, particularly when the use of such applications crosses state or national boundaries.

g. *Technology and Informed Consent.* As part of the process of establishing informed consent, counselors do the following:

1. Address issues related to the difficulty of maintaining the confidentiality of electronically transmitted communications.

2. Inform clients of all colleagues, supervisors, and employees, such as Informational Technology (IT) administrators, who might have authorized or unauthorized access to electronic transmissions.

3. Urge clients to be aware of all authorized or unauthorized users including family members and fellow employees who have access to any technology clients may use in the counseling process.

4. Inform clients of pertinent legal rights and limitations governing the practice of a profession over state lines or international boundaries.

5. Use encrypted Web sites and e-mail communications to help ensure confidentiality when possible.

6. When the use of encryption is not possible, counselors notify clients of this fact and limit electronic transmissions to general communications that are not client specific.

7. Inform clients if and for how long archival storage of transaction records are maintained.

8. Discuss the possibility of technology failure and alternate methods of service delivery.

9. Inform clients of emergency procedures, such as calling 911 or a local crisis hotline, when the counselor is not available.

10. Discuss time zone differences, local customs, and cultural or language differences that might impact service delivery.

11. Inform clients when technology assisted distance counseling services are not covered by insurance. *(See A.2.)*

h. *Sites on the World Wide Web.* Counselors maintaining sites on the World Wide Web (the Internet) do the following:

1. Regularly check that electronic links are working and professionally appropriate.

2. Establish ways clients can contact the counselor in case of technology failure.

3. Provide electronic links to relevant state licensure and professional certification boards to protect consumer rights and facilitate addressing ethical concerns.

4. Establish a method for verifying client identity.

5. Obtain the written consent of the legal guardian or other authorized legal representative prior to rendering services in the event the client is a minor child, an adult who is legally incompetent, or an adult incapable of giving informed consent.

6. Strive to provide a site that is accessible to persons with disabilities.

7. Strive to provide translation capabilities for clients who have a different primary language while also addressing the imperfect nature of such translations.

8. Assist clients in determining the validity and reliability of information found on the World Wide Web and other technology applications.

Section B: Confidentiality, Privileged Communication, and Privacy

Introduction

Counselors recognize that trust is a cornerstone of the counseling relationship. Counselors aspire to earn the trust of clients by creating an ongoing partnership, establishing and upholding appropriate boundaries, and maintaining confidentiality. Counselors communicate the parameters of confidentiality in a culturally competent manner.

B.1. Respecting Client Rights

a. *Multicultural/Diversity Considerations.* Counselors maintain awareness and sensitivity regarding cultural meanings of confidentiality and privacy. Counselors respect differing views toward disclosure of information. Counselors hold ongoing discussions with clients as to how, when, and with whom information is to be shared.

b. *Respecting Privacy.* Counselors respect client rights to privacy. Counselors solicit private information from clients only when it is beneficial to the counseling process.

c. *Respecting Confidentiality.* Counselors do not share confidential information without client consent or without sound legal or ethical justification.

d. *Explaining Limitations.* At initiation and throughout the counseling process, counselors inform clients of the limitations of confidentiality and seek to identify foreseeable situations in which confidentiality must be breached. *(See A.2.b.)*

B.2. Exceptions

a. *Danger and Legal Requirements.* The general requirement that counselors keep information confidential does not apply when disclosure is required to protect clients or identified others from serious and foreseeable harm or when legal requirements demand that confidential information must be revealed. Counselors consult with other professionals when in doubt as to the validity of an exception. Additional considerations apply when addressing end-of-life issues. *(See A.9.c.)*

b. *Contagious, Life-Threatening Diseases.* When clients disclose that they have a disease commonly known to be both communicable and life threatening, counselors may be justified in disclosing information to identifiable third parties, if they are known to be at demonstrable and high risk of contracting the disease. Prior to making a disclosure, counselors confirm that there is such a diagnosis and assess the intent of clients to inform the third parties about their disease or to engage in any behaviors that may be harmful to an identifiable third party.

c. *Court-Ordered Disclosure.* When subpoenaed to release confidential or privileged information without a client's permission, counselors obtain written, informed consent from the client or take steps to prohibit the disclosure or have it limited as narrowly as possible due to potential harm to the client or counseling relationship.

d. *Minimal Disclosure.* To the extent possible, clients are informed before confidential information is disclosed and are involved in the disclosure decision-making process. When circumstances require the disclosure of confidential information, only essential information is revealed.

B.3. Information Shared with Others

a. *Subordinates.* Counselors make every effort to ensure that privacy and confidentiality of clients are maintained by subordinates, including employees, supervisees, students, clerical assistants, and volunteers. *(See F.1.c.)*

b. *Treatment Teams.* When client treatment involves a continued review or participation by a treatment team, the client will be informed of the team's existence and composition, information being shared, and the purposes of sharing such information.

c. *Confidential Settings.* Counselors discuss confidential information only in settings in which they can reasonably ensure client privacy.

d. *Third-Party Payers.* Counselors disclose information to third-party payers only when clients have authorized such disclosure.

e. *Transmitting Confidential Information.* Counselors take precautions to ensure the confidentiality of information transmitted through the use of computers, electronic mail, facsimile machines, telephones, voicemail, answering machines, and other electronic or computer technology. *(See A.12.g.)*

f. *Deceased Clients.* Counselors protect the confidentiality of deceased clients, consistent with legal requirements and agency or setting policies.

B.4. Groups and Families

a. *Group Work.* In group work, counselors clearly explain the importance and parameters of confidentiality for the specific group being entered.

b. *Couples and Family Counseling.* In couples and family counseling, counselors clearly define who is considered "the client" and discuss expectations and limitations of confidentiality. Counselors seek agreement and document in writing such agreement among all involved parties having capacity to give consent concerning each individual's right to confidentiality and any obligation to preserve the confidentiality of information known.

B.5. Clients Lacking Capacity to Give Informed Consent

a. *Responsibility to Clients.* When counseling minor clients or adult clients who lack the capacity to give voluntary, informed consent, counselors protect the confidentiality of information received in the counseling relationship as specified by federal and state laws, written policies, and applicable ethical standards.

b. *Responsibility to Parents and Legal Guardians.* Counselors inform parents and legal guardians about the role of counselors and the confidential nature of the counseling relationship. Counselors are sensitive to the cultural diversity of families and respect the inherent rights and responsibilities of parents/guardians over the welfare of their children/charges according to law. Counselors work to establish, as appropriate, collaborative relationships with parents/guardians to best serve clients.

c. *Release of Confidential Information.* When counseling minor clients or adult clients who lack the capacity to give voluntary consent to release confidential information, counselors seek permission from an appropriate third party to disclose information. In such instances, counselors inform clients consistent with their level of understanding and take culturally appropriate measures to safeguard client confidentiality.

B.6. Records

a. *Confidentiality of Records.* Counselors ensure that records are kept in a secure location and that only authorized persons have access to records.

b. *Permission to Record.* Counselors obtain permission from clients prior to recording sessions through electronic or other means.

c. *Permission to Observe.* Counselors obtain permission from clients prior to observing counseling sessions, reviewing session transcripts, or viewing recordings of sessions with supervisors, faculty, peers, or others within the training environment.

d. *Client Access.* Counselors provide reasonable access to records and copies of records when requested by competent clients. Counselors limit the access of clients to their records, or portions of their records, only when there is compelling evidence that such access would cause harm to the client. Counselors document the request of clients and the rationale for withholding some or all of the records in the files of clients. In situations involving multiple clients, counselors provide individual clients with only those parts of records that relate directly to them and do not include confidential information related to any other client.

e. *Assistance with Records.* When clients request access to their records, counselors provide assistance and consultation in interpreting counseling records.

f. *Disclosure or Transfer.* Unless exceptions to confidentiality exist, counselors obtain written permission from clients to disclose or transfer records to legitimate third parties. Steps are taken to ensure that receivers of counseling records are sensitive to their confidential nature. *(See A.3., E.4.)*

g. *Storage and Disposal after Termination.* Counselors store records following termination of services to ensure reasonable future access, maintain records in accordance with state and federal statutes governing records, and dispose of client records and other sensitive materials in a manner that protects client confidentiality. When records are of an artistic nature, counselors obtain client (or guardian) consent with regards to handling of such records or documents. *(See A.1.b.)*

h. *Reasonable Precautions.* Counselors take reasonable precautions to protect client confidentiality in the event of the counselor's termination of practice, incapacity, or death. *(See C.2.h.)*

B.7. Research and Training

a. *Institutional Approval.* When institutional approval is required, counselors provide accurate information about their research proposals and obtain approval prior to conducting their research. They conduct research in accordance with the approved research protocol.

b. *Adherence to Guidelines.* Counselors are responsible for understanding and adhering to state, federal, agency, or institutional policies or applicable guidelines regarding confidentiality in their research practices.

c. *Confidentiality of Information Obtained in Research.* Violations of participant privacy and confidentiality are risks of participation in research involving human participants. Investigators maintain all research records in a secure manner. They explain to participants the risks of violations of privacy and confidentiality and disclose to participants any limits of confidentiality that reasonably can be expected. Regardless of the degree to which confidentiality will be maintained, investigators must disclose to participants any limits of confidentiality that reasonably can be expected. *(See G.2.e.)*

d. *Disclosure of Research Information.* Counselors do not disclose confidential information that reasonably could lead to the identification of a research participant unless they have obtained the prior consent of the person. Use of data derived from counseling relationships for purposes of training, research, or publication is confined to content that is disguised to ensure the anonymity of the individuals involved. *(See G.2.a., G.2.d.)*

e. *Agreement for Identification.* Identification of clients, students, or supervisees in a presentation or publication is permissible only when they have reviewed the material and agreed to its presentation or publication. *(See G.4.d.)*

B.8. Consultation

a. *Agreements.* When acting as consultants, counselors seek agreements among all parties involved concerning each individual's rights to confidentiality, the obligation of each individual to preserve confidential information, and the limits of confidentiality of information shared by others.

b. *Respect for Privacy.* Information obtained in a consulting relationship is discussed for professional purposes only with persons directly involved with the case. Written and oral reports present only data germane to the purposes of the consultation, and every effort is made to protect client identity and to avoid undue invasion of privacy.

c. *Disclosure of Confidential Information.* When consulting with colleagues, counselors do not disclose confidential information that reasonably could lead to the identification of a client or other person or organization with whom they have a confidential relationship unless they have obtained the prior consent of the person or organization or the disclosure cannot be avoided. They disclose information only to the extent necessary to achieve the purposes of the consultation. *(See D.2.d.)*

Section C: Professional Responsibility

Introduction

Counselors aspire to open, honest, and accurate communication in dealing with the public and other professionals. They practice in a nondiscriminatory manner within the boundaries of professional and personal competence and have a responsibility to abide by the *ACA Code of Ethics*. Counselors actively participate in local, state, and national associations that foster the development and improvement of counseling. Counselors advocate to promote change at the individual, group, institutional, and societal levels that improve the quality of life for individuals and groups and remove potential barriers to the provision or access of appropriate services being offered. Counselors have a responsibility to the public to engage in counseling practices that are based on rigorous research methodologies. In addition, counselors engage in self-care activities to maintain and promote their emotional, physical, mental, and spiritual well-being to best meet their professional responsibilities.

C.1. Knowledge of Standards

Counselors have a responsibility to read, understand, and follow the *ACA Code of Ethics* and adhere to applicable laws and regulations.

C.2. Professional Competence

a. *Boundaries of Competence.* Counselors practice only within the boundaries of their competence, based on their education, training, supervised experience, state and national professional credentials, and appropriate professional experience. Counselors gain knowledge, personal awareness, sensitivity, and skills pertinent to working with a diverse client population. *(See A.9.b., C.4.e., E.2., F.2., F.11.b.)*

b. *New Specialty Areas of Practice.* Counselors practice in specialty areas new to them only after appropriate education, training, and supervised experience. While developing skills in new specialty areas, counselors take steps to ensure the competence of their work and to protect others from possible harm. *(See F.6.f.)*

c. *Qualified for Employment.* Counselors accept employment only for positions for which they are qualified by education, training, supervised experience, state and national professional credentials, and appropriate professional experience. Counselors hire for professional counseling positions only individuals who are qualified and competent for those positions.

d. *Monitor Effectiveness.* Counselors continually monitor their effectiveness as professionals and take steps to improve when necessary. Counselors in private practice take reasonable steps to seek peer supervision as needed to evaluate their efficacy as counselors.

e. *Consultation on Ethical Obligations.* Counselors take reasonable steps to consult with other counselors or related professionals when they have questions regarding their ethical obligations or professional practice.

f. *Continuing Education.* Counselors recognize the need for continuing education to acquire and maintain a reasonable level of awareness of current scientific and professional information in their fields of activity. They take steps to maintain competence in the skills they use, are open to new procedures, and keep current with the diverse populations and specific populations with whom they work.

g. *Impairment.* Counselors are alert to the signs of impairment from their own physical, mental, or emotional problems and refrain from offering or providing professional services when such impairment is likely to harm a client or others. They seek assistance for problems that reach the level of professional impairment, and, if necessary, they limit, suspend, or terminate their professional responsibilities until such time it is determined that they may safely resume their work. Counselors assist colleagues or supervisors in recognizing their own professional impairment and provide consultation and assistance when warranted with colleagues or supervisors showing signs of impairment and intervene as appropriate to prevent imminent harm to clients. *(See A.11.b., F.8.b.)*

h. *Counselor Incapacitation or Termination of Practice.* When counselors leave a practice, they follow a prepared plan for transfer of clients and files. Counselors prepare and disseminate to an identified colleague or "records custodian" a plan for the transfer of clients and files in the case of their incapacitation, death, or termination of practice.

C.3. Advertising and Soliciting Clients

a. *Accurate Advertising.* When advertising or otherwise representing their services to the public, counselors identify their credentials in an accurate manner that is not false, misleading, deceptive, or fraudulent.

b. *Testimonials.* Counselors who use testimonials do not solicit them from current clients nor former clients nor any other persons who may be vulnerable to undue influence.

c. *Statements by Others.* Counselors make reasonable efforts to ensure that statements made by others about them or the profession of counseling are accurate.

d. *Recruiting through Employment.* Counselors do not use their places of employment or institutional affiliation to recruit or gain clients, supervisees, or consultees for their private practices.

e. *Products and Training Advertisements.* Counselors who develop products related to their profession or conduct workshops or training events ensure that the advertisements concerning these products or events are accurate and disclose adequate information for consumers to make informed choices. *(See C.6.d.)*

f. *Promoting to Those Served.* Counselors do not use counseling, teaching, training, or supervisory relationships to promote their products or training events in a manner that is deceptive or would exert undue influence on individuals who may be vulnerable. However, counselor educators may adopt textbooks they have authored for instructional purposes.

C.4. Professional Qualifications

a. *Accurate Representation.* Counselors claim or imply only professional qualifications actually completed and correct any known misrepresentations of their qualifications by others. Counselors truthfully represent the qualifications of their professional colleagues. Counselors clearly distinguish between paid and volunteer work experience and accurately describe their continuing education and specialized training. *(See C.2.a.)*

b. *Credentials* Counselors. claim only licenses or certifications that are current and in good standing.

c. *Educational Degrees.* Counselors clearly differentiate between earned and honorary degrees.

d. *Implying Doctoral-Level Competence.* Counselors clearly state their highest earned degree in counseling or closely related field. Counselors do not imply doctoral-level competence when only possessing a master's degree in counseling or a related field by referring to themselves as "Dr." in a counseling context when their doctorate is not in counseling or related field.

e. *Program Accreditation Status.* Counselors clearly state the accreditation status of their degree programs at the time the degree was earned.

f. *Professional Membership.* Counselors clearly differentiate between current, active memberships and former memberships in associations. Members of the American Counseling Association must clearly differentiate between professional membership, which implies the possession of at least a master's degree in counseling, and regular membership, which is open to individuals whose interests and activities are consistent with those of ACA but are not qualified for professional membership.

C.5. Nondiscrimination

Counselors do not condone or engage in discrimination based on age, culture, disability, ethnicity, race, religion/spirituality, gender, gender identity, sexual orientation, marital status/partnership, language preference, socioeconomic status, or any basis proscribed by law. Counselors do not discriminate against clients, students, employees, supervisees, or research participants in a manner that has a negative impact on these persons.

C.6. Public Responsibility

a. *Sexual Harassment.* Counselors do not engage in or condone sexual harassment. Sexual harassment is defined as sexual solicitation, physical advances, or verbal or nonverbal conduct that is sexual in nature, that occurs in connection with professional activities or roles, and that either

1. is unwelcome, is offensive, or creates a hostile workplace or learning environment, and counselors know or are told this; or

2. is sufficiently severe or intense to be perceived as harassment to a reasonable person in the context in which the behavior occurred. Sexual harassment can consist of a single intense or severe act or multiple persistent or pervasive acts.

b. *Reports to Third Parties.* Counselors are accurate, honest, and objective in reporting their professional activities and judgments to appropriate third parties, including courts, health insurance companies, those who are the recipients of evaluation reports, and others. *(See B.3., E.4.)*

c. *Media Presentations.* When counselors provide advice or comment by means of public lectures, demonstrations, radio or television programs, prerecorded tapes, technology-based applications, printed articles, mailed material, or other media, they take reasonable precautions to ensure that 1. the statements are based on appropriate professional counseling literature and practice, 2. the statements are otherwise consistent with the *ACA Code of Ethics,* and 3. the recipients of the information are not encouraged to infer that a professional counseling relationship has been established.

d. *Exploitation of Others.* Counselors do not exploit others in their professional relationships. *(See C.3.e.)*

e. *Scientific Bases for Treatment Modalities.* Counselors use techniques/ procedures/ modalities that are grounded in theory and/or have an empirical or scientific foundation. Counselors who do not must define the techniques/procedures as "unproven" or "developing" and explain the potential risks and ethical considerations of using such techniques/procedures and take steps to protect clients from possible harm. *(See A.4.a., E.5.c., E.5.d.)*

C.7. Responsibility to Other Professionals

a. *Personal Public Statements.* When making personal statements in a public context, counselors clarify that they are speaking from their personal perspectives and that they are not speaking on behalf of all counselors or the profession.

Section D: Relationships with Other Professionals

Introduction

Professional counselors recognize that the quality of their interactions with colleagues can influence the quality of services provided to clients. They work to become knowledgeable about colleagues within and outside the field of counseling. Counselors develop positive working relationships and systems of communication with colleagues to enhance services to clients.

D.1. Relationships with Colleagues, Employers, and Employees

a. *Different Approaches.* Counselors are respectful of approaches to counseling services that differ from their own. Counselors are respectful of traditions and practices of other professional groups with which they work.

b. *Forming Relationships.* Counselors work to develop and strengthen interdisciplinary relations with colleagues from other disciplines to best serve clients.

c. *Interdisciplinary Teamwork.* Counselors who are members of interdisciplinary teams delivering multifaceted services to clients, keep the focus on how to best serve the clients.

They participate in and contribute to decisions that affect the well-being of clients by drawing on the perspectives, values, and experiences of the counseling profession and those of colleagues from other disciplines. *(See A.1.a.)*

d. *Confidentiality.* When counselors are required by law, institutional policy, or extraordinary circumstances to serve in more than one role in judicial or administrative proceedings, they clarify role expectations and the parameters of confidentiality with their colleagues. *(See B.1.c., B.1.d., B.2.c., B.2.d., B.3.b.)*

e. *Establishing Professional and Ethical Obligations.* Counselors who are members of interdisciplinary teams clarify professional and ethical obligations of the team as a whole and of its individual members. When a team decision raises ethical concerns, counselors first attempt to resolve the concern within the team.

If they cannot reach resolution among team members, counselors pursue other avenues to address their concerns consistent with client well-being.

f. *Personnel Selection and Assignment.* Counselors select competent staff and assign responsibilities compatible with their skills and experiences.

g. *Employer Policies.* The acceptance of employment in an agency or institution implies that counselors are in agreement with its general policies and principles. Counselors strive to reach agreement with employers as to acceptable standards of conduct that allow for changes in institutional policy conducive to the growth and development of clients.

h. *Negative Conditions.* Counselors alert their employers of inappropriate policies and practices. They attempt to effect changes in such policies or procedures through constructive action within the organization. When such policies are potentially disruptive or damaging to clients or may limit the effectiveness of services provided and change cannot be effected, counselors take appropriate further action. Such action may include referral to appropriate certification, accreditation, or state licensure organizations, or voluntary termination of employment.

i. *Protection from Punitive Action.* Counselors take care not to harass or dismiss an employee who has acted in a responsible and ethical manner to expose inappropriate employer policies or practices.

D.2. Consultation

a. *Consultant Competency.* Counselors take reasonable steps to ensure that they have the appropriate resources and competencies when providing consultation services. Counselors provide appropriate referral resources when requested or needed. *(See C.2.a.)*

b. *Understanding Consultees.* When providing consultation, counselors attempt to develop with their consultees a clear understanding of problem definition, goals for change, and predicted consequences of interventions selected.

c. *Consultant Goals.* The consulting relationship is one in which consultee adaptability and growth toward self-direction are consistently encouraged and cultivated.

d. *Informed Consent in Consultation.* When providing consultation, counselors have an obligation to review, in writing and verbally, the rights and responsibilities of both counselors and consultees. Counselors use clear and understandable language to inform all parties involved about the purpose of the services to be provided, relevant costs, potential risks and benefits, and the limits of confidentiality. Working in conjunction with the consultee, counselors attempt to develop a clear definition of the problem, goals for change, and predicted consequences of interventions that are culturally responsive and appropriate to the needs of consultees. *(See A.2.a., A.2.b.)*

Section E: Evaluation, Assessment, and Interpretation

Introduction

Counselors use assessment instruments as one component of the counseling process, taking into account the client personal and cultural context. Counselors promote the well-being of individual clients or groups of clients by developing and using appropriate educational, psychological, and career assessment instruments.

E.1. General

a. *Assessment.* The primary purpose of educational, psychological, and career assessment is to provide measurements that are valid and reliable in either comparative or absolute terms. These include, but are not limited to, measurements of ability, personality, interest, intelligence, achievement, and performance. Counselors recognize the need to interpret the statements in this section as applying to both quantitative and qualitative assessments.

b. *Client Welfare.* Counselors do not misuse assessment results and interpretations, and they take reasonable steps to prevent others from misusing the information these techniques provide. They respect the client's right to know the results, the interpretations made, and the bases for counselors' conclusions and recommendations.

E.2. Competence to Use and Interpret Assessment Instruments

a. *Limits of Competence.* Counselors utilize only those testing and assessment services for which they have been trained and are competent. Counselors using technology assisted test interpretations are trained in the construct being measured and the specific instrument being used prior to using its technology based application. Counselors take reasonable measures to ensure the proper use of psychological and career assessment techniques by persons under their supervision. (See A.12.)

b. *Appropriate Use.* Counselors are responsible for the appropriate application, scoring, interpretation, and use of assessment instruments relevant to the needs of the client, whether they score and interpret such assessments themselves or use technology or other services.

c. *Decisions Based on Results.* Counselors responsible for decisions involving individuals or policies that are based on assessment results have a thorough understanding of educational, psychological, and career measurement, including validation criteria, assessment research, and guidelines for assessment development and use.

E.3. Informed Consent in Assessment

a. *Explanation to Clients.* Prior to assessment, counselors explain the nature and purposes of assessment and the specific use of results by potential recipients. The explanation will be given in the language of the client (or other legally authorized person on behalf of the client), unless an explicit exception has been agreed upon in advance. Counselors consider the client's personal or cultural context, the level of the client's understanding of the results, and the impact of the results on the client. *(See A.2., A.12.g., F.1.c.)*

b. *Recipients of Results.* Counselors consider the examinee's welfare, explicit understandings, and prior agreements in determining who receives the assessment results.

Counselors include accurate and appropriate interpretations with any release of individual or group assessment results. *(See B.2.c., B.5.)*

E.4. Release of Data to Qualified Professionals

Counselors release assessment data in which the client is identified only with the consent of the client or the client's legal representative. Such data are released only to persons recognized by counselors as qualified to interpret the data. *(See B.1., B.3., B.6.b.)*

E.5. Diagnosis of Mental Disorders

a. *Proper Diagnosis.* Counselors take special care to provide proper diagnosis of mental disorders. Assessment techniques (including personal interview) used to determine client care (e.g., locus of treatment, type of treatment, or recommended follow-up) are carefully selected and appropriately used.

b. *Cultural Sensitivity.* Counselors recognize that culture affects the manner in which clients' problems are defined. Clients' socioeconomic and cultural experiences are considered when diagnosing mental disorders. *(See A.2.c.)*

c. *Historical and Social Prejudices in the Diagnosis of Pathology.* Counselors recognize historical and social prejudices in the misdiagnosis and pathologizing of certain individuals and groups and the role of mental health professionals in perpetuating these prejudices through diagnosis and treatment.

d. *Refraining from Diagnosis.* Counselors may refrain from making and/or reporting a diagnosis if they believe it would cause harm to the client or others.

E.6. Instrument Selection

a. *Appropriateness of Instruments.* Counselors carefully consider the validity, reliability, psychometric limitations, and appropriateness of instruments when selecting assessments.

b. *Referral Information.* If a client is referred to a third party for assessment, the counselor provides specific referral questions and sufficient objective data about the client to ensure that appropriate assessment instruments are utilized. *(See A. 9.b., B.3.)*

c. *Culturally Diverse Populations.* Counselors are cautious when selecting assessments for culturally diverse populations to avoid the use of instruments that lack appropriate psychometric properties for the client population. *(See A.2.c., E.5.b.)*

E.7. Conditions of Assessment Administration
(See A.12.b., A.12.d.)

a. *Administration Conditions.* Counselors administer assessments under the same conditions that were established in their standardization. When assessments are not administered under standard conditions, as may be necessary to accommodate clients with disabilities, or when unusual behavior or irregularities occur during the administration, those conditions are noted in interpretation, and the results may be designated as invalid or of questionable validity.

b. *Technological Administration.* Counselors ensure that administration programs function properly and provide clients with accurate results when technological or other electronic methods are used for assessment administration.

c. *Unsupervised Assessments.* Unless the assessment instrument is designed, intended, and validated for self-administration and/or scoring, counselors do not permit inadequately supervised use.

d. *Disclosure of Favorable Conditions.* Prior to administration of assessments, conditions that produce most favorable assessment results are made known to the examinee.

E.8. Multicultural Issues/Diversity in Assessment

Counselors use with caution assessment techniques that were normed on populations other than that of the client. Counselors recognize the effects of age, color, culture, disability, ethnic group, gender, race, language preference, religion, spirituality, sexual orientation, and socioeconomic status on test administration and interpretation, and place test results in proper perspective with other relevant factors. *(See A.2.c., E.5.b.)*

E.9. Scoring and Interpretation of Assessments

a. *Reporting.* In reporting assessment results, counselors indicate reservations that exist regarding validity or reliability due to circumstances of the assessment or the inappropriateness of the norms for the person tested.

b. *Research Instruments.* Counselors exercise caution when interpreting the results of research instruments not having sufficient technical data to support respondent results. The specific purposes for the use of such instruments are stated explicitly to the examinee.

c. *Assessment Services.* Counselors who provide assessment scoring and interpretation services to support the assessment process confirm the validity of such interpretations. They accurately describe the purpose, norms, validity, reliability, and applications of the procedures and any special qualifications applicable to their use. The public offering of an automated test interpretations service is considered a professional-to-professional consultation. The formal responsibility of the consultant is to the consultee, but the ultimate and overriding responsibility is to the client. *(See D.2.)*

E.10. Assessment Security

Counselors maintain the integrity and security of tests and other assessment techniques consistent with legal and contractual obligations. Counselors do not appropriate, reproduce, or modify published assessments or parts thereof without acknowledgment and permission from the publisher.

E.11. Obsolete Assessments and Outdated Results

Counselors do not use data or results from assessments that are obsolete or outdated for the current purpose. Counselors make every effort to prevent the misuse of obsolete measures and assessment data by others.

E.12. Assessment Construction

Counselors use established scientific procedures, relevant standards, and current professional knowledge for assessment design in the development, publication, and utilization of educational and psychological assessment techniques.

E.13. Forensic Evaluation: Evaluation for Legal Proceedings

a. *Primary Obligations.* When providing forensic evaluations, the primary obligation of counselors is to produce objective findings that can be substantiated based on information and techniques appropriate to the evaluation, which may include examination of the individual and/or review of records. Counselors are entitled to form professional opinions based on their professional knowledge and expertise that can be supported by the data gathered in evaluations. Counselors will define the limits of their reports or testimony, especially when an examination of the individual has not been conducted.

b. *Consent for Evaluation.* Individuals being evaluated are informed in writing that the relationship is for the purposes of an evaluation and is not counseling in nature, and entities or individuals who will receive the evaluation report are identified. Written consent to be evaluated is obtained from those being evaluated unless a court orders evaluations to be conducted without the written consent of individuals being evaluated. When children or vulnerable adults are being evaluated, informed written consent is obtained from a parent or guardian.

c. *Client Evaluation Prohibited.* Counselors do not evaluate individuals for forensic purposes they currently counsel or individuals they have counseled in the past. Counselors do not accept as counseling clients individuals they are evaluating or individuals they have evaluated in the past for forensic purposes.

d. *Avoid Potentially Harmful Relationships.* Counselors who provide forensic evaluations avoid potentially harmful professional or personal relationships with family members, romantic partners, and close friends of individuals they are evaluating or have evaluated in the past.

Section F: Supervision, Training, and Teaching

Introduction

Counselors aspire to foster meaningful and respectful professional relationships and to maintain appropriate boundaries with supervisees and students. Counselors have theoretical and pedagogical foundations for their work and aim to be fair, accurate, and honest in their assessments of counselors-in-training.

F.1. Counselor Supervision and Client Welfare

a. *Client Welfare.* A primary obligation of counseling supervisors is to monitor the services provided by other counselors or counselors-in-training. Counseling supervisors monitor client welfare and supervisee clinical performance and professional development. To fulfill these obligations, supervisors meet regularly with supervisees to review case notes, samples of clinical work, or live observations. Supervisees have a responsibility to understand and follow the *ACA Code of Ethics.*

b. *Counselor Credentials.* Counseling supervisors work to ensure that clients are aware of the qualifications of the supervisees who render services to the clients. *(See A.2.b.)*

c. *Informed Consent and Client Rights.* Supervisors make supervisees aware of client rights including the protection of client privacy and confidentiality in the counseling relationship. Supervisees provide clients with professional disclosure information and inform them of how the supervision process influences the limits of confidentiality. Supervisees make clients aware of who will have access to records of the counseling relationship and how these records will be used. *(See A.2.b., B.1.d.)*

F.2. Counselor Supervision Competence

a. *Supervisor Preparation.* Prior to offering clinical supervision services, counselors are trained in supervision methods and techniques. Counselors who offer clinical supervision services regularly pursue continuing education activities including both counseling and supervision topics and skills. *(See C.2.a., C.2.f.)*

b. *Multicultural Issues/Diversity in Supervision.* Counseling supervisors are aware of and address the role of multiculturalism/diversity in the supervisory relationship.

F.3. Supervisory Relationships

a. *Relationship Boundaries with Supervisees.* Counseling supervisors clearly define and maintain ethical professional, personal, and social relationships with their supervisees. Counseling supervisors avoid nonprofessional relationships with current supervisees. If supervisors must assume other professional roles (e.g., clinical and administrative supervisor, instructor) with supervisees, they work to minimize potential conflicts and explain to supervisees the expectations and responsibilities associated with each role. They do not engage in any form of nonprofessional interaction that may compromise the supervisory relationship.

b. *Sexual Relationships.* Sexual or romantic interactions or relationships with current supervisees are prohibited.

c. *Sexual Harassment.* Counseling supervisors do not condone or subject supervisees to sexual harassment. *(See C.6.a.)*

d. *Close Relatives and Friends.* Counseling supervisors avoid accepting close relatives, romantic partners, or friends as supervisees.

e. *Potentially Beneficial Relationships.* Counseling supervisors are aware of the power differential in their relationships with supervisees. If they believe nonprofessional relationships with a supervisee may be potentially beneficial to the supervisee, they take precautions similar to those taken by counselors when working with clients. Examples of potentially beneficial interactions or relationships include attending a formal ceremony; hospital visits; providing support during a stressful event; or mutual membership in a professional association, organization, or community. Counseling supervisors engage in open discussions with supervisees when they consider entering into relationships with them outside of their roles as clinical and/or administrative supervisors. Before engaging in nonprofessional relationships, supervisors discuss with supervisees and document the rationale for such interactions, potential benefits or drawbacks, and anticipated consequences for the supervisee. Supervisors clarify the specific nature and limitations of the additional role(s) they will have with the supervisee.

F.4. Supervisor Responsibilities

a. *Informed Consent for Supervision.* Supervisors are responsible for incorporating into their supervision the principles of informed consent and participation. Supervisors inform supervisees of the policies and procedures to which they are to adhere and the mechanisms for due process appeal of individual supervisory actions.

b. *Emergencies and Absences.* Supervisors establish and communicate to supervisees procedures for contacting them or, in their absence, alternative on-call supervisors to assist in handling crises.

c. *Standards for Supervisees.* Supervisors make their supervisees aware of professional and ethical standards and legal responsibilities. Supervisors of postdegree counselors encourage these counselors to adhere to professional standards of practice. *(See C.1.)*

d. *Termination of the Supervisory Relationship.* Supervisors or supervisees have the right to terminate the supervisory relationship with adequate notice. Reasons for withdrawal are provided to the other party. When cultural, clinical, or professional issues are crucial to the viability of the supervisory relationship, both parties make efforts to resolve differences. When termination is warranted, supervisors make appropriate referrals to possible alternative supervisors.

F.5. Counseling Supervision Evaluation, Remediation, and Endorsement

a. *Evaluation.* Supervisors document and provide supervisees with ongoing performance appraisal and evaluation feedback and schedule periodic formal evaluative sessions throughout the supervisory relationship.

b. *Limitations.* Through ongoing evaluation and appraisal, supervisors are aware of the limitations of supervisees that might impede performance. Supervisors assist supervisees in securing remedial assistance when needed. They recommend dismissal from training programs, applied counseling settings, or state or voluntary professional credentialing processes when those supervisees are unable to provide competent professional services. Supervisors seek consultation and document their decisions to dismiss or refer supervisees for assistance. They ensure that supervisees are aware of options available to them to address such decisions. *(See C.2.g.)*

c. *Counseling for Supervisees.* If supervisees request counseling, supervisors provide them with acceptable referrals. Counselors do not provide counseling services to supervisees. Supervisors address interpersonal competencies in terms of the impact of these issues on clients, the supervisory relationship, and professional functioning. *(See F.3.a.)*

d. *Endorsement.* Supervisors endorse supervisees for certification, licensure, employment, or completion of an academic or training program only when they believe supervisees are qualified for the endorsement. Regardless of qualifications, supervisors do not endorse supervisees whom they believe to be impaired in any way that would interfere with the performance of the duties associated with the endorsement.

F.6. Responsibilities of Counselor Educators

a. *Counselor Educators.* Counselor educators who are responsible for developing, implementing, and supervising educational programs are skilled as teachers and practitioners. They are knowledgeable regarding the ethical, legal, and regulatory aspects of the profession, are skilled in applying that knowledge, and make students and supervisees aware of their responsibilities. Counselor educators conduct counselor education and training programs in an ethical manner and serve as role models for professional behavior. *(See C.1., C.2.a., C.2.c.)*

b. *Infusing Multicultural Issues/Diversity.* Counselor educators infuse material related to multiculturalism/diversity into all courses and workshops for the development of professional counselors.

c. *Integration of Study and Practice.* Counselor educators establish education and training programs that integrate academic study and supervised practice.

d. *Teaching Ethics.* Counselor educators make students and supervisees aware of the ethical responsibilities and standards of the profession and the ethical responsibilities of students to the profession. Counselor educators infuse ethical considerations throughout the curriculum. *(See C.1.)*

e. *Peer Relationships.* Counselor educators make every effort to ensure that the rights of peers are not compromised when students or supervisees lead counseling groups or provide clinical supervision. Counselor educators take steps to ensure that students and supervisees understand they have the same ethical obligations as counselor educators, trainers, and supervisors.

f. *Innovative Theories and Techniques.* When counselor educators teach counseling techniques/procedures that are innovative, without an empirical foundation, or without a well-grounded theoretical foundation, they define the counseling techniques/procedures as "unproven" or "developing" and explain to students the potential risks and ethical considerations of using such techniques/procedures.

g. *Field Placements.* Counselor educators develop clear policies within their training programs regarding field placement and other clinical experiences. Counselor educators provide clearly stated roles and responsibilities for the student or supervisee, the site supervisor, and the program supervisor. They confirm that site supervisors are qualified to provide supervision and inform site supervisors of their professional and ethical responsibilities in this role.

h. *Professional Disclosure.* Before initiating counseling services, counselors-in-training disclose their status as students and explain how this status affects the limits of confidentiality. Counselor educators ensure that the clients at field placements are aware of the services rendered and the qualifications of the students and supervisees rendering those services. Students and supervisees obtain client permission before they use any information concerning the counseling relationship in the training process. *(See A.2.b.)*

F.7. Student Welfare

a. *Orientation.* Counselor educators recognize that orientation is a developmental process that continues throughout the educational and clinical training of students. Counseling faculty provide prospective students with information about the counselor education program's expectations: 1. the type and level of skill and knowledge acquisition required for successful completion of the training; 2. program training goals, objectives, and mission, and subject matter to be covered; 3. bases for evaluation; 4. training components that encourage self-growth or self-disclosure as part of the training process; 5. the type of supervision settings and requirements of the sites for required clinical field experiences; 6. student and supervisee evaluation and dismissal policies and procedures; and 7. up-to-date employment prospects for graduates.

b. *Self-Growth Experiences.* Counselor education programs delineate requirements for self-disclosure or self-growth experiences in their admission and program materials. Counselor educators use professional judgment when designing training experiences they conduct that require student and supervisee self growth or self-disclosure. Students and supervisees are made aware of the ramifications their self-disclosure may have when counselors whose primary role as teacher, trainer, or supervisor requires acting on ethical obligations to the profession. Evaluative components of experiential training experiences explicitly delineate predetermined academic standards that are separate and do not depend on the student's level of self-disclosure. Counselor educators may require trainees to seek professional help to address any personal concerns that may be affecting their competency.

F.8. Student Responsibilities

a. *Standards for Students.* Counselors-in-training have a responsibility to understand and follow the *ACA Code of Ethics* and adhere to applicable laws, regulatory policies, and rules and policies governing professional staff behavior at the agency or placement setting. Students have the same obligation to clients as those required of professional counselors. *(See C.1., H.1.)*

b. *Impairment.* Counselors-in-training refrain from offering or providing counseling services when their physical, mental, or emotional problems are likely to harm a client or others. They are alert to the signs of impairment, seek assistance for problems, and notify their program supervisors when they are aware that they are unable to effectively provide services. In addition, they seek appropriate professional services for themselves to remediate the problems that are interfering with their ability to provide services to others. *(See A.1., C.2.d., C.2.g.)*

F.9. Evaluation and Remediation of Students

a. *Evaluation.* Counselors clearly state to students, prior to and throughout the training program, the levels of competency expected, appraisal methods, and timing of evaluations for both didactic and clinical competencies. Counselor educators provide students with ongoing performance appraisal and evaluation feedback throughout the training program.

b. *Limitations.* Counselor educators, throughout ongoing evaluation and appraisal, are aware of and address the inability of some students to achieve counseling competencies that might impede performance. Counselor educators

1. assist students in securing remedial assistance when needed,

2. seek professional consultation and document their decision to dismiss or refer students for assistance, and

3. ensure that students have recourse in a timely manner to address decisions to require them to seek assistance or to dismiss them and provide students with due process according to institutional policies and procedures. *(See C.2.g.)*

c. *Counseling for Students.* If students request counseling or if counseling services are required as part of a remediation process, counselor educators provide acceptable referrals.

F. 10. Roles and Relationships Between Counselor Educators and Students

a. *Sexual or Romantic Relationships.* Sexual or romantic interactions or relationships with current students are prohibited.

b. *Sexual Harassment.* Counselor educators do not condone or subject students to sexual harassment. *(See C.6.a.)*

c. *Relationships with Former Students.* Counselor educators are aware of the power differential in the relationship between faculty and students. Faculty members foster open discussions with former students when considering engaging in a social, sexual, or other intimate relationship. Faculty members discuss with the former student how their former relationship may affect the change in relationship.

d. *Nonprofessional Relationships.* Counselor educators avoid nonprofessional or ongoing professional relationships with students in which there is a risk of potential harm to the student or that may compromise the training experience or grades assigned. In addition, counselor educators do not accept any form of professional services, fees, commisions, reimbursement, or remuncration from a site for student or supervisee placement.

e. *Counseling Services.* Counselor educators do not serve as counselors to current students unless this is a brief role associated with a training experience.

f. *Potentially Beneficial Relationships.* Counselor educators are aware of the power differential in the relationship between faculty and students. If they believe a nonprofessional relationship with a student may be potentially beneficial to the student, they take precautions similar to those taken by counselors when working with clients. Examples of potentially beneficial interactions or relationships include, but are not limited to, attending a formal ceremony; hospital visits; providing support during a stressful event; or mutual membership in a professional association, organization, or community. Counselor educators engage in open discussions with students when they consider entering into relationships with students outside of their roles as teachers and supervisors. They discuss with students the rationale for such interactions, the potential benefits and drawbacks, and the anticipated consequences for the student. Educators clarify the specific nature and limitations of the additional role(s) they will have with the student prior to engaging in a nonprofessional relationship.

Nonprofessional relationships with students should be time-limited and initiated with student consent.

F.11. Multicultural/Diversity Competence in Counselor Education and Training Programs

a. *Faculty Diversity.* Counselor educators are committed to recruiting and retaining a diverse faculty.

b. *Student Diversity.* Counselor educators actively attempt to recruit and retain a diverse student body. Counselor educators demonstrate commitment to multicultural/diversity competence by recognizing and valuing diverse cultures and types of abilities students bring to the training experience. Counselor educators provide appropriate accommodations that enhance and support diverse student well-being and academic performance.

c. *Multicultural/Diversity Competence.* Counselor educators actively infuse multicultural/diversity competency in their training and supervision practices. They actively train students to gain awareness, knowledge, and skills in the competencies of multicultural practice. Counselor educators include case examples, role-plays, discussion questions, and other classroom activities that promote and represent various cultural perspectives.

Section G: Research and Publication

Introduction

Counselors who conduct research are encouraged to contribute to the knowledge base of the profession and promote a clearer understanding of the conditions that lead to a healthy and more just society. Counselors support efforts of researchers by participating fully and willingly whenever possible. Counselors minimize bias and respect diversity in designing and implementing research programs.

G.1. Research Responsibilities

a. *Use of Human Research Participants.* Counselors plan, design, conduct, and report research in a manner that is consistent with pertinent ethical principles, federal and state laws, host institutional regulations, and scientific standards governing research with human research participants.

b. *Deviation from Standard Practice.* Counselors seek consultation and observe stringent safeguards to protect the rights of research participants when a research problem suggests a deviation from standard or acceptable practices.

c. *Independent Researchers.* When independent researchers do not have access to an Institutional Review Board (IRB), they should consult with researchers who are familiar with IRB procedures to provide appropriate safeguards.

d. *Precautions to Avoid Injury.* Counselors who conduct research with human participants are responsible for the welfare of participants throughout the research process and should take reasonable precautions to avoid causing injurious psychological, emotional, physical, or social effects to participants.

e. *Principal Researcher Responsibility.* The ultimate responsibility for ethical research practice lies with the principal researcher. All others involved in the research activities share ethical obligations and responsibility for their own actions.

f. *Minimal Interference.* Counselors take reasonable precautions to avoid causing disruptions in the lives of research participants that could be caused by their involvement in research.

g. *Multicultural/Diversity Considerations in Research.* When appropriate to research goals, counselors are sensitive to incorporating research procedures that take into account cultural considerations. They seek consultation when appropriate.

G.2. Rights of Research Participants
(See A.2, A.7.)

a. *Informed Consent in Research.* Individuals have the right to consent to become research participants. In seeking consent, counselors use language that

1. accurately explains the purpose and procedures to be followed,
2. identifies any procedures that are experimental or relatively untried,

3. describes any attendant discomforts and risks,

4. describes any benefits or changes in individuals or organizations that might be reasonably expected,

5. discloses appropriate alternative procedures that would be advantageous for participants,

6. offers to answer any inquiries concerning the procedures,

7. describes any limitations on confidentiality,

8. describes the format and potential target audiences for the dissemination of research findings, and

9. instructs participants that they are free to withdraw their consent and to discontinue participation in the project at any time without penalty.

b. *Deception.* Counselors do not conduct research involving deception unless alternative procedures are not feasible and the prospective value of the research justifies the deception. If such deception has the potential to cause physical or emotional harm to research participants, the research is not conducted, regardless of prospective value. When the methodological requirements of a study necessitate concealment or deception, the investigator explains the reasons for this action as soon as possible during the debriefing.

c. *Student/Supervisee Participation.* Researchers who involve students or supervisees in research make clear to them that the decision regarding whether or not to participate in research activities does not affect one's academic standing or supervisory relationship. Students or supervisees who choose not to participate in educational research are provided with an appropriate alternative to fulfill their academic or clinical requirements.

d. *Client Participation.* Counselors conducting research involving clients make clear in the informed consent process that clients are free to choose whether or not to participate in research activities.

Counselors take necessary precautions to protect clients from adverse consequences of declining or withdrawing from participation.

e. *Confidentiality of Information.* Information obtained about research participants during the course of an investigation is confidential. When the possibility exists that others may obtain access to such information, ethical research practice requires that the possibility, together with the plans for protecting confidentiality, be explained to participants as a part of the procedure for obtaining informed consent.

f. *Persons Not Capable of Giving Informed Consent.* When a person is not capable of giving informed consent, counselors provide an appropriate explanation to, obtain agreement for participation from, and obtain the appropriate consent of a legally authorized person.

g. *Commitments to Participants.* Counselors take reasonable measures to honor all commitments to research participants. *(See A.2.c.)*

h. *Explanations After Data Collection.* After data are collected, counselors provide participants with full clarification of the nature of the study to remove any misconceptions participants might have regarding the research. Where scientific or human values justify delaying or withholding information, counselors take reasonable measures to avoid causing harm.

i. *Informing Sponsors.* Counselors inform sponsors, institutions, and publication channels regarding research procedures and outcomes. Counselors ensure that appropriate bodies and authorities are given pertinent information and acknowledgment.

j. *Disposal of Research Documents and Records.* Within a reasonable period of time following the completion of a research project or study, counselors take steps to destroy records or documents (audio, video, digital, and written) containing confidential data or information that identifies research participants.

When records are of an artistic nature, researchers obtain participant consent with regard to handling of such records or documents. *(See B.4.a, B.4.g.)*

G.3. Relationships with Research Participants (When Research Involves Intensive or Extended Interactions)

a. *Nonprofessional Relationships.* Nonprofessional relationships with research participants should be avoided.

b. *Relationships with Research Participants.* Sexual or romantic counselor-research participant interactions or relationships with current research participants are prohibited.

c. *Sexual Harassment and Research Participants.* Researchers do not condone or subject research participants to sexual harassment.

d. *Potentially Beneficial Interactions.* When a nonprofessional interaction between the researcher and the research participant may be potentially beneficial, the researcher must document, prior to the interaction (when feasible), the rationale for such an interaction, the potential benefit, and anticipated consequences for the research participant. Such interactions should be initiated with appropriate consent of the research participant. Where unintentional harm occurs to the research participant due to the nonprofessional interaction, the researcher must show evidence of an attempt to remedy such harm.

G.4. Reporting Results

a. *Accurate Results.* Counselors plan, conduct, and report research accurately. They provide thorough discussions of the limitations of their data and alternative hypotheses. Counselors do not engage in misleading or fraudulent research, distort data, misrepresent data, or deliberately bias their results. They explicitly mention all variables and conditions known to the investigator that may have affected the outcome of a study or the interpretation of data. They describe the extent to which results are applicable for diverse populations.

b. *Obligation to Report Unfavorable Results.* Counselors report the results of any research of professional value. Results that reflect unfavorably on institutions, programs, services, prevailing opinions, or vested interests are not withheld.

c. *Reporting Errors.* If counselors discover significant errors in their published research, they take reasonable steps to correct such errors in a correction erratum, or through other appropriate publication means.

d. *Identity of Participants.* Counselors who supply data, aid in the research of another person, report research results, or make original data available take due care to disguise the identity of respective participants in the absence of specific authorization from the participants to do otherwise. In situations where participants self-identify their involvement in research studies, researchers take active steps to ensure that data is adapted/changed to protect the identity and welfare of all parties and that discussion of results does not cause harm to participants.

e. *Replication Studies.* Counselors are obligated to make available sufficient original research data to qualified professionals who may wish to replicate the study.

G.5. Publication

a. *Recognizing Contributions.* When conducting and reporting research, counselors are familiar with and give recognition to previous work on the topic, observe copyright laws, and give full credit to those to whom credit is due.

b. *Plagiarism.* Counselors do not plagiarize, that is, they do not present another person's work as their own work.

c. *Review/Republication of Data or Ideas.* Counselors fully acknowledge and make editorial reviewers aware of prior publication of ideas or data where such ideas or data are submitted for review or publication.

d. *Contributors.* Counselors give credit through joint authorship, acknowledgment, footnote statements, or other appropriate means to those who have contributed significantly to research or concept development in accordance with such contributions. The principal contributor is listed first and minor technical or professional contributions are acknowledged in notes or introductory statements.

e. *Agreement of Contributors.* Counselors who conduct joint research with colleagues or students/supervisees establish agreements in advance regarding allocation of tasks, publication credit, and types of acknowledgment that will be received.

f. *Student Research.* For articles that are substantially based on students course papers, projects, dissertations or theses, and on which students have been the primary contributors, they are listed as principal authors.

g. *Duplicate Submission.* Counselors submit manuscripts for consideration to only one journal at a time. Manuscripts that are published in whole or in substantial part in another journal or published work are not submitted for publication without acknowledgment and permission from the previous publication.

h. *Professional Review.* Counselors who review material submitted for publication, research, or other scholarly purposes respect the confidentiality and proprietary rights of those who submitted it.

Counselors use care to make publication decisions based on valid and defensible standards. Counselors review article submissions in a timely manner and based on their scope and competency in research methodologies. Counselors who serve as reviewers at the request of editors or publishers make every effort to only review materials that are within their scope of competency and use care to avoid personal biases.

Section H: Resolving Ethical Issues

Introduction

Counselors behave in a legal, ethical, and moral manner in the conduct of their professional work. They are aware that client protection and trust in the profession depend on a high level of professional conduct. They hold other counselors to the same standards and are willing to take appropriate action to ensure that these standards are upheld. Counselors strive to resolve ethical dilemmas with direct and open communication among all parties involved and seek consultation with colleagues and supervisors when necessary. Counselors incorporate ethical practice into their daily professional work. They engage in ongoing professional development regarding current topics in ethical and legal issues in counseling.

H.1. Standards and the Law
(See F.9.a.)

a. *Knowledge.* Counselors understand the *ACA Code of Ethics* and other applicable ethics codes from other professional organizations or from certification and licensure bodies of which they are members. Lack of knowledge or misunderstanding of an ethical responsibility is not a defense against a charge of unethical conduct.

b. *Conflicts between Ethics and Laws.* If ethical responsibilities conflict with law, regulations, or other governing legal authority, counselors make known their commitment to the *ACA Code of Ethics* and take steps to resolve the conflict. If the conflict cannot be resolved by such means, counselors may adhere to the requirements of law, regulations, or other governing legal authority.

H.2. Suspected Violations

a. *Ethical Behavior Expected.* Counselors expect colleagues to adhere to the *ACA Code of Ethics.* When counselors possess knowledge that raises doubts as to whether another counselor is acting in an ethical manner, they take appropriate action. *(See H.2.b., H.2.c.)*

b. *Informal Resolution.* When counselors have reason to believe that another counselor is violating or has violated an ethical standard, they attempt first to resolve the issue informally with the other counselor if feasible, provided such action does not violate confidentiality rights that may be involved.

c. *Reporting Ethical Violations.* If an apparent violation has substantially harmed, or is likely to substantially harm a person or organization and is not appropriate for informal resolution or is not resolved properly, counselors take further action appropriate to the situation. Such action might include referral to state or national committees on professional ethics, voluntary national certification bodies, state licensing boards, or to the appropriate institutional authorities.

This standard does not apply when an intervention would violate confidentiality rights or when counselors have been retained to review the work of another counselor whose professional conduct is in question.

d. *Consultation.* When uncertain as to whether a particular situation or course of action may be in violation of the *ACA Code of Ethics,* counselors consult with other counselors who are knowledgeable about ethics and the *ACA Code of Ethics,* with colleagues, or with appropriate authorities

e. *Organizational Conflicts.* If the demands of an organization with which counselors are affiliated pose a conflict with the *ACA Code of Ethics,* counselors specify the nature of such conflicts and express to their supervisors or other responsible officials their commitment to the *ACA Code of Ethics.*

GLOSSARY OF TERMS

Advocacy: promotion of the well-being of individuals and groups, and the counseling profession within systems and organizations. Advocacy seeks to remove barriers and obstacles that inhibit access, growth, and development.

Assent: to demonstrate agreement, when a person is otherwise not capable or competent to give formal consent (e.g., informed consent) to a counseling service or plan.

Client: an individual seeking or referred to the professional services of a counselor for help with problem resolution or decision making.

Counselor: a professional (or a student who is a counselor-in-training) engaged in a counseling practice or other counseling-related services. Counselors fulfill many roles and responsibilities such as counselor educators, researchers, supervisors, practitioners, and consultants.

Counselor Educator: a professional counselor engaged primarily in developing, implementing, and supervising the educational preparation of counselors-in-training.

Counselor Supervisor: a professional counselor who engages in a formal relationship with a practicing counselor or counselor-in-training for the purpose of overseeing that individual's counseling work or clinical skill development.

Culture: membership in a socially constructed way of living, which incorporates collective values, beliefs, norms, boundaries, and lifestyles that are cocreated with others who share similar worldviews comprising biological, psychosocial, historical, psychological, and other factors.

Diversity: the similarities and differences that occur within and across cultures, and the intersection of cultural and social identities.

Documents: any written, digital, audio, visual, or artistic recording of the work within the counseling relationship between counselor and client.

Examinee: a recipient of any professional counseling service that includes educational, psychological, and career appraisal utilizing qualitative or quantitative techniques.

Forensic Evaluation: any formal assessment conducted for court or other legal proceedings.

Multicultural/Diversity Competence: a capacity whereby counselors possess cultural and diversity awareness and knowledge about self and others, and how this awareness and knowledge is applied effectively in practice with clients and client groups.

Multicultural/Diversity Counseling: counseling that recognizes diversity and embraces approaches that support the worth, dignity, potential, and uniqueness of individuals within their historical, cultural, economic, political, and psychosocial contexts.

Student: an individual engaged in formal educational preparation as a counselor-in-training.

Supervisee: a professional counselor or counselor-in-training whose counseling work or clinical skill development is being overseen in a formal supervisory relationship by a qualified trained professional.

Supervisor: counselors who are trained to oversee the professional clinical work of counselors and counselors-in-training.

Teaching: all activities engaged in as part of a formal educational program designed to lead to a graduate degree in counseling.

Training: the instruction and practice of skills related to the counseling profession. Training contributes to the ongoing proficiency of students and professional counselors.

American Psychological Association's *Ethical Principles of Psychologists and Code of Conduct*

INTRODUCTION AND APPLICABILITY

The American Psychological Association's (APA's) Ethical Principles of Psychologists and Code of Conduct (hereinafter referred to as the Ethics Code) consists of an Introduction, a Preamble, five General Principles (A–E), and specific Ethical Standards. The Introduction discusses the intent, organization, procedural considerations, and scope of application of the Ethics Code. The Preamble and General Principles are aspirational goals to guide psychologists toward the highest ideals of psychology. Although the Preamble and General Principles are not themselves enforceable rules, they should be considered by psychologists in arriving at an ethical course of action. The Ethical Standards set forth enforceable rules for conduct as psychologists. Most of the Ethical Standards are written broadly, in order to apply to psychologists in varied roles, although the application of an Ethical Standard may vary depending on the context. The Ethical Standards are not exhaustive. The fact that a given conduct is not specifically addressed by an Ethical Standard does not mean that it is necessarily either ethical or unethical.

This Ethics Code applies only to psychologists' activities that are part of their scientific, educational, or professional roles as psychologists. Areas covered include but are not limited to the clinical, counseling, and school practice of psychology; research; teaching; supervision of trainees; public service; policy development; social intervention; development of assessment instruments; conducting assessments; educational counseling; organizational consulting; forensic activities; program design and evaluation; and administration. This Ethics Code applies to these activities across a variety of contexts, such as in person, postal, telephone, internet, and other electronic transmissions. These activities shall be distinguished from the purely private conduct of psychologists, which is not within the purview of the Ethics Code.

Membership in the APA commits members and student affiliates to comply with the standards of the APA Ethics Code and to the rules and procedures used to enforce them. Lack of awareness or misunderstanding of an Ethical Standard is not itself a defense to a charge of unethical conduct.

The procedures for filing, investigating, and resolving complaints of unethical conduct are described in the current Rules and Procedures of the APA Ethics Committee. The APA may impose sanctions on its members for violations of the standards of the Ethics Code, including termination of APA membership, and may notify other bodies and individuals of its actions. Actions that violate the standards of the Ethics Code may also lead to the imposition of sanctions on psychologists or students whether or not they are APA members by bodies other than APA, including state psychological associations, other professional groups, psychology boards, other state or federal agencies, and payors for health services. In addition, APA may take action against a member after his or her conviction of a felony, expulsion or suspension from an affiliated state psychological association, or suspension or loss of licensure. When the sanction to be imposed by APA is less than expulsion, the 2001 Rules and Procedures do not guarantee an opportunity for an in-person hearing, but generally provide that complaints will be resolved only on the basis of a submitted record.

The Ethics Code is intended to provide guidance for psychologists and standards of professional conduct that can be applied by the APA and by other bodies that choose to adopt them. The Ethics Code is not intended to be a basis of civil liability. Whether a psychologist has violated the Ethics Code standards does not by itself determine whether the psychologist is legally liable in a court action, whether a contract is enforceable, or whether other legal consequences occur.

The modifiers used in some of the standards of this Ethics Code (e.g., *reasonably, appropriate, potentially*) are included in the standards when they would (1) allow professional judgment on the part of psychologists, (2) eliminate injustice or inequality that would occur without the modifier, (3) ensure applicability across the broad range of activities conducted by psychologists, or (4) guard against a set of rigid rules that might be quickly outdated. As used in this Ethics Code, the term *reasonable* means the prevailing professional judgment of psychologists engaged in similar activities in similar circumstances, given the knowledge the psychologist had or should have had at the time.

In the process of making decisions regarding their professional behavior, psychologists must consider this Ethics Code in addition to applicable laws and psychology board regulations. In applying the Ethics Code to their professional work, psychologists may consider other materials and guidelines that have been adopted or endorsed by scientific and professional psychological organizations and the dictates of their own conscience, as well as consult with others within the field. If this Ethics Code establishes a higher standard of conduct than is required by law, psychologists must meet the higher ethical standard. If psychologists' ethical responsibilities conflict with law, regulations, or other governing legal authority, psychologists make known their commitment to this Ethics Code and take steps to resolve the conflict in a responsible manner. If the conflict is unresolvable via such means, psychologists may adhere to the requirements of the law, regulations, or other governing authority in keeping with basic principles of human rights.

PREAMBLE

Psychologists are committed to increasing scientific and professional knowledge of behavior and people's understanding of themselves and others and to the use of such knowledge to improve the condition of individuals, organizations, and society. Psychologists respect and protect civil and human rights and the central importance of freedom of inquiry and expression in research, teaching, and publication. They strive to help the public in developing informed judgments and choices concerning human behavior. In doing so, they perform many roles, such as researcher, educator, diagnostician, therapist, supervisor, consultant, administrator, social interventionist, and expert witness.

This Ethics Code provides a common set of principles and standards upon which psychologists build their professional and scientific work.

This Ethics Code is intended to provide specific standards to cover most situations encountered by psychologists. It has as its goals the welfare and protection of the individuals and groups with whom psychologists work and the education of members, students, and the public regarding ethical standards of the discipline.

The development of a dynamic set of ethical standards for psychologists' work-related conduct requires a personal commitment and lifelong effort to act ethically; to encourage ethical behavior by students, supervisees, employees, and colleagues; and to consult with others concerning ethical problems.

GENERAL PRINCIPLES

This section consists of General Principles. General Principles, as opposed to Ethical Standards, are aspirational in nature. Their intent is to guide and inspire psychologists toward the very highest ethical ideals of the profession. General Principles, in contrast to Ethical Standards, do not represent obligations and should not form the basis for imposing sanctions. Relying upon General Principles for either of these reasons distorts both their meaning and purpose.

Principle A: Beneficence and Nonmaleficence

Psychologists strive to benefit those with whom they work and take care to do no harm. In their professional actions, psychologists seek to safeguard the welfare and rights of those with whom they interact professionally and other affected persons, and the welfare of animal subjects of research. When conflicts occur among psychologists' obligations or concerns, they attempt to resolve these conflicts in a responsible fashion that avoids or minimizes harm. Because psychologists' scientific and professional judgments and actions may affect the lives of others, they are alert to and guard against personal, financial, social, organizational, or political factors that might lead to misuse of their influence. Psychologists strive to be aware of the possible effect of their own physical and mental health on their ability to help those with whom they work.

Principle B: Fidelity and Responsibility

Psychologists establish relationships of trust with those with whom they work. They are aware of their professional and scientific responsibilities to society and to the specific communities in which they work.

Psychologists uphold professional standards of conduct, clarify their professional roles and obligations, accept appropriate responsibility for their behavior, and seek to manage conflicts of interest that could lead to exploitation or harm. Psychologists consult with, refer to, or cooperate with other professionals and institutions to the extent needed to serve the best interests of those with whom they work. They are concerned about the ethical compliance of their colleagues' scientific and professional conduct. Psychologists strive to contribute a portion of their professional time for little or no compensation or personal advantage.

Principle C: Integrity

Psychologists seek to promote accuracy, honesty, and truthfulness in the science, teaching, and practice of psychology. In these activities psychologists do not steal, cheat, or engage in fraud, subterfuge, or intentional misrepresentation of fact. Psychologists strive to keep their promises and to avoid unwise or unclear commitments. In situations in which deception may be ethically justifiable to maximize benefits and minimize harm, psychologists have a serious obligation to consider the need for, the possible consequences of, and their responsibility to correct any resulting mistrust or other harmful effects that arise from the use of such techniques.

Principle D: Justice

Psychologists recognize that fairness and justice entitle all persons to access to and benefit from the contributions of psychology and to equal quality in the processes, procedures, and services being conducted by psychologists. Psychologists exercise reasonable judgment and take precautions to ensure that their potential biases, the boundaries of their competence, and the limitations of their expertise do not lead to or condone unjust practices.

Principle E: Respect for People's Rights and Dignity

Psychologists respect the dignity and worth of all people, and the rights of individuals to privacy, confidentiality, and self-determination. Psychologists are aware that special safeguards may be necessary to protect the rights and welfare of persons or communities whose vulnerabilities impair autonomous decision making. Psychologists are aware of and respect cultural, individual, and role differences, including those based on age, gender, gender identity, race, ethnicity, culture, national origin, religion, sexual orientation, disability, language, and socioeconomic status and consider these factors when working with members of such groups. Psychologists try to eliminate the effect on their work of biases based on those factors, and they do not knowingly participate in or condone activities of others based upon such prejudices.

ETHICAL STANDARDS

1. Resolving Ethical Issues

1.01. Misuse of Psychologists' Work.

If psychologists learn of misuse or misrepresentation of their work, they take reasonable steps to correct or minimize the misuse or misrepresentation.

1.02. Conflicts Between Ethics and Law, Regulations, or Other Governing Legal Authority.

If psychologists' ethical responsibilities conflict with law, regulations, or other governing legal authority, psychologists make known their commitment to the Ethics Code and take steps to resolve the conflict. If the conflict is unresolvable via such means, psychologists may adhere to the requirements of the law, regulations, or other governing legal authority.

1.03. Conflicts Between Ethics and Organizational Demands.

If the demands of an organization with which psychologists are affiliated or for whom they are working conflict with this Ethics Code, psychologists clarify the nature of the conflict, make known their commitment to the Ethics Code, and to the extent feasible, resolve the conflict in a way that permits adherence to the Ethics Code.

1.04. Informal Resolution of Ethical Violations.

When psychologists believe that there may have been an ethical violation by another psychologist, they attempt to resolve the issue by bringing it to the attention of that individual, if an informal resolution appears appropriate and the intervention does not violate any confidentiality rights that may be involved. (See also Standards 1.02, Conflicts Between Ethics and Law, Regulations, or Other Governing Legal Authority, and 1.03, Conflicts Between Ethics and Organizational Demands.)

1.05. Reporting Ethical Violations.

If an apparent ethical violation has substantially harmed or is likely to substantially harm a person or organization and is not appropriate for informal resolution under Standard 1.04, Informal Resolution of

Ethical Violations, or is not resolved properly in that fashion, psychologists take further action appropriate to the situation. Such action might include referral to state or national committees on professional ethics, to state licensing boards, or to the appropriate institutional authorities. This standard does not apply when an intervention would violate confidentiality rights or when psychologists have been retained to review the work of another psychologist whose professional conduct is in question. (See also Standard 1.02, Conflicts Between Ethics and Law, Regulations, or Other Governing Legal Authority.)

1.06. Cooperating With Ethics Committees.

Psychologists cooperate in ethics investigations, proceedings, and resulting requirements of the APA or any affiliated state psychological association to which they belong. In doing so, they address any confidentiality issues. Failure to cooperate is itself an ethics violation. However, making a request for deferment of adjudication of an ethics complaint pending the outcome of litigation does not alone constitute noncooperation.

1.07. Improper Complaints.

Psychologists do not file or encourage the filing of ethics complaints that are made with reckless disregard for or willful ignorance of facts that would disprove the allegation.

1.08. Unfair Discrimination Against Complainants and Respondents.

Psychologists do not deny persons employment, advancement, admissions to academic or other programs, tenure, or promotion, based solely upon their having made or their being the subject of an ethics complaint. This does not preclude taking action based upon the outcome of such proceedings or considering other appropriate information.

2. Competence

2.01. Boundaries of Competence.

(a) Psychologists provide services, teach, and conduct research with populations and in areas only within the boundaries of their competence, based on their education, training, supervised experience, consultation, study, or professional experience.

(b) Where scientific or professional knowledge in the discipline of psychology establishes that an understanding of factors associated with age, gender, gender identity, race, ethnicity, culture, national origin, religion, sexual orientation, disability, language, or socioeconomic status is essential for effective implementation of their services or research, psychologists have or obtain the training, experience, consultation, or supervision necessary to ensure the competence of their services, or they make appropriate referrals, except as provided in Standard 2.02, Providing Services in Emergencies.

(c) Psychologists planning to provide services, teach, or conduct research involving populations, areas, techniques, or technologies new to them undertake relevant education, training, supervised experience, consultation, or study.

(d) When psychologists are asked to provide services to individuals for whom appropriate mental health services are not available and for which psychologists have not obtained the competence necessary, psychologists with closely related prior training or experience may provide such services in order to ensure that services are not denied if they make a reasonable effort to obtain the competence required by using relevant research, training, consultation, or study.

(e) In those emerging areas in which generally recognized standards for preparatory training do not yet exist, psychologists nevertheless take reasonable steps to ensure the competence of their work and to protect clients/patients, students, supervisees, research participants, organizational clients, and others from harm.

(f) When assuming forensic roles, psychologists are or become reasonably familiar with the judicial or administrative rules governing their roles.

2.02. Providing Services in Emergencies.

In emergencies, when psychologists provide services to individuals for whom other mental health services are not available and for which psychologists have not obtained the necessary training, psychologists may provide such services in order to ensure that services are not denied. The services are discontinued as soon as the emergency has ended or appropriate services are available.

2.03. Maintaining Competence.

Psychologists undertake ongoing efforts to develop and maintain their competence.

2.04. Bases for Scientific and Professional Judgments.

Psychologists' work is based upon established scientific and professional knowledge of the discipline. (See also Standards 2.01e, Boundaries of Competence, and 10.01b, Informed Consent to Therapy.)

2.05. Delegation of Work to Others.

Psychologists who delegate work to employees, supervisees, or research or teaching assistants or who use the services of others, such as interpreters, take reasonable steps to (1) avoid delegating such work to persons who have a multiple relationship with those being served that would likely lead to exploitation or loss of objectivity; (2) authorize only those responsibilities that such persons can be expected to perform competently on the basis of their education, training, or experience, either independently or with the level of supervision being provided; and (3) see that such persons perform these services competently. (See also Standards 2.02, Providing Services in Emergencies; 3.05, Multiple Relationships; 4.01, Maintaining Confidentiality; 9.01, Bases for Assessments; 9.02, Use of Assessments; 9.03, Informed Consent in Assessments; and 9.07, Assessment by Unqualified Persons.)

2.06. Personal Problems and Conflicts.

(a) Psychologists refrain from initiating an activity when they know or should know that there is a substantial likelihood that their personal problems will prevent them from performing their work-related activities in a competent manner.

(b) When psychologists become aware of personal problems that may interfere with their performing work-related duties adequately, they take appropriate measures, such as obtaining professional consultation or assistance, and determine whether they should limit, suspend, or terminate their work-related duties. (See also Standard 10.10, Terminating Therapy.)

3. Human Relations

3.01. Unfair Discrimination.

In their work-related activities, psychologists do not engage in unfair discrimination based on age, gender, gender identity, race, ethnicity, culture, national origin, religion, sexual orientation, disability, socioeconomic status, or any basis proscribed by law.

3.02. Sexual Harassment.

Psychologists do not engage in sexual harassment. Sexual harassment is sexual solicitation, physical advances, or verbal or nonverbal conduct that is sexual in nature, that occurs in connection with the psychologist's activities or roles as a psychologist, and that either (1) is unwelcome, is offensive, or creates a hostile workplace or educational environment, and the psychologist knows or is told this or (2) is sufficiently severe or intense to be abusive to a reasonable person in the context. Sexual harassment can consist of a single intense or severe act or of multiple persistent or pervasive acts. (See also Standard 1.08, Unfair Discrimination Against Complainants and Respondents.)

3.03. Other Harassment.

Psychologists do not knowingly engage in behavior that is harassing or demeaning to persons with whom they interact in their work based on factors such as those persons' age, gender, gender identity, race, ethnicity, culture, national origin, religion, sexual orientation, disability, language, or socioeconomic status.

3.04. Avoiding Harm.

Psychologists take reasonable steps to avoid harming their clients/patients, students, supervisees, research participants, organizational clients, and others with whom they work, and to minimize harm where it is foreseeable and unavoidable.

3.05. Multiple Relationships.

(a) A multiple relationship occurs when a psychologist is in a professional role with a person and (1) at the same time is in another role with the same person, (2) at the same time is in a relationship with a person closely associated with or related to the person with whom the psychologist has the professional relationship, or (3) promises to enter into another relationship in the future with the person or a person closely associated with or related to the person.

A psychologist refrains from entering into a multiple relationship if the multiple relationship could reasonably be expected to impair the psychologist's objectivity, competence, or effectiveness in performing his or her functions as a psychologist, or otherwise risks exploitation or harm to the person with whom the professional relationship exists.

Multiple relationships that would not reasonably be expected to cause impairment or risk exploitation or harm are not unethical.

(b) If a psychologist finds that, due to unforeseen factors, a potentially harmful multiple relationship has arisen, the psychologist takes reasonable steps to resolve it with due regard for the best interests of the affected person and maximal compliance with the Ethics Code.

(c) When psychologists are required by law, institutional policy, or extraordinary circumstances to serve in more than one role in judicial or administrative proceedings, at the outset they clarify role expectations and the extent of confidentiality and thereafter as changes occur. (See also Standards 3.04, Avoiding Harm, and 3.07, Third-Party Requests for Services.)

3.06. Conflict of Interest.

Psychologists refrain from taking on a professional role when personal, scientific, professional, legal, financial, or other interests or relationships could reasonably be expected to (1) impair their objectivity, competence, or effectiveness in performing their functions as psychologists or (2) expose the person or organization with whom the professional relationship exists to harm or exploitation.

3.07. Third-Party Requests for Services.

When psychologists agree to provide services to a person or entity at the request of a third party, psychologists attempt to clarify at the outset of the service the nature of the relationship with all individuals or organizations involved. This clarification includes the role of the psychologist (e.g., therapist, consultant, diagnostician, or expert witness), an identification of who is the client, the probable uses of the services provided or the information obtained, and the fact that there may be limits to confidentiality. (See also Standards 3.05, Multiple Relationships, and 4.02, Discussing the Limits of Confidentiality.)

3.08. Exploitative Relationships.

Psychologists do not exploit persons over whom they have supervisory, evaluative, or other authority such as clients/patients, students, supervisees, research participants, and employees. (See also Standards 3.05, Multiple Relationships; 6.04, Fees and Financial Arrangements; 6.05, Barter With Clients/Patients; 7.07, Sexual Relationships With Students and Supervisees; 10.05, Sexual Intimacies With Current Therapy Clients/Patients; 10.06, Sexual Intimacies With Relatives or Significant Others of Current Therapy Clients/Patients; 10.07, Therapy With Former Sexual Partners; and 10.08, Sexual Intimacies With Former Therapy Clients/Patients.)

3.09. Cooperation with Other Professionals.

When indicated and professionally appropriate, psychologists cooperate with other professionals in order to serve their clients/patients effectively and appropriately. (See also Standard 4.05, Disclosures.)

3.10. Informed Consent.

(a) When psychologists conduct research or provide assessment, therapy, counseling, or consulting services in person or via electronic transmission or other forms of communication, they obtain the informed consent of the individual or individuals using language that is reasonably understandable to that person or persons except when conducting such activities without consent is mandated by law or governmental regulation or as otherwise provided in this Ethics Code. (See also Standards 8.02, Informed Consent to Research; 9.03, Informed Consent in Assessments; and 10.01, Informed Consent to Therapy.)

(b) For persons who are legally incapable of giving informed consent, psychologists nevertheless (1) provide an appropriate explanation, (2) seek the individual's assent, (3) consider such persons' preferences and best interests, and (4) obtain appropriate permission from a legally authorized person, if such substitute consent is permitted or required by law. When consent by a legally authorized person is not permitted or required by law, psychologists take reasonable steps to protect the individual's rights and welfare.

(c) When psychological services are court ordered or otherwise mandated, psychologists inform the individual of the nature of the anticipated services, including whether the services are court ordered or mandated and any limits of confidentiality, before proceeding.

(d) Psychologists appropriately document written or oral consent, permission, and assent. (See also Standards 8.02, Informed Consent to Research; 9.03, Informed Consent in Assessments; and 10.01, Informed Consent to Therapy.)

3.11. Psychological Services Delivered to or through Organizations.

(a) Psychologists delivering services to or through organizations provide information beforehand to clients and when appropriate those directly affected by the services about (1) the nature and objectives of the services, (2) the intended recipients, (3) which of the individuals are clients, (4) the relationship the psychologist will have with each person and the organization, (5) the probable uses of services provided and information obtained, (6) who will have access to the information, and (7) limits of confidentiality. As soon as feasible, they provide information about the results and conclusions of such services to appropriate persons.

(b) If psychologists will be precluded by law or by organizational roles from providing such information to particular individuals or groups, they so inform those individuals or groups at the outset of the service.

3.12. Interruption of Psychological Services.

Unless otherwise covered by contract, psychologists make reasonable efforts to plan for facilitating services in the event that psychological services are interrupted by factors such as the psychologist's illness, death, unavailability, relocation, or retirement or by the client's/patient's relocation or financial limitations. (See also Standard 6.02c, Maintenance, Dissemination, and Disposal of Confidential Records of Professional and Scientific Work.)

4. Privacy and Confidentiality

4.01. Maintaining Confidentiality.

Psychologists have a primary obligation and take reasonable precautions to protect confidential information obtained through or stored in any medium, recognizing that the extent and limits of confidentiality may be regulated by law or established by institutional rules or professional or scientific relationship. (See also Standard 2.05, Delegation of Work to Others.)

4.02. Discussing the Limits of Confidentiality.

(a) Psychologists discuss with persons (including, to the extent feasible, persons who are legally incapable of giving informed consent and their legal representatives) and organizations with whom they establish a scientific or professional relationship (1) the relevant limits of confidentiality and (2) the foreseeable uses of the information generated through their psychological activities. (See also Standard 3.10, Informed Consent.)

(b) Unless it is not feasible or is contraindicated, the discussion of confidentiality occurs at the outset of the relationship and thereafter as new circumstances may warrant.

(c) Psychologists who offer services, products, or information via electronic transmission inform clients/patients of the risks to privacy and limits of confidentiality.

4.03. Recording.

Before recording the voices or images of individuals to whom they provide services, psychologists obtain permission from all such persons or their legal representatives. (See also Standards 8.03, Informed Consent for Recording Voices and Images in Research; 8.05, Dispensing With Informed Consent for Research; and 8.07, Deception in Research.)

4.04. Minimizing Intrusions on Privacy.

(a) Psychologists include in written and oral reports and consultations, only information germane to the purpose for which the communication is made.

(b) Psychologists discuss confidential information obtained in their work only for appropriate scientific or professional purposes and only with persons clearly concerned with such matters.

4.05. Disclosures.

(a) Psychologists may disclose confidential information with the appropriate consent of the organizational client, the individual client/patient, or another legally authorized person on behalf of the client/patient unless prohibited by law.

(b) Psychologists disclose confidential information without the consent of the individual only as mandated by law, or where permitted by law for a valid purpose such as to (1) provide needed professional services; (2) obtain appropriate professional consultations; (3) protect the client/patient, psychologist, or others from harm; or (4) obtain payment for services from a client/patient, in which instance disclosure is limited to the minimum that is necessary to achieve the purpose. (See also Standard 6.04e, Fees and Financial Arrangements.)

4.06. Consultations.

When consulting with colleagues, (1) psychologists do not disclose confidential information that reasonably could lead to the identification of a client/patient, research participant, or other person or organization with whom they have a confidential relationship unless they have obtained the prior consent of the person or organization or the disclosure cannot be avoided, and (2) they disclose information only to the extent necessary to achieve the purposes of the consultation. (See also Standard 4.01, Maintaining Confidentiality.)

4.07. Use of Confidential Information for Didactic or Other Purposes.

Psychologists do not disclose in their writings, lectures, or other public media, confidential, personally identifiable information concerning their clients/patients, students, research participants, organizational clients, or other recipients of their services that they obtained during the course of their work, unless (1) they take reasonable steps to disguise the person or organization, (2) the person or organization has consented in writing, or (3) there is legal authorization for doing so.

5. Advertising and Other Public Statements

5.01. Avoidance of False or Deceptive Statements.

(a) Public statements include but are not limited to paid or unpaid advertising, product endorsements, grant applications, licensing applications, other credentialing applications, brochures, printed matter, directory listings, personal resumes or curricula vitae, or comments for use in media such as print or electronic transmission, statements in legal proceedings, lectures and public oral presentations, and published materials. Psychologists do not knowingly make public statements that are false, deceptive, or fraudulent concerning their research, practice, or other work activities or those of persons or organizations with which they are affiliated.

(b) Psychologists do not make false, deceptive, or fraudulent statements concerning (1) their training, experience, or competence; (2) their academic degrees; (3) their credentials; (4) their institutional or association affiliations; (5) their services; (6) the scientific or clinical basis for, or results or degree of success of, their services; (7) their fees; or (8) their publications or research findings.

(c) Psychologists claim degrees as credentials for their health services only if those degrees (1) were earned from a regionally accredited educational institution or (2) were the basis for psychology licensure by the state in which they practice.

5.02. Statements by Others.

(a) Psychologists who engage others to create or place public statements that promote their professional practice, products, or activities retain professional responsibility for such statements.

(b) Psychologists do not compensate employees of press, radio, television, or other communication media in return for publicity in a news item. (See also Standard 1.01, Misuse of Psychologists' Work.)

(c) A paid advertisement relating to psychologists' activities must be identified or clearly recognizable as such.

5.03. Descriptions of Workshops and Non-Degree-Granting Educational Programs.

To the degree to which they exercise control, psychologists responsible for announcements, catalogs, brochures, or advertisements describing workshops, seminars, or other non-degree-granting educational programs ensure that they accurately describe the audience for which the program is intended, the educational objectives, the presenters, and the fees involved.

5.04. Media Presentations.

When psychologists provide public advice or comment via print, internet, or other electronic transmission, they take precautions to ensure that statements (1) are based on their professional knowledge, training, or experience in accord with appropriate psychological literature and practice; (2) are otherwise consistent with this Ethics Code; and (3) do not indicate that a professional relationship has been established with the recipient. (See also Standard 2.04, Bases for Scientific and Professional Judgments.)

5.05. Testimonials.

Psychologists do not solicit testimonials from current therapy clients/patients or other persons who because of their particular circumstances are vulnerable to undue influence.

5.06. In-Person Solicitation.

Psychologists do not engage, directly or through agents, in uninvited in-person solicitation of business from actual or potential therapy clients/patients or other persons who because of their particular circumstances are vulnerable to undue influence. However, this prohibition does not preclude (1) attempting to implement appropriate collateral contacts for the purpose of benefiting an already engaged therapy client/patient or (2) providing disaster or community outreach services.

6. Record Keeping and Fees

6.01. Documentation of Professional and Scientific Work and Maintenance of Records.

Psychologists create, and to the extent the records are under their control, maintain, disseminate, store, retain, and dispose of records and data relating to their professional and scientific work in order to (1) facilitate provision of services later by them or by other professionals, (2) allow for replication of research design and analyses, (3) meet institutional requirements, (4) ensure accuracy of billing and payments, and (5) ensure compliance with law. (See also Standard 4.01, Maintaining Confidentiality.)

6.02. Maintenance, Dissemination, and Disposal of Confidential Records of Professional and Scientific Work

(a) Psychologists maintain confidentiality in creating, storing, accessing, transferring, and disposing of records under their control, whether these are written, automated, or in any other medium. (See also Standards

4.01, Maintaining Confidentiality, and 6.01, Documentation of Professional and Scientific Work and Maintenance of Records.)

(b) If confidential information concerning recipients of psychological services is entered into databases or systems of records available to persons whose access has not been consented to by the recipient, psychologists use coding or other techniques to avoid the inclusion of personal identifiers.

(c) Psychologists make plans in advance to facilitate the appropriate transfer and to protect the confidentiality of records and data in the event of psychologists' withdrawal from positions or practice. (See also Standards 3.12, Interruption of Psychological Services, and 10.09, Interruption of Therapy.)

6.03. Withholding Records for Nonpayment.

Psychologists may not withhold records under their control that are requested and needed for a client's/patient's emergency treatment solely because payment has not been received.

6.04. Fees and Financial Arrangements.

(a) As early as is feasible in a professional or scientific relationship, psychologists and recipients of psychological services reach an agreement specifying compensation and billing arrangements.

(b) Psychologists' fee practices are consistent with law.

(c) Psychologists do not misrepresent their fees.

(d) If limitations to services can be anticipated because of limitations in financing, this is discussed with the recipient of services as early as is feasible. (See also Standards 10.09, Interruption of Therapy, and 10.10, Terminating Therapy.)

(e) If the recipient of services does not pay for services as agreed, and if psychologists intend to use collection agencies or legal measures to collect the fees, psychologists first inform the person that such measures will be taken and provide that person an opportunity to make prompt payment. (See also Standards 4.05, Disclosures; 6.03, Withholding Records for Nonpayment; and 10.01, Informed Consent to Therapy.)

6.05. Barter with Clients/Patients.

Barter is the acceptance of goods, services, or other nonmonetary remuneration from clients/patients in return for psychological services. Psychologists may barter only if (1) it is not clinically contraindicated, and (2) the resulting arrangement is not exploitative. (See also Standards 3.05, Multiple Relationships, and 6.04, Fees and Financial Arrangements.)

6.06. Accuracy in Reports to Payors and Funding Sources.

In their reports to payors for services or sources of research funding, psychologists take reasonable steps to ensure the accurate reporting of the nature of the service provided or research conducted, the fees, charges, or payments, and where applicable, the identity of the provider, the findings, and the diagnosis. (See also Standards 4.01, Maintaining Confidentiality; 4.04, Minimizing Intrusions on Privacy; and 4.05, Disclosures.)

6.07. Referrals and Fees.

When psychologists pay, receive payment from, or divide fees with another professional, other than in an employer-employee relationship, the payment to each is based on the services provided (clinical, consultative, administrative, or other) and is not based on the referral itself. (See also Standard 3.09, Cooperation With Other Professionals.)

7. Education and Training

7.01. Design of Education and Training Programs.

Psychologists responsible for education and training programs take reasonable steps to ensure that the programs are designed to provide the appropriate knowledge and proper experiences, and to meet the requirements for licensure, certification, or other goals for which claims are made by the program. (See also Standard 5.03, Descriptions of Workshops and Non-Degree-Granting Educational Programs.)

7.02. Descriptions of Education and Training Programs.

Psychologists responsible for education and training programs take reasonable steps to ensure that there is a current and accurate description of the program content (including participation in required course- or program-related counseling, psychotherapy, experiential groups, consulting projects, or community service), training goals and objectives, stipends and benefits, and requirements that must be met for satisfactory completion of the program. This information must be made readily available to all interested parties.

7.03. Accuracy in Teaching.

(a) Psychologists take reasonable steps to ensure that course syllabi are accurate regarding the subject matter to be covered, bases for evaluating progress, and the nature of course experiences. This standard does not preclude an instructor from modifying course content or requirements when the instructor considers it pedagogically necessary or desirable, so long as students are made aware of these modifications in a manner that enables them to fulfill course requirements. (See also Standard 5.01, Avoidance of False or Deceptive Statements.)

(b) When engaged in teaching or training, psychologists present psychological information accurately. (See also Standard 2.03, Maintaining Competence.)

7.04. Student Disclosure of Personal Information.

Psychologists do not require students or supervisees to disclose personal information in course- or program-related activities, either orally or in writing, regarding sexual history, history of abuse and neglect, psychological treatment, and relationships with parents, peers, and spouses or significant others except if (1) the program or training facility has clearly identified this requirement in its admissions and program materials or (2) the information is necessary to evaluate or obtain assistance for students whose personal problems could reasonably be judged to be preventing them from performing their training- or professionally related activities in a competent manner or posing a threat to the students or others.

7.05. Mandatory Individual or Group Therapy.

(a) When individual or group therapy is a program or course requirement, psychologists responsible for that program allow students in undergraduate and graduate programs the option of selecting such therapy from practitioners unaffiliated with the program. (See also Standard 7.02, Descriptions of Education and Training Programs.)

(b) Faculty who are or are likely to be responsible for evaluating students' academic performance do not themselves provide that therapy. (See also Standard 3.05, Multiple Relationships.)

7.06. Assessing Student and Supervisee Performance.

(a) In academic and supervisory relationships, psychologists establish a timely and specific process for providing feedback to students and supervisees. Information regarding the process is provided to the student at the beginning of supervision.

(b) Psychologists evaluate students and supervisees on the basis of their actual performance on relevant and established program requirements.

7.07. Sexual Relationships With Students and Supervisees.

Psychologists do not engage in sexual relationships with students or supervisees who are in their department, agency, or training center or over whom psychologists have or are likely to have evaluative authority. (See also Standard 3.05, Multiple Relationships.)

8. Research and Publication

8.01. Institutional Approval.

When institutional approval is required, psychologists provide accurate information about their research proposals and obtain approval prior to conducting the research. They conduct the research in accordance with the approved research protocol.

8.02. Informed Consent to Research.

(a) When obtaining informed consent as required in Standard 3.10, Informed Consent, psychologists inform participants about (1) the purpose of the research, expected duration, and procedures; (2) their right to decline to participate and to withdraw from the research once participation has begun; (3) the foreseeable consequences of declining or withdrawing; (4) reasonably foreseeable factors that may be expected to influence their willingness to participate such as potential risks, discomfort, or adverse effects; (5) any prospective research benefits; (6) limits of confidentiality; (7) incentives for participation; and (8) whom to contact for questions about the research and research participants' rights. They provide opportunity for the prospective participants to ask questions and receive answers. (See also Standards 8.03, Informed Consent for Recording Voices and Images in Research; 8.05, Dispensing With Informed Consent for Research; and 8.07, Deception in Research.)

(b) Psychologists conducting intervention research involving the use of experimental treatments clarify to participants at the outset of the research (1) the experimental nature of the treatment; (2) the services that will or will not be available to the control group(s) if appropriate; (3) the means by which assignment to treatment and control groups will be made; (4) available treatment alternatives if an individual does not wish to participate in the research or wishes to withdraw once a study has begun; and (5) compensation for or monetary costs of participating including, if appropriate, whether reimbursement from the participant or a third-party payor will be sought. (See also Standard 8.02a, Informed Consent to Research.)

8.03. Informed Consent for Recording Voices and Images in Research.

Psychologists obtain informed consent from research participants prior to recording their voices or images for data collection unless (1) the research consists solely of naturalistic observations in public places, and it is not anticipated that the recording will be used in a manner that could cause personal identification or harm, or (2) the research design includes deception, and consent for the use of the recording is obtained during debriefing. (See also Standard 8.07, Deception in Research.)

8.04. Client/Patient, Student, and Subordinate Research Participants.

(a) When psychologists conduct research with clients/patients, students, or subordinates as participants, psychologists take steps to protect the prospective participants from adverse consequences of declining or withdrawing from participation.

(b) When research participation is a course requirement or an opportunity for extra credit, the prospective participant is given the choice of equitable alternative activities.

8.05. Dispensing With Informed Consent for Research.

Psychologists may dispense with informed consent only (1) where research would not reasonably be assumed to create distress or harm and involves (a) the study of normal educational practices, curricula, or classroom management methods conducted in educational settings; (b) only anonymous questionnaires, naturalistic observations, or archival research for which disclosure of responses would not place participants at risk of criminal or civil liability or damage their financial standing, employability, or reputation, and confidentiality is protected; or (c) the study of factors related to job or organization effectiveness conducted in organizational settings for which there is no risk to participants' employability, and confidentiality is protected or (2) where otherwise permitted by law or federal or institutional regulations.

8.06. Offering Inducements for Research Participation.

(a) Psychologists make reasonable efforts to avoid offering excessive or inappropriate financial or other inducements for research participation when such inducements are likely to coerce participation.

(b) When offering professional services as an inducement for research participation, psychologists clarify the nature of the services, as well as the risks, obligations, and limitations. (See also Standard 6.05, Barter With Clients/Patients.)

8.07. Deception in Research.

(a) Psychologists do not conduct a study involving deception unless they have determined that the use of deceptive techniques is justified by the study's significant prospective scientific, educational, or applied value and that effective nondeceptive alternative procedures are not feasible.

(b) Psychologists do not deceive prospective participants about research that is reasonably expected to cause physical pain or severe emotional distress.

(c) Psychologists explain any deception that is an integral feature of the design and conduct of an experiment to participants as early as is feasible, preferably at the conclusion of their participation, but no later than at the conclusion of the data collection, and permit participants to withdraw their data. (See also Standard 8.08, Debriefing.)

8.08. Debriefing.

(a) Psychologists provide a prompt opportunity for participants to obtain appropriate information about the nature, results, and conclusions of the research, and they take reasonable steps to correct any misconceptions that participants may have of which the psychologists are aware.

(b) If scientific or humane values justify delaying or withholding this information, psychologists take reasonable measures to reduce the risk of harm.

(c) When psychologists become aware that research procedures have harmed a participant, they take reasonable steps to minimize the harm.

8.09. Humane Care and Use of Animals in Research.

(a) Psychologists acquire, care for, use, and dispose of animals in compliance with current federal, state, and local laws and regulations, and with professional standards.

(b) Psychologists trained in research methods and experienced in the care of laboratory animals supervise all procedures involving animals and are responsible for ensuring appropriate consideration of their comfort, health, and humane treatment.

(c) Psychologists ensure that all individuals under their supervision who are using animals have received instruction in research methods and in the care, maintenance, and handling of the species being used, to the extent appropriate to their role. (See also Standard 2.05, Delegation of Work to Others.)

(d) Psychologists make reasonable efforts to minimize the discomfort, infection, illness, and pain of animal subjects.

(e) Psychologists use a procedure subjecting animals to pain, stress, or privation only when an alternative procedure is unavailable and the goal is justified by its prospective scientific, educational, or applied value.

(f) Psychologists perform surgical procedures under appropriate anesthesia and follow techniques to avoid infection and minimize pain during and after surgery.

(g) When it is appropriate that an animal's life be terminated, psychologists proceed rapidly, with an effort to minimize pain and in accordance with accepted procedures.

8.10. Reporting Research Results.

(a) Psychologists do not fabricate data. (See also Standard 5.01a, Avoidance of False or Deceptive Statements.)

(b) If psychologists discover significant errors in their published data, they take reasonable steps to correct such errors in a correction, retraction, erratum, or other appropriate publication means.

8.11. Plagiarism.

Psychologists do not present portions of another's work or data as their own, even if the other work or data source is cited occasionally.

8.12. Publication Credit.

(a) Psychologists take responsibility and credit, including authorship credit, only for work they have actually performed or to which they have substantially contributed. (See also Standard 8.12b, Publication Credit.)

(b) Principal authorship and other publication credits accurately reflect the relative scientific or professional contributions of the individuals involved, regardless of their relative status. Mere possession of an institutional position, such as department chair, does not justify authorship credit. Minor contributions to the research or to the writing for publications are acknowledged appropriately, such as in footnotes or in an introductory statement.

(c) Except under exceptional circumstances, a student is listed as principal author on any multiple-authored article that is substantially based on the student's doctoral dissertation. Faculty advisors discuss publication credit with students as early as feasible and throughout the research and publication process as appropriate. (See also Standard 8.12b, Publication Credit.)

8.13. Duplicate Publication of Data.

Psychologists do not publish, as original data, data that have been previously published. This does not preclude republishing data when they are accompanied by proper acknowledgment.

8.14. Sharing Research Data for Verification.

(a) After research results are published, psychologists do not withhold the data on which their conclusions are based from other competent professionals who seek to verify the substantive claims through reanalysis and who intend to use such data only for that purpose, provided that the confidentiality of the participants can be protected and unless legal rights concerning proprietary data preclude their release. This does not preclude psychologists from requiring that such individuals or groups be responsible for costs associated with the provision of such information.

(b) Psychologists who request data from other psychologists to verify the substantive claims through reanalysis may use shared data only for the declared purpose. Requesting psychologists obtain prior written agreement for all other uses of the data.

8.15. Reviewers.

Psychologists who review material submitted for presentation, publication, grant, or research proposal review respect the confidentiality of and the proprietary rights in such information of those who submitted it.

9. Assessment

9.01. Bases for Assessments.

(a) Psychologists base the opinions contained in their recommendations, reports, and diagnostic or evaluative statements, including forensic testimony, on information and techniques sufficient to substantiate their findings. (See also Standard 2.04, Bases for Scientific and Professional Judgments.)

(b) Except as noted in 9.01c, psychologists provide opinions of the psychological characteristics of individuals only after they have conducted an examination of the individuals adequate to support their statements or conclusions. When, despite reasonable efforts, such an examination is not practical, psychologists document the efforts they made and the result of those efforts, clarify the probable impact of their limited information on the reliability and validity of their opinions, and appropriately limit the nature and extent of their conclusions or recommendations. (See also Standards 2.01, Boundaries of Competence, and 9.06, Interpreting Assessment Results.)

(c) When psychologists conduct a record review or provide consultation or supervision and an individual examination is not warranted or necessary for the opinion, psychologists explain this and the sources of information on which they based their conclusions and recommendations.

9.02. Use of Assessments.

(a) Psychologists administer, adapt, score, interpret, or use assessment techniques, interviews, tests, or instruments in a manner and for purposes that are appropriate in light of the research on or evidence of the usefulness and proper application of the techniques.

(b) Psychologists use assessment instruments whose validity and reliability have been established for use with members of the population tested. When such validity or reliability has not been established, psychologists describe the strengths and limitations of test results and interpretation.

(c) Psychologists use assessment methods that are appropriate to an individual's language preference and competence, unless the use of an alternative language is relevant to the assessment issues.

9.03. Informed Consent in Assessments.

(a) Psychologists obtain informed consent for assessments, evaluations, or diagnostic services, as described in Standard 3.10, Informed Consent, except when (1) testing is mandated by law or governmental regulations; (2) informed consent is implied because testing is conducted as a routine educational, institutional, or organizational activity (e.g., when participants voluntarily agree to assessment when applying for a job); or (3) one purpose of the testing is to evaluate decisional capacity. Informed consent includes an explanation of the nature and purpose of the assessment, fees, involvement of third parties, and limits of confidentiality and sufficient opportunity for the client/patient to ask questions and receive answers.

(b) Psychologists inform persons with questionable capacity to consent or for whom testing is mandated by law or governmental regulations about the nature and purpose of the proposed assessment services, using language that is reasonably understandable to the person being assessed.

(c) Psychologists using the services of an interpreter obtain informed consent from the client/patient to use that interpreter, ensure that confidentiality of test results and test security are maintained, and include in their recommendations, reports, and diagnostic or evaluative statements, including forensic testimony, discussion of any limitations on the data obtained. (See also Standards 2.05, Delegation of Work to Others; 4.01, Maintaining Confidentiality; 9.01, Bases for Assessments; 9.06, Interpreting Assessment Results; and 9.07, Assessment by Unqualified Persons.)

9.04. Release of Test Data.

(a) The term *test data* refers to raw and scaled scores, client/patient responses to test questions or stimuli, and psychologists' notes and recordings concerning client/patient statements and behavior during an examination. Those portions of test materials that include client/patient responses are included in the definition of *test data*. Pursuant to a client/patient release, psychologists provide test data to the client/patient or other persons identified in the release. Psychologists may refrain from releasing test data to protect a client/patient or others from substantial harm or misuse or misrepresentation of the data or the test, recognizing that in many instances release of confidential information under these circumstances is regulated by law. (See also Standard 9.11, Maintaining Test Security.)

(b) In the absence of a client/patient release, psychologists provide test data only as required by law or court order.

9.05. Test Construction.

Psychologists who develop tests and other assessment techniques use appropriate psychometric procedures and current scientific or professional knowledge for test design, standardization, validation, reduction or elimination of bias, and recommendations for use.

9.06. Interpreting Assessment Results.

When interpreting assessment results, including automated interpretations, psychologists take into account the purpose of the assessment as well as the various test factors, test-taking abilities, and other characteristics of the person being assessed, such as situational, personal, linguistic, and cultural differences, that might affect psychologists' judgments or reduce the accuracy of their interpretations. They indicate any significant limitations of their interpretations. (See also Standards 2.01b and c, Boundaries of Competence, and 3.01, Unfair Discrimination.)

9.07. Assessment by Unqualified Persons.

Psychologists do not promote the use of psychological assessment techniques by unqualified persons, except when such use is conducted for training purposes with appropriate supervision. (See also Standard 2.05, Delegation of Work to Others.)

9.08. Obsolete Tests and Outdated Test Results.

(a) Psychologists do not base their assessment or intervention decisions or recommendations on data or test results that are outdated for the current purpose.

(b) Psychologists do not base such decisions or recommendations on tests and measures that are obsolete and not useful for the current purpose.

9.09. Test Scoring and Interpretation Services

(a) Psychologists who offer assessment or scoring services to other professionals accurately describe the purpose, norms, validity, reliability, and applications of the procedures and any special qualifications applicable to their use.

(b) Psychologists select scoring and interpretation services (including automated services) on the basis of evidence of the validity of the program and procedures as well as on other appropriate considerations. (See also Standard 2.01b and c, Boundaries of Competence.)

(c) Psychologists retain responsibility for the appropriate application, interpretation, and use of assessment instruments, whether they score and interpret such tests themselves or use automated or other services.

9.10. Explaining Assessment Results.

Regardless of whether the scoring and interpretation are done by psychologists, by employees or assistants, or by automated or other outside services, psychologists take reasonable steps to ensure that explanations of results are given to the individual or designated representative unless the nature of the relationship precludes provision of an explanation of results (such as in some organizational consulting, pre-employment or security screenings, and forensic evaluations), and this fact has been clearly explained to the person being assessed in advance.

9.11. Maintaining Test Security.

The term *test materials* refers to manuals, instruments, protocols, and test questions or stimuli and does not include *test data* as defined in Standard 9.04, Release of Test Data. Psychologists make reasonable efforts to maintain the integrity and security of test materials and other assessment techniques consistent with law and contractual obligations, and in a manner that permits adherence to this Ethics Code.

10. Therapy

10.01. Informed Consent to Therapy.

(a) When obtaining informed consent to therapy as required in Standard 3.10, Informed Consent, psychologists inform clients/patients as early as is feasible in the therapeutic relationship about the nature and anticipated course of therapy, fees, involvement of third parties, and limits of confidentiality and provide sufficient opportunity for the client/patient to ask questions and receive answers. (See also Standards 4.02, Discussing the Limits of Confidentiality, and 6.04, Fees and Financial Arrangements.)

(b) When obtaining informed consent for treatment for which generally recognized techniques and procedures have not been established, psychologists inform their clients/patients of the developing nature of the treatment, the potential risks involved, alternative treatments that may be available, and the voluntary nature of their participation. (See also Standards 2.01e, Boundaries of Competence, and 3.10, Informed Consent.)

(c) When the therapist is a trainee and the legal responsibility for the treatment provided resides with the supervisor, the client/patient, as part of the informed consent procedure, is informed that the therapist is in training and is being supervised and is given the name of the supervisor.

10.02. Therapy Involving Couples or Families.

(a) When psychologists agree to provide services to several persons who have a relationship (such as spouses, significant others, or parents and children), they take reasonable steps to clarify at the outset (1) which of the individuals are clients/patients and (2) the relationship the psychologist will have with each person. This clarification includes the psychologist's role and the probable uses of the services provided or the information obtained. (See also Standard 4.02, Discussing the Limits of Confidentiality.)

(b) If it becomes apparent that psychologists may be called on to perform potentially conflicting roles (such as family therapist and then witness for one party in divorce proceedings), psychologists take reasonable steps to clarify and modify, or withdraw from, roles appropriately. (See also Standard 3.05c, Multiple Relationships.)

10.03. Group Therapy.

When psychologists provide services to several persons in a group setting, they describe at the outset the roles and responsibilities of all parties and the limits of confidentiality.

10.04. Providing Therapy to Those Served by Others.

In deciding whether to offer or provide services to those already receiving mental health services elsewhere, psychologists carefully consider the treatment issues and the potential client's/patient's welfare. Psychologists discuss these issues with the client/patient or another legally authorized person on behalf of the client/patient in order to minimize the risk of confusion and conflict, consult with the other service providers when appropriate, and proceed with caution and sensitivity to the therapeutic issues.

10.05. Sexual Intimacies With Current Therapy Clients/Patients.

Psychologists do not engage in sexual intimacies with current therapy clients/patients.

10.06. Sexual Intimacies With Relatives or Significant Others of Current Therapy Clients/Patients.

Psychologists do not engage in sexual intimacies with individuals they know to be close relatives, guardians, or significant others of current clients/patients. Psychologists do not terminate therapy to circumvent this standard.

10.07. Therapy with Former Sexual Partners.

Psychologists do not accept as therapy clients/patients persons with whom they have engaged in sexual intimacies.

10.08. Sexual Intimacies with Former Therapy Clients/Patients.

(a) Psychologists do not engage in sexual intimacies with former clients/patients for at least two years after cessation or termination of therapy.

(b) Psychologists do not engage in sexual intimacies with former clients/patients even after a two-year interval except in the most unusual circumstances. Psychologists who engage in such activity after the two years following cessation or termination of therapy and of having no sexual contact with the former client/patient bear the burden of demonstrating that there has been no exploitation, in light of all relevant factors, including (1) the amount of time that has passed since therapy terminated; (2) the nature, duration, and intensity of the therapy; (3) the circumstances of termination; (4) the client's/patient's personal history; (5) the client's/patient's current mental status; (6) the likelihood of adverse impact on the client/patient; and (7) any statements or actions made by the therapist during the course of therapy suggesting or inviting the possibility of a posttermination sexual or romantic relationship with the client/patient. (See also Standard 3.05, Multiple Relationships.)

10.09. Interruption of Therapy.

When entering into employment or contractual relationships, psychologists make reasonable efforts to provide for orderly and appropriate resolution of responsibility for client/patient care in the event that the employment or contractual relationship ends, with paramount consideration given to the welfare of the client/patient. (See also Standard 3.12, Interruption of Psychological Services.)

10.10. Terminating Therapy.

(a) Psychologists terminate therapy when it becomes reasonably clear that the client/patient no longer needs the service, is not likely to benefit, or is being harmed by continued service.

(b) Psychologists may terminate therapy when threatened or otherwise endangered by the client/patient or another person with whom the client/patient has a relationship.

(c) Except where precluded by the actions of clients/patients or third-party payors, prior to termination psychologists provide pretermination counseling and suggest alternative service providers as appropriate.

HISTORY AND EFFECTIVE DATE FOOTNOTE

This version of the APA Ethics Code was adopted by the American Psychological Association's Council of Representatives during its meeting, August 21, 2002, and is effective beginning June 1, 2003. Inquiries concerning the substance or interpretation of the APA Ethics Code should be addressed to the Director, Office of Ethics, American Psychological Association, 750 First Street, NE, Washington, DC 20002-4242. The Ethics Code and information regarding the Code can be found on the APA web site, http://www.apa.org/ethics. The standards in this Ethics Code will be used to adjudicate complaints brought concerning alleged conduct occurring on or after the effective date. Complaints regarding conduct occurring prior to the effective date will be adjudicated on the basis of the version of the Ethics Code that was in effect at the time the conduct occurred.

The APA has previously published its Ethics Code as follows:

American Psychological Association. (1953). Ethical standards of psychologists. Washington, DC: Author.

American Psychological Association. (1959). Ethical standards of psychologists. *American Psychologist, 14*, 279–282.

American Psychological Association. (1963). Ethical standards of psychologists. *American Psychologist, 18*, 56–60.

American Psychological Association. (1968). Ethical standards of psychologists. *American Psychologist, 23*, 357–361.

American Psychological Association. (1977, March). Ethical standards of psychologists. *APA Monitor*, 22–23.

American Psychological Association. (1979). Ethical standards of psychologists. Washington, DC: Author.

American Psychological Association. (1981). Ethical principles of psychologists. *American Psychologist, 36*, 633–638.

American Psychological Association. (1990). Ethical principles of psychologists (Amended June 2, 1989). *American Psychologist, 45,* 390–395.

American Psychological Association. (1992). Ethical principles of psychologists and code of conduct. *American Psychologist, 47,* 1597–1611.

Request copies of the APA's Ethical Principles of Psychologists and Code of Conduct from the APA Order Department, 750 First Street, NE, Washington, DC 20002-4242, or phone (202) 336-5510.

Index

CPSIA information can be obtained
at www.ICGtesting.com
Printed in the USA
FFOW03n1829230713
1460FF